Sophie Richards is a women's health practitioner who shares her expertise and insights from her own health journey in order to help and inspire others. She runs the women's health community Found and is the host of the *Finally Found* podcast.

After suffering for ten years with chronic pain, bloating, and fatigue, and being told by medical professionals that no solution was available to her—even after being formally diagnosed with endometriosis—Sophie set out to find her own way to alleviate her debilitating symptoms and completely transformed her life.

Sophie Richards

The Anti-Inflammatory 30-DAY RESET

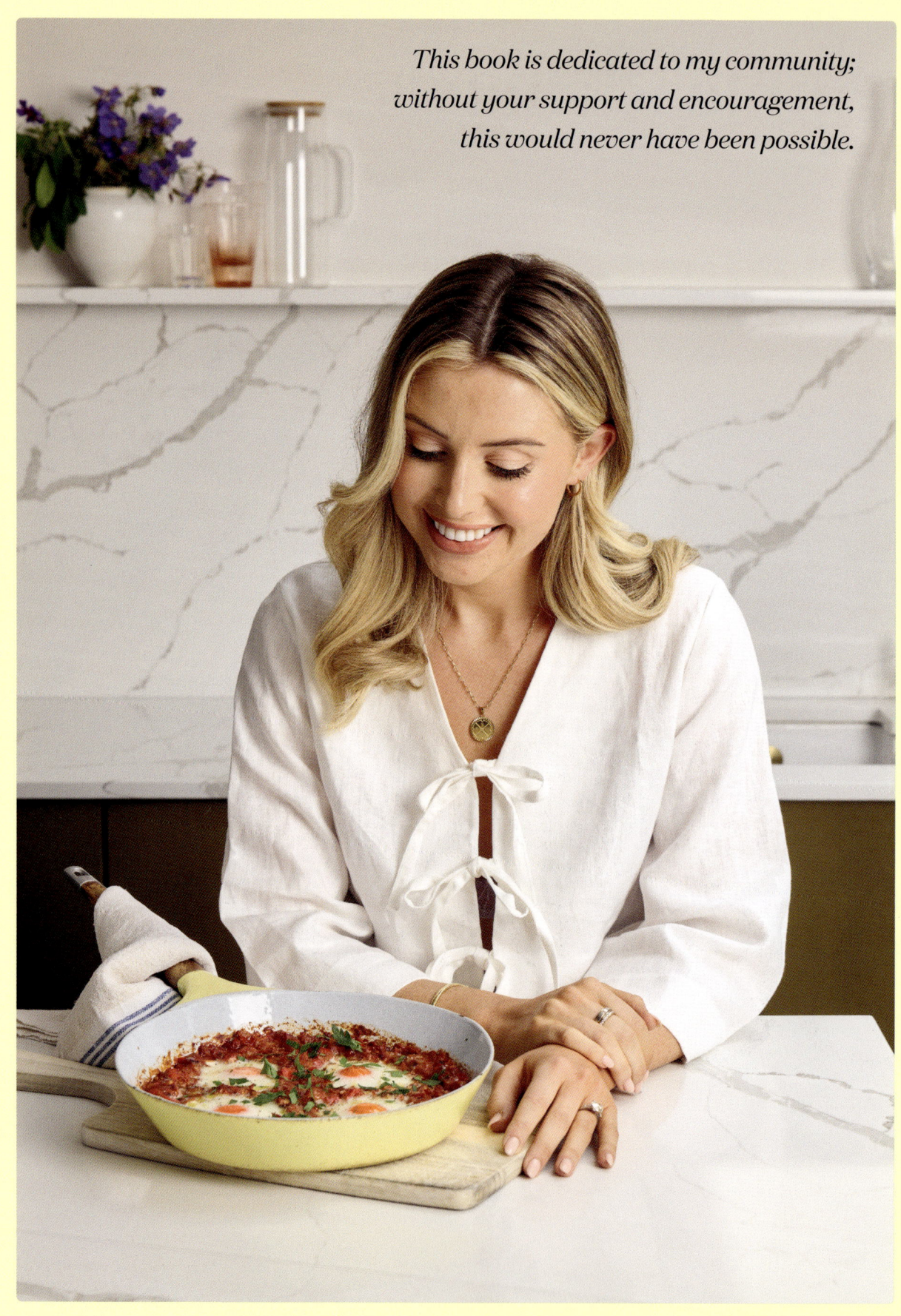

This book is dedicated to my community; without your support and encouragement, this would never have been possible.

Sophie Richards

The Anti-Inflammatory 30-Day Reset

Simple Steps to *Transform Your Health* for Good

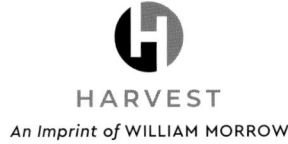

Contents

01
Introduction	6
My Journey & Discovering Inflammation	8
All About Inflammation	16
Hormones	22
Blood Sugar	36
What Comes Next?	40

02
The Six Pillars of Inflammation

Pillar 1: Food Is More than Fuel	42
Pillar 2: Gut Health	70
Pillar 3: Detoxification	86
Pillar 4: Sleep	98
Pillar 5: Stress	108
Pillar 6: Movement	120

03
Your 30-Day Reset Plan	132

04
Breakfast	142
Lunch	170
Main Meals	200
Dessert	232
Savory Snacks	252
Sweet Snacks	262
Pantry	288
Drinks	306

Universal Conversion Chart	323
References	324
Index	326
Acknowledgments	334

Introduction

For nearly a decade I was drained of energy, exhausted, in pain, and completely confused about my own body.

I was told it was "normal" to bloat, suffer unbearable period pain, and feel tired all the time. I was made to believe it was just "part of being a woman," and when I broke down and cried for help, I was labeled dramatic and hysterical, dismissed, and misdiagnosed for years, and given pills over answers at every opportunity.

And the worst part of this is that my story is far from unique. It's happening to millions of women right now . . . and if you're reading this, I'm guessing this might feel familiar to you, too, and I'm sorry. It's not fair, but I hope this book will improve things.

> *So many women put up with symptoms like:*
>
> - **Constant bloating**
> - **Fatigue**
> - **Weight gain**
> - **Acne**
> - **Brain fog**
> - **Mood swings**
> - **Anxiety**
> - **Depression**
> - **Hormonal imbalances**
> - **Skin problems**

All of these symptoms are too often labeled as "normal." That needs to stop right now. Yes, these might be common, but they aren't normal.

Recognizing that distinction changed my life and made me realize that change is possible and if I could get to the bottom of my symptoms, I might get my life back.

After years of being misdiagnosed and let down by the medical system, I was finally diagnosed with endometriosis. But then I was given the wrong surgery and told my best chance at a relatively pain-free life was to have a hysterectomy, or have a baby . . . at the age of twenty-one. More invasive surgeries followed, alongside egg freezing to preserve the little hope I had. But even after all of this, my symptoms were still there, still causing me daily misery.

So, I stopped asking for answers and went looking for them myself. I made it my life mission to get to the bottom of my symptoms, and I promised that if I ever found the answers, I'd share every single detail so that others could benefit, too.

What changed everything for me was discovering "inflammation" and how it can be linked to almost every symptom we experience, from hormonal fluctuations and period pain to chronic health issues like PCOS, endometriosis, and autoimmune conditions.

This book is the result of everything I've lived through, studied, experienced, and tested via surgeries, setbacks, hormonal chaos, and ultimately rebuilding my body (and my life) from the inside out. And now it's all here for you, too!

And if you're reading this, I already know one thing . . . you're ready. You're tired of feeling lost in your body, tired of "doing everything right" and yet still feeling wrong . . . you want clarity, control, and most of all, you want to feel happy and healthy again.

This isn't a fad, it isn't a cleanse, it isn't a diet . . . it's a chance to hit the RESET button on your life.

In these pages, you'll discover how inflammation can sit at the root of so many symptoms, from painful periods to gut issues, fatigue, skin flare-ups, anxiety, and more. You'll learn everything you need to know about the foundations of inflammation, hormones, and balancing blood sugar (the foundations of health!), followed by a deep dive into the six pillars we can use to live an anti-inflammatory life and manage our symptoms for good. These pillars are: food, gut health, detoxification, sleep, stress, and movement. My biggest struggle on this journey was figuring out what I could eat that actually tasted GOOD, and finding creative meals and recipes with those anti-inflammatory ingredients . . . which is exactly why I've included more than eighty step-by-step recipes right here in this book, so that you'll never feel at a loss for what to cook and eat.

No perfection is required and no immediate action either! The first half of this book will help everything make sense, and then, when you're ready, you can start your 30-day reset. A practical, empowering, step-by-step challenge that will help you feel better right now, and set you up for a lifetime of health and happiness.

If you've been longing for answers, clarity, and a body that finally makes sense . . . you're in the right place. Because once you understand what's really going on inside, the overwhelm disappears, the shame lifts, and you'll finally get your energy, confidence, and health back.

This is your turning point. You're not broken or lazy, you just need the answers. This was my road map out of a lifetime of pain and into an abundance of health, longevity, and more—and now it can be yours, too!

Let's do it together,

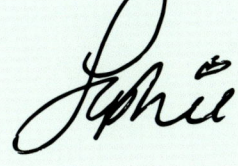

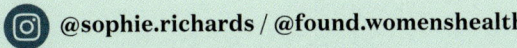
@sophie.richards / @found.womenshealth

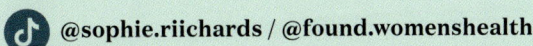
@sophie.riichards / @found.womenshealth

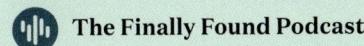
The Finally Found Podcast

My Journey & Discovering Inflammation

I still remember the day my doctor told me that my constantly bloated belly and horrendous period pain were just me putting on weight and being dramatic. The words every seventeen-year-old wants to hear . . . ! I'd gone to the doctor desperate for help, but the pain I was in was labeled as "normal" and the message I came away with was clear: I needed to toughen up and get on with it (and of course take the pill—because that solves everything, right?). Well, sadly that wasn't the case for me. Nor, I know, for a lot of others, too.

I was very late getting my period. I was sixteen turning seventeen, a crucial age when it comes to school, friendships, thinking about college or university, and of course . . . boys, and absolutely NOT a time when I had envisaged becoming chronically ill for the next decade of my life. We usually say hindsight is a wonderful thing, but in this instance I'm quite glad I didn't know then that my next ten years would be spent arguing with doctors, being dismissed, misdiagnosed, and undergoing the wrong surgery. It was not the future I was dreaming of, and if I'm honest I still mourn my late teens and early twenties, picturing what life could have been like. However, I'm also a firm believer that everything happens for a reason, and right now, I'm living a life beyond my wildest dreams. All because I found an anti-inflammatory way of living, which tackled my symptoms, stopped my endless surgeries, and introduced me to my real passion, helping other women feel their best selves.

Growing up, my life was pretty normal. I was raised on a farm, which meant I was always outdoors, always moving, and had a fairly standard diet of home-cooked meat, fish, and vegetables. I was active as a child and constantly on the go, doing various jobs around the farm, including feeding the baby cows, my favorite! Although my meals were generally healthy, I had the biggest sweet tooth you can imagine. I'd bake cakes just to eat the batter, scoff a whole family-sized pack of custard creams, and never really saw any issue with it. It was all just part of my day-to-day life, and I never gave it a second thought.

As a family, we have suffered some unlucky turns when it comes to health, and especially in our experience with serious symptoms being ignored. My mum was severely unwell from her late teens to mid-thirties, constantly fatigued and low in iron, which turned out to be celiac disease, an autoimmune condition where the immune system attacks the lining of the small intestine when gluten is consumed. She can't eat any wheat either! Her symptoms were obvious, but she was dismissed for years before having the help she needed. My brother became seriously ill from the age of seven, and when he turned ten a mysterious lump appeared on his neck. Doctors said it would go away on its own, or at worst be TB. Sadly this lump wasn't going anywhere: it turned out to be cancer. Thankfully, my mum pushed on for answers and demanded further investigation, which is how my brother received the diagnosis, had timely treatment, and thankfully made a full recovery. Then there's my journey . . . I had a particularly nasty cough when I was a baby, and my mum with her "mother's instinct" took me straight to the doctor, who shockingly dismissed her pleading for further investigation. What was really going on was pneumonia, which, by the time it was finally diagnosed, had spread to both lungs, and became so serious that my entire family was called to say their goodbyes. That was my first brush with death, but sadly not my last.

Even as a child I always struggled with constipation, which I carried with me until my mid-twenties, and had a gluten and dairy intolerance, which wasn't a surprise given my mother's celiac diagnosis and my brother's lactose allergy—it's in the genes, sadly. However, other than these pretty serious "one-off" incidents for myself and my brother growing up, day-to-day we were all pretty healthy!

Then came my first period, and everything changed.

Almost overnight, I went from being a normal teen, full of life, to being regularly doubled over in pain. I developed extreme bloating, all my energy disappeared, and I just felt like I'd been taken hostage by my own body. I simply wasn't myself any more; my life had completely changed and I spent most of my time exhausted but unable to sleep, in pain, and feeling embarrassed about my symptoms. Eventually, after a couple of months of struggling, I decided enough was enough and I went to the doctor, which felt incredibly daunting at the time because communicating that I was having problems "down there" was difficult and nerve-racking! But I plucked up the courage, telling the doctor that I was in a lot of pain and (TMI incoming! get ready, this book is full of it!) that I was bleeding from my butt as well as my vagina while on my period, and also that I had this sharp tugging pain that felt like someone was plunging a corkscrew into my lower tummy! However, I experienced what sadly most women do when they go to the doctor with "pain down there," and was told the same thing over and over again . . . "It's normal. Periods are painful, and you'll probably just grow out of it anyway." But the pain I felt didn't seem normal. I was missing school, fainting, struggling to function, and the saddest part of it all was that eventually I started believing what I was being told: that maybe I was just too sensitive, maybe I just wasn't built to cope? To this day, the most offensive misdiagnosis I was given was "phantom symptoms," meaning the symptoms were quite literally in my head . . . which didn't explain the amounts of blood I was bleeding each month.

Years later, after endless appointments and still no answers, I ended up having emergency surgery. They found cysts on my ovaries and commented that some of my organs were stuck together, too—but nothing to worry about, of course: all "normal" according to the surgeon, which I now know was completely untrue. This "gluing" of organs is called adhesion, when one organ sticks to another, and is a very common sign of endometriosis, but it was never picked up.

The distinction between "normal" and "common" may seem trivial, but it's not, it's life-changing.

"It's common, not normal"

It's common for people to be unwell. It's common to struggle with our periods. It's common to feel tired, in pain, constantly bloated, and burned out. But none of that is normal, and the more I was told otherwise, the more I started questioning everything.

Going to university was the tipping point. I was thrown into a world of late nights, cheap food, alcohol, high stress, and minimal sleep, and my body just couldn't cope. In continuous pain and discomfort, I started to crumble, my relationships suffered, my mental health was in the trenches, and I felt completely out of control. I still had no answers, despite pleading with doctors for five years for help. I felt like I was losing everything, including my dignity! The conversation changed from "It's just painful periods" at school, to now, at university, "It must be an STI"—because of course all women with pelvic pain at university **MUST** be having unprotected casual sex on all occasions. The irony was, I had one boyfriend at uni, and my endometriosis was so bad that sex became almost impossible, so the endless STI tests, all of which proved it was not an STI, were a waste of time.

I got very close to giving up, until finally a trusted and brilliant doctor mentioned the word "endometriosis." Shortly after, I had another operation, an exploratory laparoscopy (a fancy way of saying they'll have a look in your tummy to see what's going on!), and from this I received my formal diagnosis. You'd think things would have gotten better from this point, but all my main symptoms came rushing back and I was told I had two choices: have a baby or have a hysterectomy, as these were supposed to "cure" my endometriosis and take away all the pain. I was twenty-one, felt like a baby myself, and was in a very new relationship, too, so having a baby was not in the cards! A hysterectomy, however? It was an extreme option, but it was presented to me as the ticket to a pain-free life, and so that's what I began to accept would be in my future after I graduated from university. I didn't want it immediately because it was a major operation that would have disrupted my studies, and there was no way in hell I was going to let that happen, as I was determined to achieve first-class honors, no matter what.

What saved me was a placement year in London. While there, I went to a GP purely to ask for stronger pain meds, but this doctor did something no one else had done before: she actually listened! She acknowledged the years of pain, dismissal, surgeries, and misdiagnoses I had suffered and referred me to an endometriosis specialist. (I didn't even know they existed until that point.) This specialist told me three things that changed my life:

1. **A hysterectomy does not cure endometriosis.**
2. **Having a baby does not cure endometriosis.**
3. **I'd had the wrong surgery. I'd had ablation, and I should have had excision surgery. Ablation is like cutting a weed, excision is like ripping it out at the root. The weeds will grow back with both, but excision is much more effective long-term.**

My next step was having my third surgery at twenty-two, with the endometriosis specialist, when she performed the correct procedure, excision. She found endometriosis in far more areas than my previous surgeon had, mainly between my rectum and vagina (rectal-vaginal endometriosis), which explained why I was bleeding from my rectum (sexy, I know!) and had this horrid tugging pain there before my period. My pain improved after this surgery, and although she mentioned I'd possibly need one more operation to really get to the bottom of the damage endometriosis had done, overall I should feel better. Unfortunately, this did mean I had to quit my highly sought-after placement year at Aldi. Despite it all being out of my control, and my being genuinely in too much pain to work and needing time for the surgery and recovery, I just felt like I had failed. I remember feeling I should have tried harder, or should even have delayed the surgery so that I could prove myself at work, but in reality my body couldn't cope and my mental health wasn't in a great place either.

After the third surgery, life was slightly easier. I was still getting daily pain and bloating, and my periods were a dark hole in my diary each month, but the excruciating emergency room trips stopped, which was success in my eyes. I was able to attend most of my lectures in person, there were no more missed exams, and thanks to Covid making all lectures virtual, I was able to catch up easily on the lessons I missed because of flare-ups.

This new way of working, an accessible work-from-home model, allowed me to achieve my dream of getting a first-class degree, something I still feel immensely proud of.

I then secured my dream graduate role, account management with Procter & Gamble. It was in Yorkshire during lockdown, which meant a six-hour move away from family and friends, but I was excited about the opportunity. I loved working with retailers, and my manager, Jonathan Olding, was the most wonderful human inside and out. I explained my medical history and we made an agreement that if I was having an "endo day"—meaning I needed to work from home or take time off—he had my back, and I will forever be grateful for the time we worked together.

Sadly, the pain that surgery had once helped was coming back thick and fast, and a terrifying trip to the emergency room found me back on the operating table after a week-long flare-up had aggravated my appendix into full-blown appendicitis. I struggle to talk about the forty-eight hours prior to this surgery because, in truth, I almost died. This particular flare-up wasn't anything special, it was very "normal," but it became concerning after I passed out a few times. Writing this now, I can't believe I didn't take this seriously, but bear in mind this was almost a monthly occurrence, so for me it was "normal." I thought I could sleep this one off, but that's not how appendicitis works, sadly, and I was in real trouble. An ambulance came to my rescue, and I was immediately on the operating table faced with one of the most painful ultimatums of my life. Due to my medical history, the surgeon said there was a real possibility of needing to remove both ovaries due to cysts complicating the operation. I was twenty-four, facing my fourth surgery, on my own and having to decide whether I should have life-saving surgery and risk my ovaries (and, as a result, my dreams of becoming a mom), or hope my appendicitis would stop, which wasn't really an option. I woke up from surgery screaming, not from the pain, but from wanting an answer—Did I still have my ovaries? The longest thirty minutes of my life went by until I was told, "You have your ovaries." The surgery had been successful.

After almost saying goodbye to my possibility of having a family, I changed my job to move to London, where I went straight to a fertility clinic to ensure I was protected if this situation ever happened again. I had always been told prior to this situation that I was ridiculous, I was young and would be fine! However, that last surgery proved that youth wasn't helping me and I needed to take action. I did two rounds of egg-freezing, one I self-funded and the second round was paid for by my parents. A privilege I will never forget, as the NHS typically won't fund fertility treatment unless you're trying and failing to get pregnant, or going through chemotherapy. Something I hope to change one day!

It was during my egg-freezing journey that I started to take my "hobby blog" seriously. After getting the news that a hysterectomy and a baby do **NOT** cure endometriosis, I didn't want anyone else to go through what I had. I also wanted a space to raise awareness and track progress (if any), to hopefully inspire others going on the same journey as me. So I started an Instagram page, previously called "The Endo Spectrum." Truthfully, the name was chosen because I wanted to hide behind it because of what I was posting about! Sex, periods, problems with having a poo . . . it wasn't exactly dinner-table chat for my family, but I had a fire in me to make a change that thankfully my cousin Jess fueled to no end! I often had doubts about what I was sharing, which wasn't helped by the whispers of how "cringe" my posts were from even those close to me. However, Jess filled me with the confidence I needed to persist, as did other wonderful friends I made along the way, notably Sevs . . . and now that online account is proudly changed to my name: **@sophie.richards**!

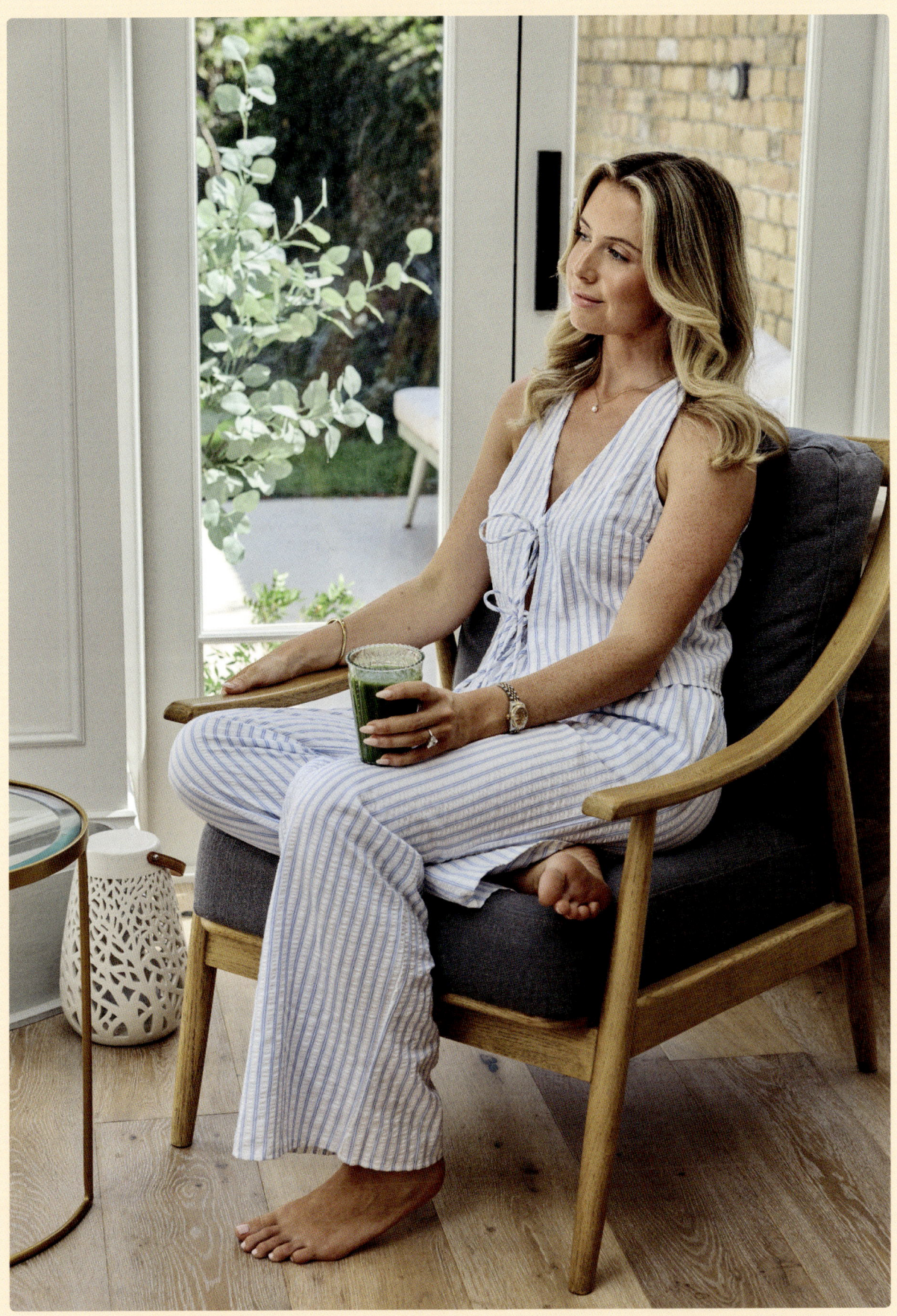

Despite all this, I still wasn't really getting anywhere with my health. Even after all the surgeries, the diagnosis, the treatments, etc., I still didn't feel good, and I was battling inflammation every day. My bloating was out of control, my weight was skyrocketing, my hormones were all over the place, and I just didn't recognize myself. My emotions didn't feel like my own, and neither did my appearance. I'd look into the mirror, and looking back at me would be this bloated, puffy, sore, sad girl who had no idea what was going on or how things were ever going to change. I was also working in a corporate job, sitting at a desk all day, pushing myself beyond what my body could manage. I felt misunderstood and exhausted, constantly fighting flare-ups with no idea why they were happening.

In desperation, I started researching, learning, and investigating; reading anything relevant I could lay my hands on. Hormones, inflammation, and balancing blood sugar kept coming up time and time again, and so did "managing your cycle," which I'd been told was best to stop altogether, whether through the pill or a hysterectomy . . . neither of which I wanted.

Realizing I needed to change my lifestyle, I quit my job. And inspired by the research I'd been doing, I signed up for a women's health practitioner course with certification in menstrual health, to try to learn all the things I didn't yet understand about what living a truly healthy life looks like and, most important, **HOW** to do it.

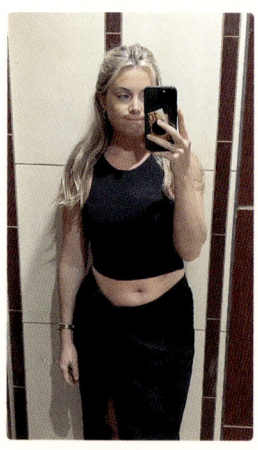
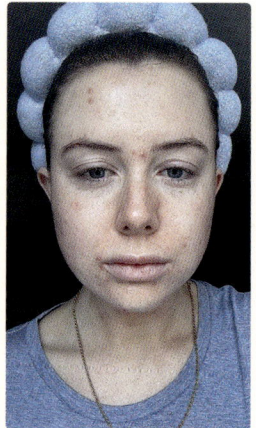
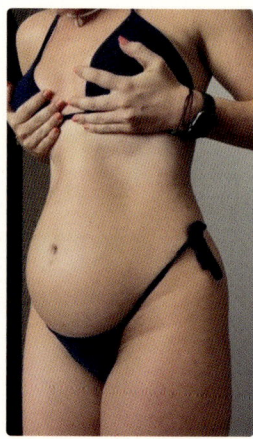

Interestingly, although my mission was to fix my endometriosis, I soon realized that it wasn't the root of the problem. The real issue was what was *triggering* my endometriosis flare-ups, as well as my other symptoms, like acne, brain fog, nausea, constipation, mood swings . . . everything! And that, I discovered, was inflammation!

At first it seemed simple. I knew my bloating was inflammation because it was easy to see—I looked nine months pregnant! I also knew that certain foods triggered a reaction, because when I ate particular meals, all of a sudden I blew up like a balloon (usually meals containing dairy and gluten, but there were unknowns, too). My confusion around food became clearer after following a very strict anti-inflammatory diet (called the AIP). It helped me, but it didn't fix everything, because food was only one piece of the puzzle. Even when my diet was "perfect," I'd still have big flare-ups, often when periods of stress came around, or when my sleep was off. My face would swell up, I'd catch colds constantly, and bad period pain would come flooding back, too.

This personal experience, along with what I learned while studying hormonal health, made me realize that inflammation can affect the whole body. That it isn't just about food; other lifestyle factors are equally important. Food, gut health, detoxification, sleep, stress, movement . . . the six core pillars of inflammation.

Understanding those six pillars is what finally helped me reduce inflammation in a meaningful way, and when I say reduce inflammation, I don't just mean less bloating or fewer flare-ups. I mean fewer symptoms across the board. I started to feel more balanced, my mental health stabilized, my energy came back, and as a result my spark for life did, too. My skin also started to improve after ten years of painful acne, and most important, my cycle stabilized. My periods weren't painful any more, and my endometriosis felt non-existent—I was finally symptom-free, and I still am, when I follow an anti-inflammatory way of living. I say this, rather than "I'm cured forever," because health will always be a work in progress. No one is perfect and life throws curve balls along the way. Our bodies respond to real-life events, so when life gets in the way, our health can be thrown off balance, too. However, following this anti-inflammatory way of living 80 percent of the time has changed my life 100 percent.

It's not a quick fix, and long-term health requires long-term consistency. However, the changes you can see in just thirty days can be astronomical. Just by changing my diet, I got rid of ten years of symptoms in a matter of months.

I still live with endometriosis, but it no longer rules my life. I now understand my body, I know what triggers symptoms, and I know how to support myself. When a flare-up happens, 99.9 percent of the time I can trace it back to one of those pillars being off—and THAT is control I never thought I'd have.

This book exists because I never want anyone else to feel the way I did: confused, overwhelmed, and alone. It's why I began blogging about my experiences on my Instagram page, and now with this book I want to give you the road map to health that I never had. The **WHY** behind your symptoms and the **HOW** to manage them. Always discuss your symptoms with your trusted medical provider but never underestimate the power you have to improve your health through lifestyle tweaks.

I truly hope you find the help you need in this book, and that sharing what I've learned from my research and personal experience can help you avoid what I went through. For those who are reading this, in the depths of your journey with pain and inflammation, feeling like there's no hope, I am living proof that things can get better, that life can be not only pain-free but full of excitement and opportunity, too.

If I can do it, I know you can, too. I can't wait for you to start your 30-day reset, and would love to support you on your journey, so make sure to use the hashtag **#30DAYRESET** and join our community at **@found.womenshealth** where the Found team and I will be hosting challenges and events and you can meet like-minded people on the same path.

All About Inflammation

What is inflammation? And why is it such a big deal?

We often hear people say they feel puffy, bloated, or sluggish—these are all signs of inflammation. It doesn't just show up in one area. It can affect your face, tummy, arms, legs... and often it's happening internally, where you can't even see it.

Inflammation is a full-body response, so symptoms can pop up anywhere, even if the root cause is one specific issue such as an injury or condition. That's why healing it takes a full-body approach. You can't just spot-treat one area, you need to support your whole system—and that's what we're going to do in this book!

> *Inflammation definition:* Inflammation is an important biological response induced by various harmful stimuli, like viruses, bacterial infections, toxins, toxic compounds, tissue injury.[1]

Inflammation is like your body's emergency services team. Imagine having paramedics, firefighters, policemen, and bodyguards all on standby, ready to act when something goes wrong. When we suffer an injury, infection, or even a spike in stress, the team rushes to the scene with sirens going off! Think of the last time you cut your finger—you probably got a little bit of swelling and redness, right? That's inflammation doing its job: the security team has rushed to the cut, is clearing out the bacteria and damaged cells, and is starting the healing process (nail-biters, you'll know this feeling well!). Once the situation is under control, the emergency team packs up and heads home, as if nothing had ever happened... that is IF everything's working well. If everything's good, your emergency team efficiently clocks on when there's trouble, and clocks off once it's tackled. This short-term inflammation (or "acute" inflammation) is there to protect and heal us. So short-term (acute) inflammation is actually a **GOOD** thing.

So why does inflammation have such a bad rep?

When the inflammatory response is constant (chronic), this is when problems start to occur. It's like when a friend asks to stay the night; it's not a problem for one or two days. But fast forward a few months to when they've completely taken over your house and brought all their friends with them. They're making a mess in the kitchen, the living room's a dump, the sofa's covered in stains, and don't even **START** on the bathroom situation... and the worst part? You were there all along, watching it happen! You just didn't realize how bad it was getting until all of a sudden your house is burning down and you've been brought to tears! This is what happens when inflammation lingers for too long—it can wreak havoc on your body, weakening your immune system, because it's so busy fighting off these unwanted guests that it doesn't have time to function properly, leaving you feeling sick, tired, and even more exposed to other illnesses.

But here's the good news—it's never too late to make a change. All we need to do is find the troublemakers, kick them (and their friends) out of the house, and start the clean-up process. Before you know it, you'll be sitting on your fresh clean sofa with a cup of tea enjoying your peaceful home.

That is our mission. Your body is your home, and we need to get to the root of your chronic inflammation, so that you can live a healthy, happy, pain-free life. We want to find the right balance of inflammation, as we will always need our GOOD short-term inflammatory response, but not to the point where it's destroying us.

Signs and symptoms of *chronic* inflammation

I just mentioned how chronic (long-term) inflammation causes havoc in our body, but it does so in such a slow way that we often don't see the signs until something serious happens. Additionally, we've been taught that inflammation or pain are localized and contained where the immediate problem is; however, this is not the case. My wake-up call happened during my first surgery at nineteen, when I was in excruciating agony with a twisted cyst (unrelated to my endometriosis) that was ready to burst. BUT there were signs for years before this happened. Below are a list of some potential signs of chronic inflammation. Remember, you don't need all of these to qualify.

» Digestive issues: bloating, IBS, constipation, or food intolerances.
» Joint pain and stiffness: achey, swollen, or stiff joints.
» Skin problems: acne, eczema, psoriasis, premature aging.
» Brain fog and fatigue: feeling sluggish, forgetful, or always exhausted.
» Weight gain or trouble losing weight: especially around the belly.
» Autoimmune conditions: when the body mistakenly attacks itself.
» Mood swings and anxiety: inflammation can throw off brain chemicals.

After reading those, were you nodding along? Personally, I had a delightful combination of almost all of these. Constipation, food intolerances that seemed to come out of nowhere, stiff hands, raging acne, weight fluctuations, endometriosis (although not classified as an autoimmune condition, many experts believe it should be because of its characteristics), and the mood swings were all in full sway!

Genetics and chronic conditions:
why some of us are more prone to inflammation

We're all born with a deck of cards we can't change—our genetics. And some of us have unfortunately been dealt a hand that means we're more prone to inflammation than others. This explains why your best friend can smash an almond croissant for breakfast, pasta for lunch, and a chocolate bar later on and still have washboard abs! I am unfortunately not that person, and I'm guessing—if you're reading this book—neither are you, but that's OK, this book will help.

Carbs often have a bad reputation, and for some people there is a genetic reason why they don't fully "agree" with us. There's a gene called "AMY1," which plays a big role in how we digest carbs. We all have between two and fifteen copies of this gene; some people even have up to twenty. The more AMY1 you have, the better you process carbohydrates. So that friend who eats anything and stays lean probably has loads of AMY1 genes. However, this absolutely does **NOT** mean we need to cut carbs; they're very important. The fewer AMY1 genes you have, the less efficient your body will be at digesting carbs, which is why it's important to pick the right type of carbs for you. You'll learn all about why carbs are essential and wholefoods vs. ultra-processed foods in the Food Pillar (see page 42).

When it comes to chronic conditions, there's often a genetic link, so once again this is out of our control. I have endometriosis, which is thought to have a strong hereditary link, and for those of you who have chronic or autoimmune conditions, your body is already exhausting its bodyguards by fighting these conditions, not only meaning you have chronic inflammation, but also making you more susceptible to catching coughs, colds, and flu because your immune system is preoccupied with chronic issues, leaving fewer resources to fight infections.

So what do we do? Does this mean we're destined for a life of inflammation? Absolutely **NOT**, and I'm living proof of it. There's a quote I live by that goes:

Genetics load the gun but lifestyle pulls the trigger.

Yes, our genetics are out of our control, but our lifestyle dictates how these genes present themselves. Let me explain . . .

My endometriosis and inflammation symptoms started when I was turning seventeen. Prior to that, I lived on cookies, processed foods and, when I was old enough to discover it, alcohol . . . yes, I was a big fan of that, too. If I had carried on with those as my staples, it wouldn't have mattered if I had the **PERFECT** genetics, I'd still be on the road to type 2 diabetes and a world of pain and inflammation. It's why I've come to see endometriosis as a good thing in my life—it forced me to wake up to the unhealthy inflammatory lifestyle I was living, whereas now I live healthily and symptom-free!

So, genetically blessed <u>or not</u>, our lifestyle holds the key to how we feel, and that's why we should all be focusing on managing inflammation. Understanding the pillars that drive inflammation is important for each and every one of us, chronic condition or not, as once we understand what the triggers are, and most important how we can take **ACTION** to overcome them, we can take control of our health, and—regardless of genes—feel the best we've ever felt!

The six key pillars that drive inflammation

1. **Food and nutrition**

   What you eat can either fuel or fight inflammation.

2. **Gut health**

   A healthy gut barrier keeps inflammation in check; a damaged gut leads to trouble!

3. **Detoxification**

   Your body's ability to get rid of toxins effectively and the toxic load it's dealing with.

4. **Sleep**

   Poor sleep fuels inflammation; quality sleep calms it.

5. **Stress**

   Both physical and emotional stress drive inflammation, and it's a very common trigger in today's world!

6. **Exercise and movement**

   The right movement reduces inflammation, but overtraining makes it worse.

These six pillars are the foundation of what drives inflammation and our overall health. You may be familiar with these pillars as they often form the foundation of health-based advice—for good reason! In my conversation with Dr. Nitu Bajekal on the *Finally Found* podcast, she refers to evidence-based lifestyle medicine and explains the scientific research supporting such pillars. Yes, lifestyle changes can feel insignificant compared to taking medication, but the research speaks for itself and so do the results!

Take a second now and with **NO** judgment, ask yourself: are you sleeping enough; have you been stressed recently (or just constantly); are you consistently eating well; are you moving your body? Whatever your answers, don't worry, we will go through all this step-by-step together, and by the end of the book you'll have all the answers you've been looking for and an action plan that will get you to where you want to be.

Working on these pillars completely changed my life—and it will change yours, too! By now, you've read about how much I struggled before figuring out what was driving my inflammation. I won't sit here and say my life and health are perfect now, because they're not. Life happens, and sometimes we focus too much on one thing while neglecting others (for me, it's stress). But when you understand why each pillar matters, and, most important, when you know how to fix things, you'll be blown away by the changes you start to see and feel, some of which will be immediate!

Before we dive into the pillars, it's important to know that there are two key themes that flow through all of them, shaping everything along the way like the bedrock beneath a building. I like to think of these as the foundation that holds the pillars up. So before we break down each pillar, let's get really clear on these two themes. They are: hormones and blood sugar. They're especially important for women, and understanding them will make everything else fall into place so much more easily.

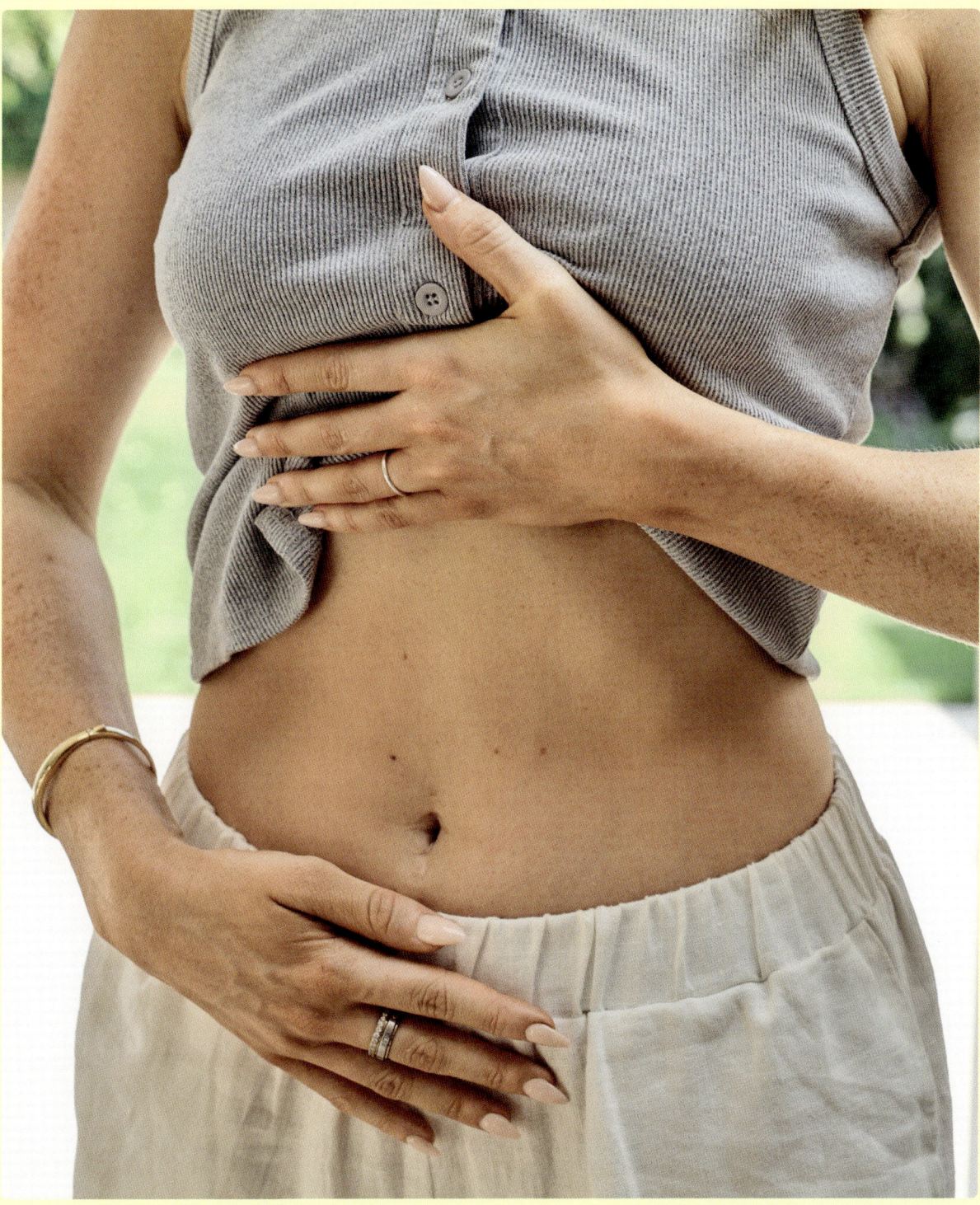

Hormones

Hormones, inflammation and the menstrual cycle:
the keys to long-term health

Whether you're having periods (or maybe they've gone missing due to hormonal imbalances or chronic conditions like endometriosis and polycystic ovary syndrome, known as PCOS), going through perimenopause, or you've crossed over to menopause, I want you to remember that managing inflammation is the foundation of hormone health, and therefore the foundation of whatever phase of life you're in. It's the difference between thriving in every phase of life or feeling like your body is working against you.

There's a misconception that when you're young, anything goes. That you can treat your body like crap and, by some magic, you just "bounce back." I wish this was true, but sadly, as a lot of women are realizing, it is not the case. We think that our painful periods, bloating, acne, and so on are just "normal" parts of being a woman . . . but actions have consequences, and how we treat our health, and specifically our menstrual health, has a **HUGE** ripple effect. So the aim of the game is to make sure this ripple effect is a good one, and—spoiler—we're going to learn how to do that by working through the six pillars of inflammation (see page 42 onward).

Now, if you're sitting there reading this and thinking, "Well, I'm already peri- or menopausal, so I'm screwed!" then think again! We have so much power when it comes to our health, power I've witnessed firsthand—so all is not lost. It's all about putting in the right effort, right now, which can completely change your life. The reason I highlight the importance of respecting our cycle as early as we can is that the greater our menstrual health, the easier we transition into perimenopause and menopause. But it's important to also remember it's never too late to make a positive change.

How you experience your menstrual cycle, perimenopause, and menopause is governed by hormones. When your hormones are balanced, you feel energized, clear-headed, emotionally stable, and physically strong. When they're not? Fatigue, painful periods, anxiety, bloating, cravings, heavy bleeding, and mood swings become your new "normal"—although remember this is **NOT** normal, it's a physical manifestation of what's going on with your hormones—and you don't have to accept it.

Inflammation is a key driver of hormonal imbalances, which is why it's so important to get it under control. Whether you're navigating your cycle, preparing for perimenopause or already in menopause, the key to feeling good is hormonal balance, and that starts with reducing inflammation through the six wonderful pillars of inflammation, which you'll know inside and out by the end of this book. But first of all, I want to share what I **WISH** we were taught about our cycles and about the transition to menopause, and how inflammation hanging around can be a nightmare.

Hormones and inflammation: the constant loop

Hormones are chemical messengers that tell your body what to do. They control everything from mood, metabolism, and sleep to digestion, energy, and fertility. But they don't work in isolation. They work together, just like a group of perfectly choreographed dancers. They must all follow their routine, come on and off stage at the right time, and jump to the right height (not too high or for too long) in order to pull off their very important performance.

Sadly, we've all seen a dance routine that has resembled more of a car crash. I remember an unpleasant experience I once had in a disco-dancing competition, in which a last-minute costume change led to the lead dancers not being able to see properly, causing them to fall flat on their faces, bringing down the rest of us with them! We all scrambled back to our feet, desperately trying to recover, but we were out of sync, out of luck . . . and scored zeros across the board.

As in my short and tragic dance debut, once one of the main dancers (or, in this case, hormones) tumbles, the rest follow. This is exactly what happens when we have chronic inflammation in the body that impacts our key hormones: it has a domino effect on the rest of our hormones, causing chaos with our menstrual cycle or our transition through perimenopause and menopause.

The hormonal hierarchy

If there's one thing I want you to take away from this entire section on hormones, it's this: all hormones are important, but not all hormones are created equal. There is a hierarchy. And at the very top? Insulin and cortisol.

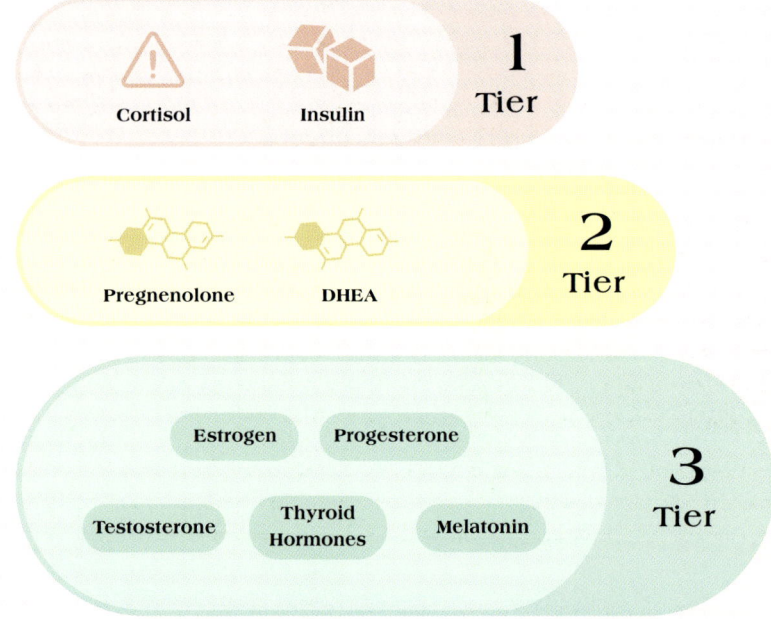

I imagine the hormonal hierarchy as like the structure of a company with two CEOs. Cortisol and insulin are the CEOs of your body, overseeing everything from your energy levels and metabolism to your menstrual cycle, mood, and inflammation. When they're working as they should, everything below them follows suit. But when they're out of balance (like a CEO that doesn't properly support its staff), all the hormones beneath the CEOs run amok, including key hormones like estrogen, progesterone, and thyroid hormones, which then affects how you feel every single day, as these are the hormones that manage your menstrual cycle, and later your transition through perimenopause and menopause.

So, when we talk about balancing our hormones, we HAVE to focus on the tier 1 hormones (your CEO hormones) first. Inflammation fuels the imbalance of both these hormones, and it becomes a vicious cycle whereby inflammation causes chaos, and the chaos causes more inflammation. One of the biggest disruptors and causes of inflammation is blood sugar dysregulation, which can happen when any of the six pillars we will explore in this book are impacted. So, before we get into the pillars, we also need to discuss blood sugar so that you know exactly what's going on, and you'll find this in the next section of the book (see page 37). But for now, just know that when your blood sugar is off, it directly impacts both your insulin and your cortisol, which as we can see from the hormonal hierarchy will have a disastrous impact on the rest of your hormones. So managing your blood sugar is absolutely key.

The menstrual cycle:
your monthly health report card

After leaving my corporate job, I knew I wanted to learn more about women's health and put myself through formal training, not only for my own knowledge but also to help give thoroughly researched information online. I trained to become a women's health practitioner, with a certificate specifically in menstrual health. My favorite part of the training was learning that our menstrual cycle is a direct reflection of our overall health, and as such, our monthly cycle acts like a monthly health report card. Dr. Mary Claire, a board-certified obstetrics and gynecology specialist, describes it as paying into your health pension each month, because how you treat your cycle now determines how smooth your transition into perimenopause and menopause will be. This **DEFINITELY** should have been on the curriculum at school, but sadly, as with anything related to women's health, it was brushed aside.

A healthy cycle is regular, pain-free, and predictable . . . dreamy, right? If yours is all over the place, heavy, painful, irregular, or comes with intense PMS (premenstrual symptoms), it could be your body telling you something is off. This was me for almost ten years. Every month was filled with dread, bleeding through pads, brain fog, fatigue—not to mention the fact that I felt like someone had stuck two corkscrews into my ovaries and was rotating them for what felt like a lifetime. Only for all that to repeat itself the following month (that is, when my periods were regular . . .)!

I **WISH** someone had explained to me back then that there are four phases to our menstrual cycle, which you can use to understand how your body is working, what it needs, and how to optimize it. Holistic wellness practices often liken the four phases of the menstrual cycle to the four seasons, which I think is such a beautiful way of imagining this dance of the hormones, and so much more nuanced than the black and white of either being on your period or not on it.

I'll break down these four phases across the next few pages, but remember, there's no such thing as a perfect cycle, particularly when it comes to its length! There's a myth that the ideal cycle is twenty-eight days, but in reality it can be anywhere from twenty-one to thirty-five days, according to the NHS, so take these time frames as a guide.

Understanding your menstrual cycle

Your menstrual cycle isn't just your period; it's a finely tuned hormonal routine that happens every month and can dictate how you feel, how much energy you have, and even how productive or social you want or are able to be. So when you're feeling the highs or the lows, it can be largely to do with your hormones and where you are in your cycle. If you don't believe me, I don't blame you . . . I laughed at this, too, until I started tracking my cycle and felt like I'd become a psychic overnight! Suddenly I could predict when my period would come, how I would feel, when I would have more or less energy—everything.

Each phase of our cycle has its own hormonal shifts, which naturally trigger a more or less inflammatory response in the body. When everything is in balance, people often feel in rhythm with their energy, mood, and body. But when our hormones are out of sync due to inflammation, stress, blood-sugar imbalances, etc., these shifts can feel extreme. Symptoms I used to experience and that are common with cycles that are "off" include:

- » Intense PMS
- » Painful periods
- » Mood swings
- » Bloating
- » Fatigue
- » Anxiety
- » Depression
- » Weight fluctuations

The menstrual cycle's hormonal fluctuations can be particularly challenging for those with autoimmune conditions and chronic health issues. If you already have a heightened immune system, you may be more sensitive to these fluctuations, which can make inflammation-related symptoms feel much more extreme.

As I mentioned, the best way to think about your cycle is like the four seasons. Just as nature moves through winter, spring, summer, and fall, your body follows its own changes. Just like the seasons, when everything is working well, each phase transitions smoothly and naturally into the next. But when hormones are off? You get stuck in an endless winter, an overwhelming summer, or an unpredictable autumn . . . which nobody wants!

The four phases of your cycle

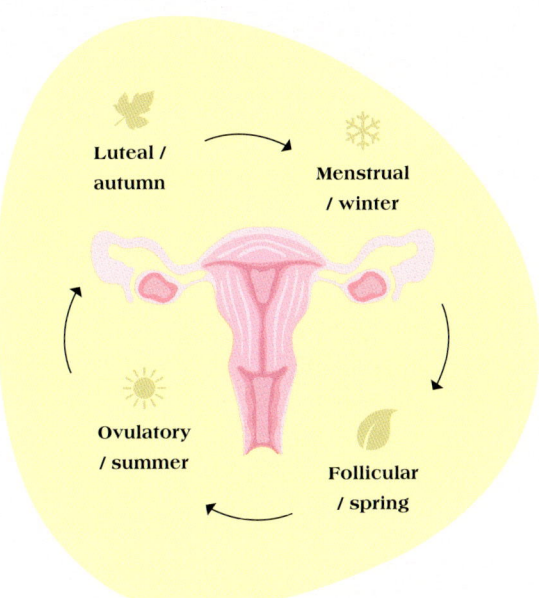

Menstrual phase (days 1–5): your inner winter

This is the start of your cycle and is when you have your period. Day 1 of your cycle is day 1 of your period. Hormones are at their lowest, and it is normal to feel a little tired, introverted, and craving warmth and rest. If you have a chronic health condition, such as endometriosis, PCOS, or even asthma or arthritis, you may notice the worsening of symptoms around this time due to increased inflammation in this phase. Menstruation itself is associated with increased inflammation, though there is not a clear understanding of how or why (as always, more funding is needed for researching women's health!). So be kind to yourself in this phase as it's normal to feel a bit "meh." Your body is shedding the uterine lining, which I like to think of as a natural monthly detox.

> *Out of balance?*
>
> *When hormones are out of balance, things can look VERY different! Your period can be incredibly painful, with intense cramping, heavy bleeding, and extreme fatigue. Why? We have things called prostaglandins, which are hormone-like compounds that trigger inflammation and help the uterus contract (a good thing!); however, too many prostaglandins can cause intense cramping and even radiate out of the pelvis, causing bowel contractions and those "period poos" that see us running to the bathroom! Other signs our hormones are out of balance are skipped periods, and, sadly, just because the period has skipped it doesn't always mean the symptoms will. Inflammation can be a huge driver of hormonal imbalances, which can be a result of lifestyle as well as underlying conditions like endometriosis, PCOS, and fibroids.*

Follicular phase (days 6–14): your inner spring

Estrogen, which women's health coach Zoe Antonia calls our "Beyoncé hormone," begins to rise, and you might have newfound energy and motivation and feel overall like your mood is much brighter. This is a great time to get creative, start new projects, and socialize. However, the increase in estrogen also increases our inflammatory response, which means if our immune system is already heightened and we are dealing with lots of inflammation we may not feel as good as we should in this phase.

> *Out of balance?*
>
> *If estrogen doesn't rise enough you might still feel flat or foggy. If it rises too high, or isn't processed properly by the body, symptoms like bloating, breast tenderness, or mood swings can show up. This is sometimes called estrogen dominance . . . and it can leave you feeling anything but Beyoncé!*

Ovulation (days 14–16): your inner summer

Estrogen peaks (Beyoncé's out in full force!), testosterone surges, and LH (luteinizing hormone) triggers ovulation. This is your most magnetic phase: your libido, energy, and confidence are sky-high and you probably feel you could take over the world! Fun fact: you are at your most attractive during ovulation, as your fertility is at its peak and so attracting a "mate" is the body's goal. So if you feel like your skin is glowing and your hair is shinier . . . it probably is! Meanwhile, if you struggle with ovulation pain, it could be those pesky prostaglandins rearing their heads again if you are a little too inflamed, as they are partially responsible for releasing the egg to be ovulated.

> *Out of balance?*
>
> *If ovulation doesn't happen, it not only impacts your mood, but also your fertility, and you won't produce any of your cool, calm, and collected hormone progesterone. Without enough progesterone you'll likely notice more PMS, anxiety, and irregular menstrual cycles. Without regular ovulation, our estrogen and testosterone will also be low, which has a wider impact on bone and muscle health. Progesterone is naturally anti-inflammatory but too much stress and inflammation in the body can block ovulation altogether. We want all of those positive benefits of ovulation on our health and longevity— so managing inflammation to ensure we ovulate as regularly as possible is as important as paying into a retirement fund.*

Luteal phase (days 17–28): your inner autumn

Progesterone rises to calm the nervous system and prepare the body for either pregnancy or your next period. This is a slower, more reflective phase, so you typically don't feel like going "out out" or starting any new projects.

> *Out of balance?*
>
> *When your progesterone levels are optimal, it's a naturally anti-inflammatory phase but when progesterone is low you may struggle. PMS can hit very hard, making you more irritable, anxious, and susceptible to mood swings. You'll get cravings for all the wrong stuff, and sleeping soundly will feel like a thing of the past.*

Your cycle is so much more than your period! And remember that these cycle phases are only a guide to offer some useful context as to when and why you may be feeling differently during your cycle—there are no strict rules!

Hopefully, from learning about the four phases of the menstrual cycle, you can see how your period is only **ONE** part of it. Nicole Jardim, a certified women's health coach, highlights ovulation as the real star of the show: this is not only when fertility peaks, but also when other key hormones like progesterone are influenced, as well as when bone density, insulin sensitivity, and other vital body processes are supported and managed. When we go through the transition to menopause, this is when we lose our monthly ovulation and estrogen drops, so those symptoms we commonly think of as part of getting older, like brain fog, poor sleep, low mood, and stubborn weight gain, are often rooted in this hormonal shift. It's not just about losing your period, it's about the ripple effect that the loss of ovulation has across your whole body.

Perimenopause: the real menopause?

I used to think that menopause was the scary thing I needed to prepare for, but what people describe as "menopause" is in fact usually perimenopause. This is the messy middle, the transition that can last anywhere from four to ten-plus years before menopause actually happens. It's the storm before the calm, when hormone levels can fluctuate wildly before eventually stabilizing.

What most women fear—the hot flashes, mood swings, weight gain, heavy periods, and brain fog—is actually perimenopause. However, just as I was wrong about menopause, I was also wrong in thinking I would one day need to be scared of this transition, and I hope once you read more you will realize this, too. Whether you're looking ahead or going through it right now, I want you to know that just as lifestyle "pulls the trigger" when it comes to genetics, it's also the case for the transition through perimenopause and menopause. These periods of our lives do **NOT** have to be this "hell" that we've come to accept as normal; there's so much we can do to prepare for it and gracefully transition through it.

In terms of preparation, you'll be happy to know it's the same steps as those we need to take to manage our menstrual cycle! When you take steps to lower inflammation and control blood sugar, stress, and so on, you will be setting yourself up for success when it comes to your transition into perimenopause. Kirsty Smith, a hormone coach I adore, always says that the smoother your cycles are, the smoother your transition will be. If your body is inflamed, stressed, and out of balance, perimenopause will come crashing down and indeed feel like the "hell" we've been warned about.

What's happening in perimenopause?

As women enter this time of their life, the first hormones to decline are progesterone and testosterone, which is exactly why so many women feel frazzled, flat, and fatigued. Here's why:

» **Progesterone** is your "keep calm and collected" hormone. It helps with mood stability, deep sleep, and lowering inflammation. When it starts to drop, you might feel more anxious, irritable, restless, and inflamed. Sleep can also go out the window, making everything feel ten times harder.

» **Testosterone** is often forgotten in women's health, but we NEED it. It gives us energy, motivation, confidence, and libido. When testosterone dips, you can feel flat, unmotivated, and weaker, like you've lost your spark. Muscle mass starts to decline, which we will explore in more depth when we reach the section about the Movement Pillar, but for now, you just need to know that muscle is fantastic at helping you regulate your blood sugar, metabolism, and overall longevity. So losing muscle should not be on anyone's wish list.

Later on, estrogen starts fluctuating wildly. One month perhaps it's too high . . . leading to heavy periods, bloating, mood swings, and sore breasts. The next, it plummets . . . causing hot flashes, dry skin, vaginal dryness, and disturbed sleep.

Even weirder, your cycle can start speeding up before it disappears completely. Some women get multiple cycles in one month because the body is engineering more chances to get pregnant before it's "too late." Although this is very clever and quite interesting (at least to me!), it's not exactly pleasant to go through.

Why does managing inflammation help?

This is the most important thing to understand—inflammation makes perimenopause much worse. This is why reducing inflammation is an essential part of a healthy perimenopause transition.

And if you're already in perimenopause and struggling, don't panic. We now know that if the hormones at the bottom of the hierarchy are causing issues, the fastest way to get them back under control is by supporting cortisol and insulin, the CEO hormones. When you do this, your body starts working with you, not against you.

This is why the six pillars of inflammation are the key to navigating perimenopause with as much ease as possible.

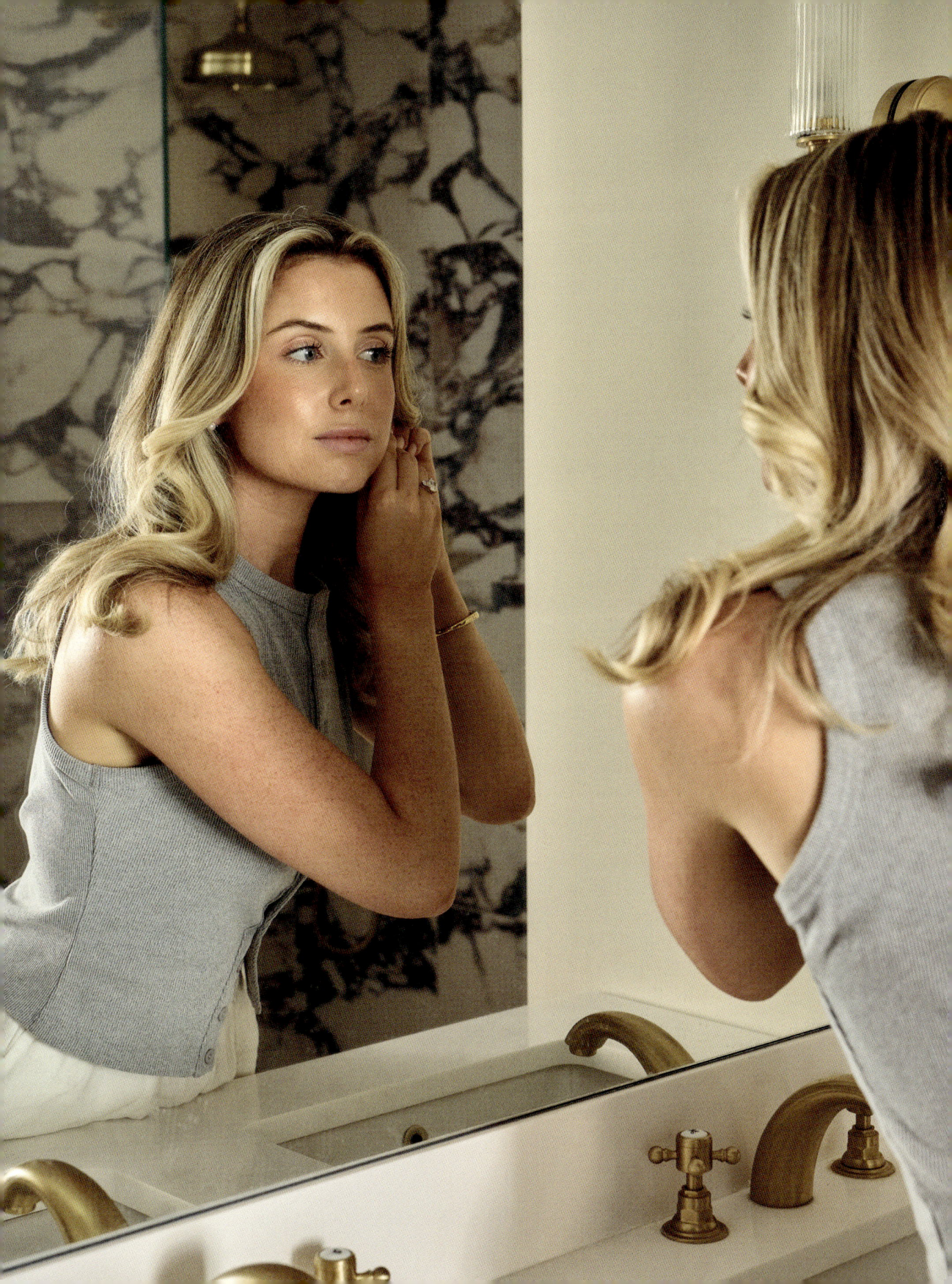

Menopause: a new beginning *(not the end!)*

If you'd asked me a few years ago what I thought menopause was, I probably would've said something like "hot flashes, mood swings, and the beginning of the end." Because that's exactly how people talk about it. It's the dreaded "change" that's always spoken about in secret, and joked about as the end of your "womanhood." What total rubbish! You are not defined by which phase of your life you are in, and being a "woman" is so much more than that.

Another thing that blew my mind, and I was quite embarrassed that I didn't know this before my training, is that menopause itself is only **ONE DAY!**

Menopause is the exact day when you've gone twelve consecutive months without a period. That's it. After that, you're officially in postmenopause, where your hormones finally stabilize at lower levels. The chaos you might have experienced during perimenopause settles, and your body adjusts to its new normal. Yes, menopause does mark the end of your reproductive years, but it doesn't mean the end of feeling strong, confident, and full of life. In fact, for many women, this phase is where they finally feel FREE. No more worrying about cycles, pregnancy, or hormonal rollercoasters ... just a new chapter, with a new set of rules.

But (and this is a big but) how well you feel in menopause depends on how well you've taken care of your hormones beforehand. Just as with how you'll feel going through perimenopause: if you've managed inflammation, kept blood sugar stable, and supported your gut and stress levels, you're far more likely to transition into menopause feeling strong, calm, and in control. But remember: it's never too late to make a positive change!

What's happening in menopause?

Menopause is when your ovaries stop releasing eggs, and your estrogen and progesterone levels drop significantly. This hormonal shift can bring about a range of changes, including:

- » **Hot flashes and night sweats:** that sudden wave of heat that feels like you've been thrown into a sauna.
- » **Sleep disturbances:** whether it's struggling to fall asleep, waking up drenched in sweat, or just feeling wired for no reason.
- » **Vaginal dryness:** caused by lower estrogen levels which can reduce natural lubrication, leading to discomfort (this can happen to non-menopausal women, too, by the way).
- » **Mood changes:** from feeling totally fine one minute to wanting to cry into your tea the next.
- » **Metabolism shifts:** weight might redistribute (especially around your tummy), and muscle mass can decline if you're not actively working to maintain it.

Sounds intense, I know, but once again . . . inflammation can be a huge contributor to the severity of these symptoms. High inflammation levels can:

- Trigger more intense hot flashes.
- Worsen sleep problems.
- Contribute to weight gain and blood-sugar issues.
- Make mood swings more extreme.

Perspective on menopause

When researching menopause, I found it fascinating how different cultures view menopause. In the Western world, we either dread it, mock it, or avoid talking about it completely, and women over a certain age may well be "written off." This is often due to uncontrollable symptoms making traditional work impossible, and so day-to-day tasks that used to be easy now become crippling. However, is this just because of the Western culture we have? Is there a place where not only are menopausal women symptom free, they're also respected?

- *Japanese women often report fewer menopausal symptoms, and menopause (konenki) is seen as a natural life transition, not a medical condition to "fix" (abs-cbn.com).*
- *Among Mayan women, menopause is almost symptom-free and is actually viewed as a time of increased wisdom and social status (mindsethealth.com).*
- *In some indigenous cultures, postmenopausal women are considered spiritual leaders and the wise matriarchs of their communities.*

How different is that from the Western approach, where menopause is often seen as something to dread and "fix"?

This perspective shift is so important. Menopause isn't an ending, it's a rebirth into a new phase of life. And when you take care of your body, it can be a time of power, confidence, and strength.

So, whether it's in your future, or you're right in the middle of menopause, I hope I've convinced you that it truly is something to be celebrated and respected, not feared or be ashamed of.

Why all this matters

As women, we've been told that painful or missing periods, fatigue, bloating, unpredictable weight changes, and difficult transitions through perimenopause and menopause are normal. Yes they *are* common, but they are not normal! But with the right steps and guidance, things can change.

When we understand the foundations of inflammation and our hormones, and most important take action to support them (exactly what this reset is designed to do), you won't just feel the results, you'll see them, too! In your energy, focus, workouts, cycles, skin, weight, and in the way you move through every stage of life. This is the power of viewing your body as a whole, treating your health as one connected picture, and supporting it from the inside out.

This matters for everyone, but especially if you live with chronic conditions, or autoimmune conditions or those alike, e.g., endometriosis, PCOS (polycystic ovary syndrome), IBS (irritable bowel syndrome), gut problems, or food intolerances. Even without a diagnosis, daily inflammation takes its toll. It is not just about being tired of the pain and exhaustion, it's about the knock-on effect these symptoms have on our cycles and the way we transition through perimenopause and menopause. The menstrual cycle is one of the clearest reflections of overall health, and managing inflammation through the CEO hormones (cortisol and insulin) is key to restoring balance.

I know all of this firsthand! Before tackling inflammation, my periods were unbearable, and pain, bloating, and exhaustion controlled my life. Once I focused on inflammation, hormones, and balancing blood sugar, everything changed.

> **No more crippling cramps.**
>
> **No more relentless bloating.**
>
> **No more feeling like my body was fighting me.**

It's never too late to take back control

Something I wish every woman knew is that it is never too late to change. In an ideal world, we would all have been taught to understand and care for our cycle from our very first period. Instead, many of us were encouraged to simply ignore it until fertility or pregnancy became a focus.

Wherever you are in life—whether you're just starting your period, in your reproductive years, navigating perimenopause, or in menopause—the tools and practices in this book will help you to feel better now and also to prepare for your future self.

The six pillars of inflammation are at the heart of this. When we lower inflammation, we stop chasing symptoms and begin addressing root causes. That is when real, lasting change happens.

Before we delve into the six pillars of inflammation, there's one more quick but essential topic we all need to understand first: blood-sugar balancing. Now that you know that keeping your CEO hormones (cortisol and insulin) in check is key to hormonal harmony, it's important to know that blood sugar has an enormous impact on them both. It's the thread that runs through each pillar. If we can keep our blood sugar steady, we keep the CEOs happy, and that sets the stage for balanced hormones and a more anti-inflammatory life. Read on, and you'll understand why.

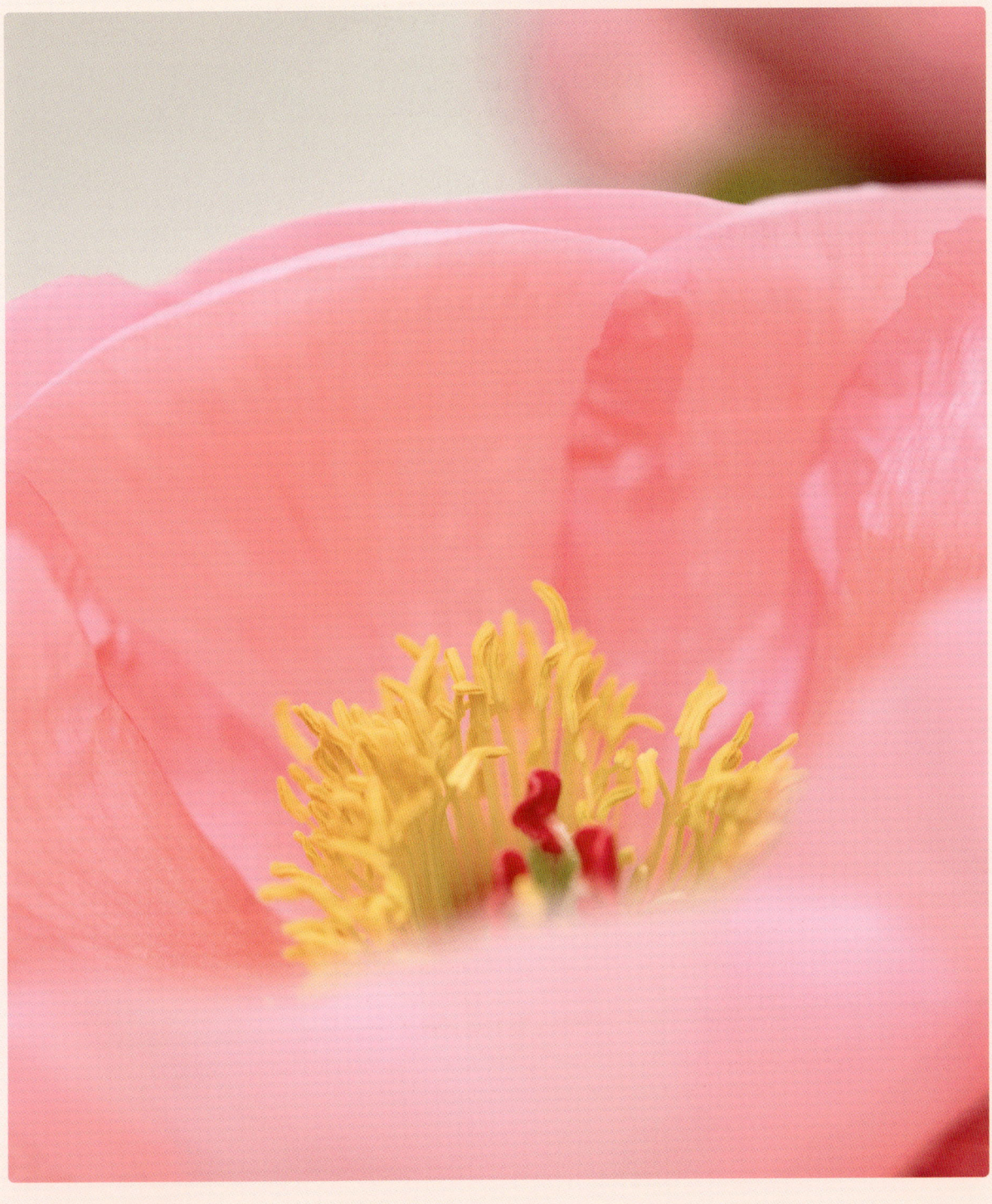

Blood Sugar

If there's one thing I wish I'd known sooner about inflammation and women's health, it's how important blood sugar is, and that it's about SO much more than just table sugar, weight, or diabetes, it's about everything! Blood sugar is one of the major reasons you wake up energized or exhausted, why you get hangry, why your skin flares up out of nowhere, why your cravings feel impossible to control, and why you either feel cool, calm, and collected . . . or all over the place.

I am someone who has always struggled with intense sugar cravings, and I used to blame it on my genetics because my mum struggles with them, too. I used to describe it as this annoying devil on my shoulder nagging at me, reminding me of all the little treats tucked away in the cupboard. My mum was exactly the same, so we concluded we had a "sweet gene" in the family!

On top of blaming this imaginary sweet gene, I also used to put it down to willpower . . . or rather, a lack of it! I used to think I just had the willpower of a toddler and that there was no point avoiding it because I'd give in eventually anyway . . . and cookies and cakes taste so good, so why not? One won't hurt, right? The issue is that this magical sugar high we feel in the moment always ends the same way. As our blood sugar drops back down, we feel tired, sluggish, and filled with guilt. To make matters worse, the sugar crash brings with it a desperate need to come back to balance, so your body starts screaming out for more sugar, and before you know it, you're back on the sofa, custard creams in hand, making and breaking that promise to yourself that you'll "just have the one."

This blood-sugar roller coaster doesn't just make you feel rubbish. It's also a major driver of inflammation—the very reason you're here reading this book. And one of the biggest reasons for that is what it does to your hormones.

What blood sugar actually is

Every time you eat carbohydrates, your body breaks them down into glucose (a type of sugar), which enters your bloodstream. Blood sugar is just the level of glucose in your blood at any given time. To keep that level balanced, your body releases insulin (one of your tier 1 CEO hormones), which acts like a taxi, carrying glucose into your cells, where it can be used for energy.

In a balanced body, this process is smooth sailing. Your cells get the energy they need, and you feel stable, clear-headed, and fueled. No intrusive sugar craving thoughts or wild moods . . . cool, calm, and collected!

But when blood sugar is constantly spiking and crashing, whether that's because of the type of food you eat, skipping meals, stress, poor sleep, or any of the other pillars in this book, that balance gets thrown off. This causes a stress response in the body, triggering an increased production of cortisol, too—and because insulin and cortisol are the CEO hormones sitting at the top of your hormonal hierarchy, this imbalance kicks off a domino effect that disrupts everything underneath. Reminder: those wonderful hormones underneath control your menstrual cycle and your transition through perimenopause and menopause. So balancing blood sugar is VERY important for keeping all your hormones doing what they are meant to.

How blood sugar affects your hormones
(and drives inflammation)

Insulin

When you're constantly eating foods that spike blood sugar, like refined carbs, sugary snacks, or ultra-processed fod, insulin goes into overdrive, producing far more than usual to keep up with the demand from all this extra sugar. If this is a regular occurrence, it can lead to insulin resistance, where your cells stop responding properly. Imagine your cells are like a house, and insulin comes knocking on your door a couple of times a day, asking you to let sugar in . . . not a problem. However . . . now imagine that insulin was ringing your doorbell 24/7. You'd get fed up and stop answering the door! **THAT** is insulin resistance. Not only does this affect metabolism, but it also has a domino effect on your hormones, and throws off estrogen, progesterone, and testosterone, which is why conditions like PCOS are so often tied to blood-sugar imbalances. Symptoms like irregular cycles, acne, unwanted hair growth or loss, weight gain, and mood swings can all be a result of unbalanced blood sugar and can be incredibly frustrating, upsetting, and debilitating to live with. My endometriosis always flares up when my blood sugar is out of balance, something I **WISH** I'd known sooner.

Cortisol

Cortisol is your stress hormone, but it also plays a key role in blood-sugar regulation. When your blood sugar drops too low, like when you skip meals or fast for too long, cortisol steps in to help. It triggers the liver to release stored glucose (called glycogen), pulling it back into the bloodstream to provide a quick burst of energy for your body. This is helpful in the short term (for example, if your body thinks you're under attack you need quick access to energy [sugar] in your bloodstream), but when it happens all the time, it keeps cortisol high and that's when inflammation creeps in. Your body recognizes high levels of cortisol as a stressor and sends the bodyguards in to help, triggering the immune response and inflammation.

> Constant cortisol and insulin dysregulation can lead to:
>
> » Low progesterone = PMS, anxiety, sleep problems.
>
> » High or low estrogen = heavy periods, bloating, mood swings.
>
> » Sluggish thyroid = low energy, poor digestion, slow metabolism.

And, of course, all of this contributes to the exact symptoms so many of us are trying to fix . . . fatigue that sleep doesn't solve, hormonal acne, weight gain especially around the tummy, irregular and painful periods, and a confused foggy brain that doesn't seem to clear.

This is why blood sugar is at the root of inflammation, hormone imbalance, and pretty much everything else we'll explore in this book.

What happens when blood sugar is out of balance

This is what unbalanced blood sugar looks like, and how those roller-coaster highs and lows show up in everyday life:

Blood-sugar spikes

When you eat a meal high in refined carbs, glucose floods the bloodstream. Insulin steps in to remove it quickly, which causes a crash. That's when fatigue, cravings, and brain fog hit. The body wants balance, so it pushes you to grab something sugary again . . . and the cycle continues.

Blood-sugar dips

When you go too long without eating, or don't eat enough carbs, your blood sugar drops too low. The body releases cortisol to bring it back up by pulling sugar from the liver. That constant cortisol release keeps you in fight-or-flight (aka stress mode) and ramps up inflammation.

Whether it's a spike or a crash, both patterns stress the body, activate the immune system unnecessarily, and fuel the inflammatory fire. And over time, that starts to affect everything from your mood and energy to your periods and skin.

Why this matters

No matter what life stage you're in, whether it's monthly cycles, the ups and downs of perimenopause, or navigating menopause, your hormones rely on insulin and cortisol being in balance, and when blood sugar is stable:

- » Your body can better regulate estrogen, progesterone, and thyroid hormones.
- » Inflammation stays low.
- » Hormonal transitions feel smoother, more manageable, and less chaotic.

This is why balancing blood sugar is one of the most powerful ways to support your hormones at every stage of life, and why each pillar I discuss in the next section of the book is explored with this in mind—to ensure your CEO hormones always stay in check.

What comes next?

When it comes to making a change, I know you're probably eager and ready to start right NOW, and that's great... but I'd recommend you read about all six pillars before embarking on the 30-day reset. Allow the information to sink in, understand how all these pillars are showing up in your life, and THEN pick the reset that works for you.

My goal (and life mission) is to help people understand the how and why behind inflammation, and that regardless of genes, chronic health conditions, or unfortunate life events that have knocked us off track, we're all capable of drawing a line and overcoming these health challenges we're facing day in, day out. We don't need to suffer in silence or put it down to just "being a woman"—rubbish! We have one life, and we're here to make it a good one!

You've learned how your hormones don't just control your mood or periods, they govern your entire health, and when they're off (especially your CEO hormones, cortisol and insulin), the ripple effect can be enormous: painful heavy periods, mood swings, acne, hair loss (or unwanted growth), and constant flare-ups of conditions like PCOS, endometriosis, and other chronic or autoimmune diseases. And blood sugar? It's right at the center of all of it. When blood sugar isn't stable, cortisol and insulin suffer, and when they suffer, your whole hormonal system comes tumbling down, driving inflammation up, and fueling a vicious unbalanced hormonal hierarchy.

That's why hormones and blood sugar aren't part of the six pillars I explore in this book, they're the entire foundation beneath them. They show up in every area of your life, from how you eat to how you move, how you sleep, how you handle stress, how well your gut is working, and how effectively your body can detox. They're not something to "work on" once and tick off, they're areas that need to be understood and supported consistently. That's exactly what the six pillars will help you to do.

Now for the exciting part! It's time to get into the juicy section of this book, which is the six pillars of inflammation. Here you'll find practical, proven advice you can focus on to support your body, calm inflammation, and finally feel like yourself again. Not only are the suggestions here rooted in science and research, but they're also tried and tested by me. I got my life back, and I'm making it my mission to share EVERYTHING so that you can, too.

Let's say goodbye to inflammation... forever!

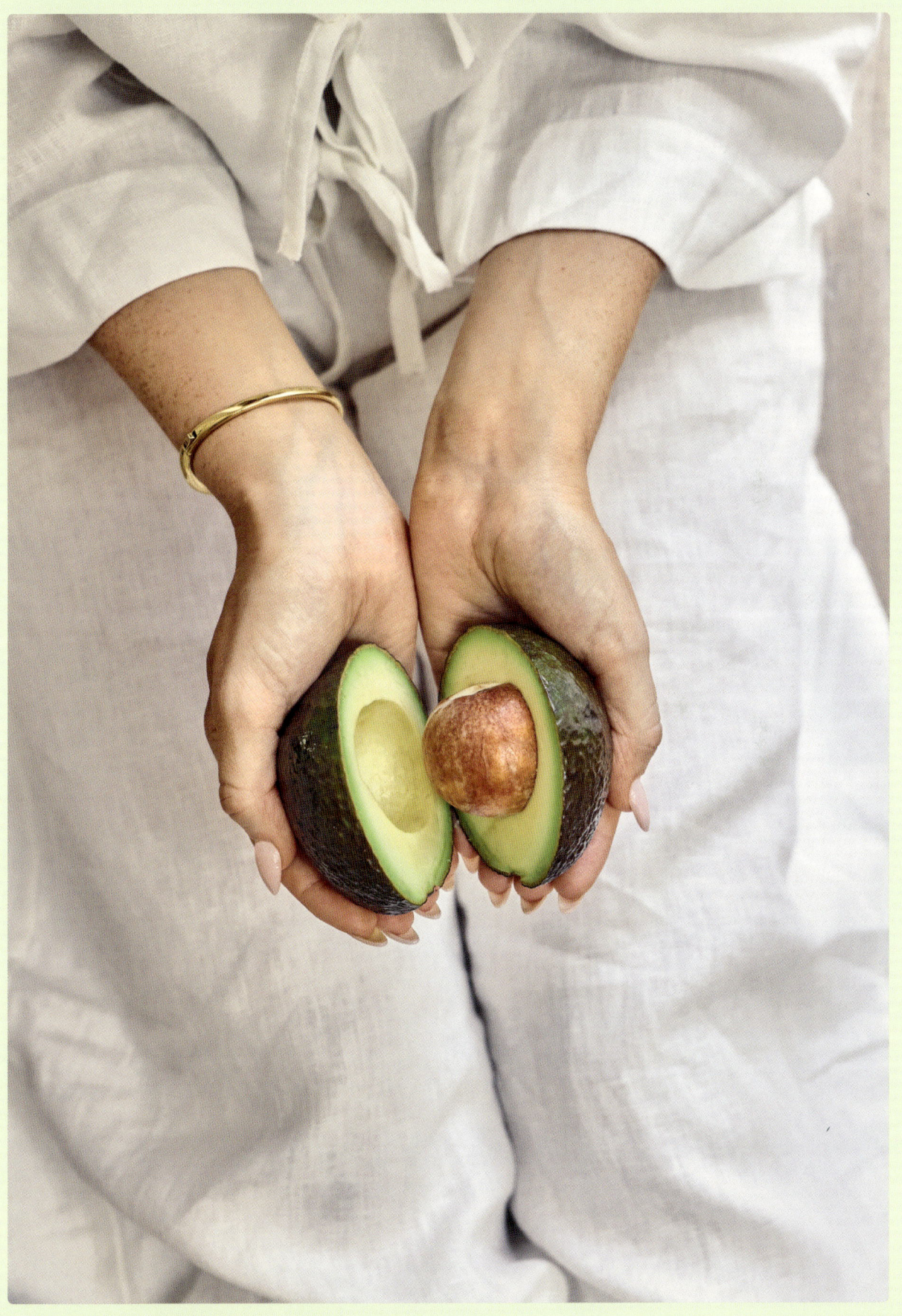

Pillar 1: Food Is More Than Fuel

Food has somehow become controversial. With the rise of social media, more than ever we're subjected to a confusion of wildly different diets, all claiming to be the "cure" or "fix" we're looking for. Before we get into the myths, fads, and most important the **TRUTH** about food, it's important to know that food is more than just fuel. While this pillar explores how food does, of course, fuel us to feel our best (or worst) self, there's so much more to food than simply what it does to our bodies.

Growing up in a Welsh family, I used to love making Welsh cakes with my nana (think half cake half cookie—a delightful combination), and baking in general was a huge part of my childhood—memories I will cherish forever. As I got older, this wholesome love for baking changed to boozy bottomless brunches with the girls, which I look back on and still laugh hysterically at the terrible decisions we used to make after a bucket of margaritas. Cakes, cookies, and alcohol are all things that I indulged in in the past, and occasionally eat now, but the reason I mention this is that our relationship with food, especially "treats" like sugary snacks and alcohol, is more complicated than just what we put in our mouth. It's the celebrations we share, the love we give, and the memories we have with our families and friends that often revolve around a feast. So you can breathe a big sigh of relief that I'm not going to take any of that away from you.
 I am, however, going to reveal which foods are going to make you feel your best, explain exactly what they do for your body, and show how filling up your plate with **nutritious** food is the answer, crowding out the non-nutritious to better serve your health.

Ultra-processed foods

Let's get one thing straight: you are not broken for craving sugar. As humans, we're hard-wired to seek it out. Thousands of years ago, sweet foods like ripe fruit or honey were rare and precious—a quick source of energy that could mean the difference between surviving or not. So our brains evolved to light up when we found sugar . . . and to eat as much of it as possible, because who knew when we'd find it again?

But answer this . . . when was the last time you had to hunt for sugar? I can guarantee that if you pause for a moment right now, and think about something sweet, you'll quickly remember where your sweet treats are hidden, and your mouth might even start salivating, too. This evolutionary sweet tooth, which once helped keep us alive, has been taken advantage of in a world driven by money, which profits off our overconsumption, and makes decisions based on the health of our economy instead of our bodies.

The emotional connection we have with food has been hijacked by scientists working 24/7 to make sure that what we put in our mouth is ludicrously tasty, addictive, and binge-worthy. These foods have been scientifically engineered to be this way, to make it almost impossible to stop eating . . . so when you're beating yourself up for accidentally eating ten cookies even though you **SWORE** it would just be one, just remember there's a team of scientists working against you. If you don't believe me, Chris Van Tulleken has written an entire book called *Ultra-Processed People,* which delves into how companies are engineering their food to have the perfect crunch, texture, and even the perfect smell from the puff of opening a package of chips.

More than 50 percent of the UK diet is now made up of ultra-processed foods (UPFs), packed with preservatives, additives, and unpronounceable ingredients. These foods hijack your hunger signals, spike your blood sugar, and keep you craving more and more . . . It's not a personal failure or lack of willpower, it's a clever business model.

> *Not all processed foods are bad. Chopping, blending, and cooking = fine. But **ultra-processed foods (UPFs)** are in a different league, chemically altered, stripped of nutrients, and pumped full of preservatives and additives that your body doesn't recognize, e.g., protein bars, cookies, sweets, most packaged breads, and anything with a long list of ingredients.*
>
> ***How to spot a UPF:***
>
> » Long ingredient list
> » Words you can't pronounce
> » Designed to be addictive (hyper palatable = can't stop eating)
> » Artificial ingredients and chemicals

So if willpower is useless in these scenarios—surely we're all doomed? Well, I am living proof that once you know **WHY** food matters, and how it connects with inflammation, you'll have the power to build meals that fuel your health, and not inflammation. As I've mentioned, I used to polish off a family-size pack of custard creams with two coffees in **ONE** sitting, and that was just the start! I was addicted to sugar, constantly thinking about it, and even had anxiety about not satisfying my cravings. What was actually happening wasn't poor willpower. It was clever packaging and addictive ingredients, and once I started I couldn't stop. Once you're on the blood-sugar roller coaster, it's hard to get off. The answer is either not getting on the roller coaster in the first place, or if you do fancy a "sweet" ride, pick one with fewer ups and downs, that satisfies your cravings and nourishes you at the same time, like the delicious sweet treats and desserts later in this book! You'll feel a lot better for it.

The "perfect" diet

If you're anything like me, I'm guessing this isn't your first rodeo when it comes to changing the way you eat. We're all looking for a better way to manage our health, reduce our symptoms, and finally feel less bloated. Perhaps, like me, you'll have tried various polarizing diets that promise the world and deliver mixed results. Such as:

» Vegan diet
» Carnivore diet
» Keto diet
» Celery juice cleanse
» Gluten-free diet
» Dairy-free diet

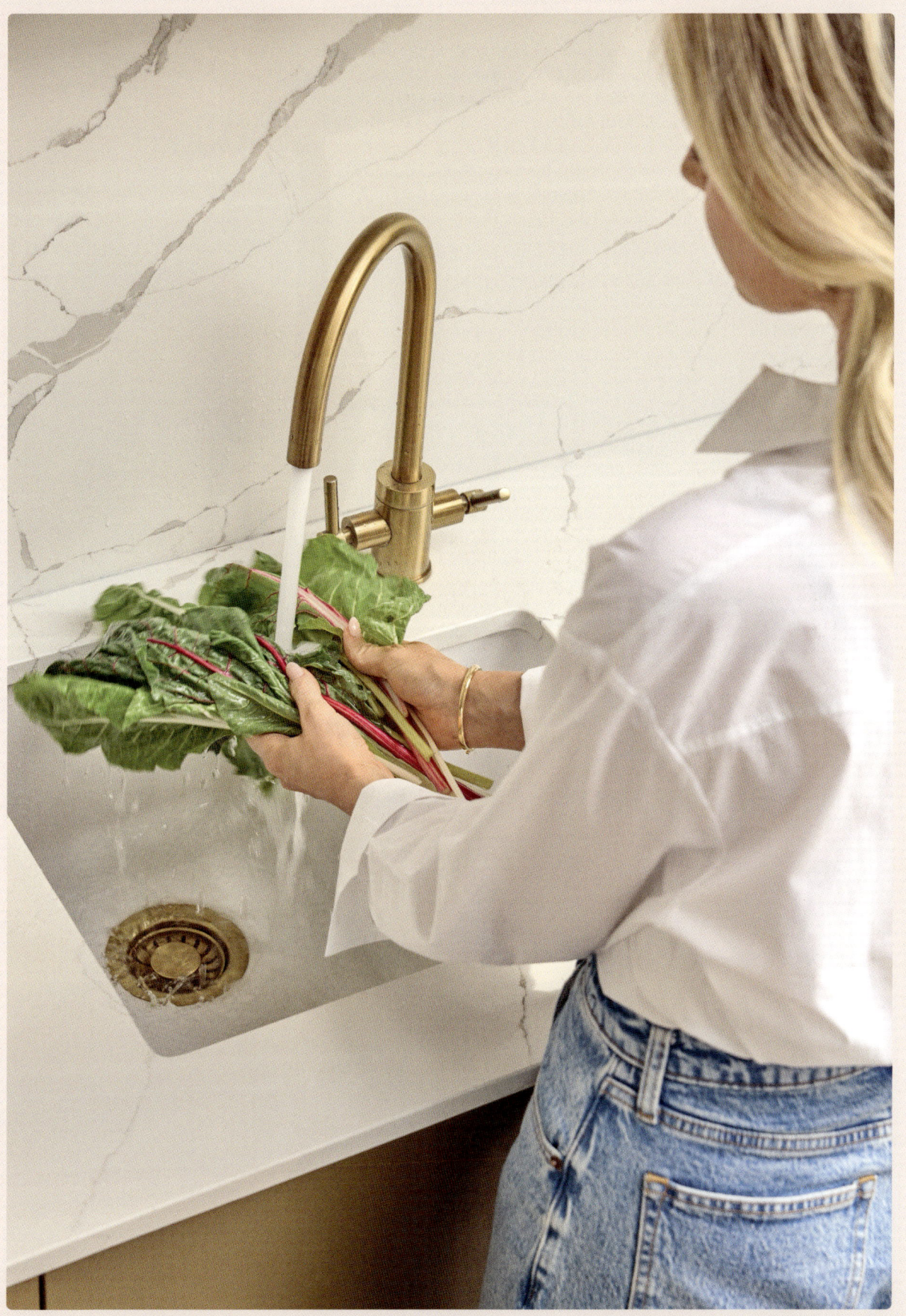

When it comes to extreme diets, I'd be a hypocrite to say they don't work because I've tried them ALL, and actually they all did help, to varying degrees, at least in the short term. However, I came to realize that it wasn't the diet itself that helped... because both the vegan AND carnivore diets reduced my bloating and pain, and yet with one banishing meat, and the other requiring me to live ONLY on meat, how was it possible that they both had the same effect? It was because I followed each diet with a non-processed food rule. On the carnivore diet, I was focusing only on organic grass-fed meat, and on the vegan diet I focused on organic vegetables—on both occasions I said goodbye to processed foods!

I wish I'd realized back then that it wasn't fats or carbs that were making me unwell—it was largely down to ultra-processed foods, and so ANY diet that cut them out left me feeling better! This realization came when I tried the Autoimmune Protocol (AIP), a strict short-term elimination diet. On this plan you eat only meat, fish, fruit, and vegetables (no grains, legumes, nuts, seeds, or nightshades) until symptoms settle. Then you reintroduce foods one at a time, every few days, to see what brings symptoms back.

Within thirty days, almost all my symptoms disappeared: no more period pain, heavy bleeding, or cramping, and I lost over fourteen pounds in weight that I'd previously thought was stubborn fat. I felt incredible, had more energy than I'd had for years, and friends couldn't believe my physical transformation either. I was eager to see what my trigger foods were, and when I started reintroducing, it was clear that ultra-processed foods were a big NO for my body. This cemented my suspicions and I have adopted a 80–90 percent whole-food diet ever since, which has also set the foundations for this book.

Something that was interesting, though, was that some whole foods, like chile and certain grains, triggered symptoms, too. How could this be? The answer lies in the difference between food intolerances and a compromised gut, which I dive deeper into on page 64. Some people do react to specific foods, but often our bodies respond negatively because the gut is inflamed or imbalanced, not because the food itself is "bad." Have you ever had a meal one day and felt fine, but on a different day the same meal gave you a bad belly? Well... stress, poor sleep, and other lifestyle factors can add to this, making even nutritious foods hard to tolerate.

For those with food intolerances, a short-term protocol like AIP can be useful to uncover true intolerances (see page 64). But for most people, inflammation is driven by ultra-processed foods and/or a gut that could do with love and support. So, when whole foods cause problems, it's often more about gut health than the food itself.

This is why it's so important to start with the foundations. Before cutting out long lists of foods because you think your body doesn't like them, focus on the six pillars of inflammation: nutrition, gut health, detoxification, stress, sleep, and movement. When these are supported, your body is far better able to enjoy a wide variety of nourishing foods.

Food is our foundation. By reducing ultra-processed foods and strengthening the six pillars, you can achieve many of the benefits of an anti-inflammatory protocol without the extremes or the feeling of restriction.

Food is our foundation!

The food we put into our system is what sets our body up for success. It influences our blood sugar, hormones, gut health, immune system . . . and of course, as a result, determines whether we're fighting or *fixing* inflammation. Once you understand what a truly anti-inflammatory diet looks like, you might start to see where your choices could be tripping you up, and that's a **GOOD** thing. There's no judgment here, it's just about learning the facts and gently holding them up next to your current habits to see where things might need a little realignment. I also want to remind you that this is **NOT** a diet in the sense of weight loss. Yes, you may lose weight: I lost fourteen pounds very quickly because I didn't realize the extent to which processed foods were impacting my body. However, when I use the term "diet," I'm referring to the way we eat rather than the calorie restriction definition we're so used to reading about. There's no calorie counting or restriction here—just eating real foods, and plenty of them!

How foods fight or fuel inflammation

When I started my "health" journey, I didn't realize that most of the healthy products I was eating were in fact causing inflammation. So when I say we're fueling inflammation unknowingly, I'm not just talking about the obvious things like fast food, sugary frappuccinos, or packets of cookies, I'm including all sorts of foods labeled as "healthy," too . . . and they are much more sneaky than the obvious unhealthy treats.

Ultra-processed foods (UPFs) make up more than half the average UK diet. As I've mentioned, these aren't just convenient or tasty; they're chemically engineered to be addictive, hyper-palatable, and designed to override your body's natural hunger cues. It's no wonder we're stuck in a cycle of cravings, crashes, and inflammation. Our biology is being manipulated by a business model that profits from keeping us hooked. UPFs fuel oxidative stress, disrupt gut health, spike blood sugar, and demand constant clean-up work from organs such as our liver . . . which puts more pressure on the body, leaving us with chronic inflammation. This messes with our hormones, energy, mood, and immune system . . . and leaves us feeling sick, bloated, and unhappy, with our weight creeping up and up, even when we are restricting calories.

However, this doesn't have to be the case. When you eat **REAL** food that is rich in nutrients, fiber, antioxidants, and healthy fats, your body will start to change and you'll feel the difference. You'll regulate your blood sugar, your gut will get what it needs to work *with* you, not against you, and your immune system won't be constantly firing . . . leaving your hormones to stabilize, and keeping unwelcome symptoms at bay.

None of this is about being perfect, it's just about understanding how powerful food can be, and how to use this to your advantage. I know changes to what we eat can be the most overwhelming step when it comes to tackling health challenges, so it's why I've included in this book more than eighty healthy and delicious anti-inflammatory recipes for you to cook your way through. However, I want you to first understand the **WHY** behind the ingredients and combinations you will see, so that you can make great choices with or without this book.

What to eat:
real food, macronutrients, micronutrients, supplements, and more!

½ Nonstarchy Carbohydrates

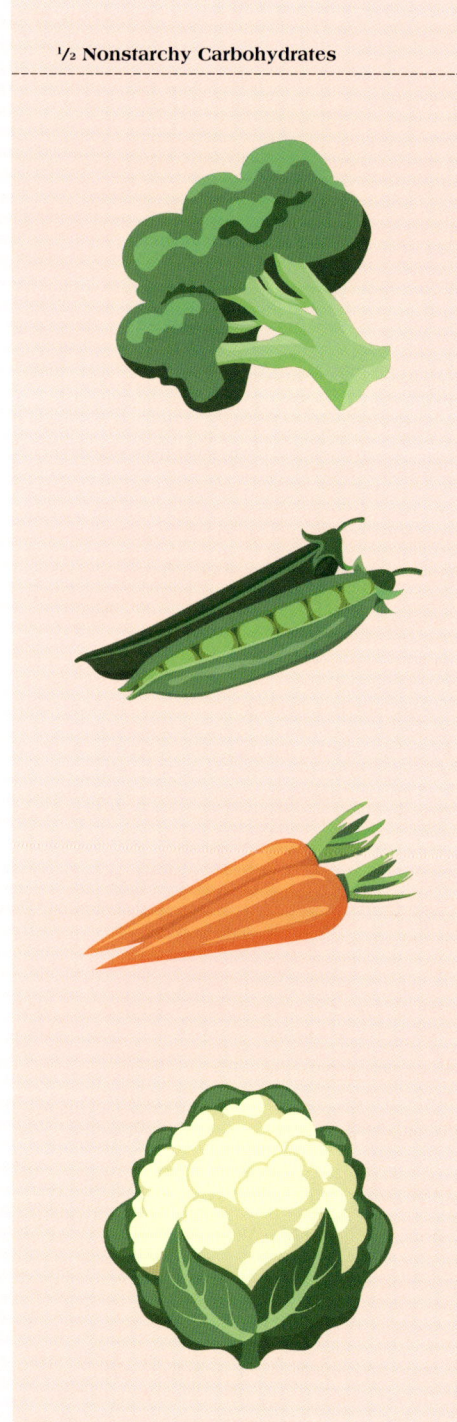

¼ Starchy Carbohydrates
(fruits, vegetables, and grains)

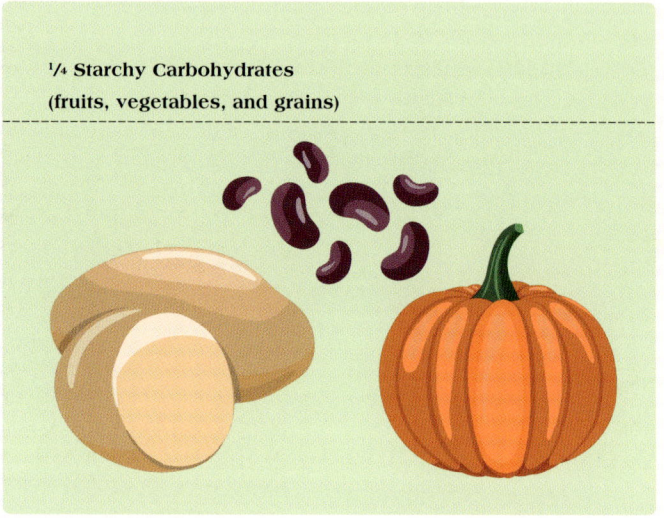

¼ Protein

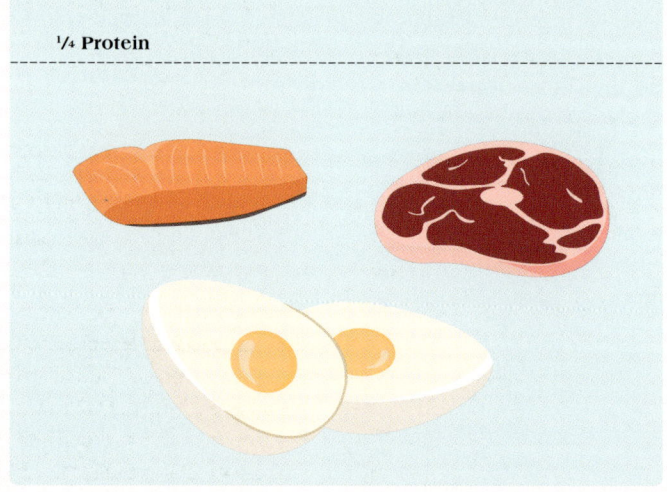

Healthy Fats

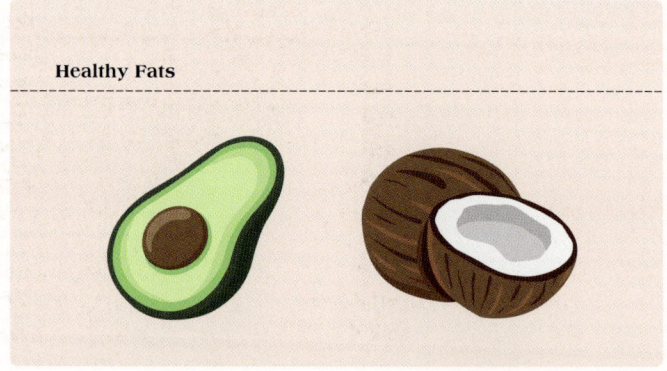

Macronutrients

Macronutrients, or "macros" for short, are the three main nutrients your body needs in large amounts to function. These are:

- » Fat
- » Protein
- » Carbohydrates

They're called "macro" because you need a lot of them (as opposed to micronutrients like vitamins and minerals, which you need in smaller amounts). Each macro plays a key role in how you feel, how much energy you have, how efficiently your hormones are produced, how quickly (or slowly) your metabolism is running . . . and as a result your overall health. When all three are balanced correctly, they are the ultimate anti-inflammatory trio.

Learning the WHY behind the Big Three is what made me stop fasting and following a low-carbohydrate diet. Both had helped my inflammation in the short term, but long-term they brought unwanted gut symptoms and low energy, and I had started developing a poor relationship with food. Thankfully, when I started studying hormones, I quickly learned the importance of all three macronutrients. I learned how they function in the body, and what happens if you don't have enough of each . . . and the reality was shocking. So I want to share the wisdom I learned, which helps me live an anti-inflammatory lifestyle and has changed my life not just in the short term, but forever!

Fat: your hormones' favorite fuel

Fat has been one of the most misunderstood foods on this planet. For a long time we were told it was the enemy, blamed for everything from heart disease to weight gain, and as a result we were fed the narrative that "fat-free" everything was a good idea. As a child who grew up drinking full-fat milk straight from the farm, this was heartbreaking! The reality, however, is that not only is fat essential for making some of our hormones, but also the fat that is removed from food to make it "healthier" is often substituted with sugar for flavor, and more recently, with sweeteners, causing chaos to our blood sugar and gut health. Without fat, your body literally can't function properly, because fat is the foundation of some of the most VIP hormones in your body, the very hormones that control your cycle, health, and metabolism and manage inflammation. So, FAT IS BACK ON THE MENU. Focusing on high-quality, whole-food sources of fat is key to living an anti-inflammatory life.

Fat + hormones

Your hormones aren't made out of thin air, they need raw materials. Fat (or rather the cholesterol that comes from fat) is one of the main raw materials required for making those key hormones in the hormonal hierarchy.

The main hormones that rely on cholesterol from dietary fat are:

» **Cortisol:** one of your CEO hormones, it helps your body respond to stress and recover from it. When cortisol is out of balance, it can feel like burnout, constantly feeling run down, less stress resilience, and "tired but wired" energy, which can lead to feeling tired even after a full night's sleep.

» **Estrogen:** supports brain function, bone strength, mood, and cycle health. Without enough fat we are at risk of slipping into a low-estrogen state which can bring with it a range of symptoms such as brain fog, weight changes, low mood, or irregular cycles.

» **Progesterone:** your calming, balancing hormone, important for sleep, mood, and cycle regulation. Without enough fat, we may experience symptoms of low progesterone, which can include poor sleep, mood issues, spotting, infertility, and many more.

» **Testosterone:** without enough fat we may notice that our sex drive plummets, along with our motivation and confidence, and our ability to build muscle and lose stubborn weight around our tummy.

I hope you can now see how important fat is to support overall hormone regulation so that you can finally ditch symptoms like PMS, poor sleep, mood swings, low libido, fertility issues, and inflammation. Eating healthy fats isn't just supportive, it's non-negotiable if you want to feel balanced, energized, and inflammation-free.

Fat quality matters

Not all fats are created equal. It's why I don't like the "traffic light" system we have on the UK's food labeling system. UPF food can often be given green lights across the board, which is very misleading. For example, a processed protein bar could be green across all these "health" labels as it's low in sugar; however, these are often high in preservatives, additives, and chemicals that aren't monitored on this basic out-of-date traffic-light system. This misleading tool drives people who want to improve their health, like me and you, to pick up this bar and munch away, not realizing we would have been better off having a regular chocolate bar in some cases! Instead, we should be focusing on the *quality* of our ingredients, and the quality of fat really does matter.

High-quality fats:

These are the fats that help reduce inflammation, balance hormones, and support your metabolism:

» **Omega-3s** from wild salmon, sardines, mackerel, walnuts, flaxseeds, chia.
» **Mono-unsaturated fats** from extra-virgin olive oil, avocado, nuts, and seeds.
» **Saturated fats** (in moderation) from grass-fed butter, ghee, and high-quality animal products.

Lower-quality fats:

These are the ones that drive inflammation and disrupt your hunger hormones, such as leptin (more about this hormone below):

» **Highly processed oils** like sunflower, soybean, rapeseed (known as canola in the US), and corn oil—found in most UPFs.
» **Factory-farmed animal fats** (due to poor omega-3 to omega-6 ratios—see the box below for more info on this).

> *What's the deal with omegas?!*
>
> *Simply put, omegas are healthy fats that your body can't make on its own, so you need to get them from food, which is why they're called "essential fatty acids." The main ones are omega-3 and omega-6, and keeping them in balance is KEY!*
>
> *Omega-3s are anti-inflammatory, and omega-6s are pro-inflammatory . . . but you need a balance of both. Most UPFs are packed with omega-6s and barely any omega-3s, throwing this ratio way off.*
>
> *A fascinating study has shown that eggs from pasture-raised chickens had three times more omega-3s and up to ten times better omega-6 to omega-3 ratios compared to caged hens.*

Fat and hunger: the leptin connection

Fat also helps regulate leptin, the hunger hormone that tells your brain when you're full. However, when you eat too many inflammatory fats (like those in UPFs), this signal can go all over the place, leading to overeating, sugar cravings, and constant hunger . . . sound familiar?

When you prioritize high-quality fats, you naturally feel more satisfied, balanced, and in control of your appetite.

So yes, fat is fabulous . . . when it comes from the right sources.

> *Quick win swaps:*
> » *Cook with olive oil, avocado oil, or ghee instead of vegetable oil.*
> » *Add avocado to toast, salads, and smoothies.*
> » *Sprinkle flax or chia seeds on porridge or yogurt.*

Protein: the non-negotiable macronutrient

For years, I thought protein was just for those men who would grunt every time they took a step in the gym . . . or for that one time my brother decided he wanted to "bulk up" and started living off protein powder. Either way, my perception of protein was that it was mainly for men, and for those who wanted to get big bulky muscles, so protein was NEVER a focus for me. I just stuck to the calorie count of whatever snack I was picking up, and as long as it said "healthy" on the label somewhere and was under 100 calories—I was sold. I had no consideration for the macronutrients, or indeed the micronutrients, which we'll come to shortly. I didn't care about the chemicals either, just the calories. I wish I could go back and give my old self a shake, because I was completely wrong about protein, and as a result I made less than ideal choices.

Protein isn't just for bulking up or getting big muscles. It's the foundation of everything from your hair, skin, and nails to your hormones, mood, metabolism, and immune system, so YES, it's even the foundation of inflammation, too. If you're constantly tired, craving sugar, breaking out, or feeling like your body's not bouncing back . . . protein (or lack of it) could be the missing piece. It certainly was for me.

Why protein is essential (especially for women)

Protein is your body's number one building material: every cell in your body needs it and when you don't get enough, your body starts borrowing it from your own tissues (clever, I know, but not ideal). The knock-on impact this has doesn't just mean you lose important tissue like muscle, but it sends your hormones into chaos (insulin—your CEO hormone—is a protein-based hormone!), so inflammation, sugar cravings, muscle loss, and a sluggish metabolism are all on the cards if you're not eating enough protein.

Protein + hormones

Protein acts as an essential building block for key hormones and a lack of protein can disrupt basic functions, including:

- » **Insulin:** helps to regulate blood sugar.
- » **Thyroid hormones:** these control your appetite, metabolism, and energy.
- » **Growth hormone:** aids recovery from inflammation or illness and supports healthy aging.
- » **Glucagon:** works with insulin to prevent crashes and regulate blood sugar.

Basically: all the things that make you feel and look your best rely on protein!

Not all hormones are protein-based—some, like estrogen, progesterone, cortisol, and testosterone, are made from fat (specifically cholesterol). However, hormones don't work in isolation, they need to be in balance. That's why it's just as important to support your protein-based hormones, too, because they all work as a team!

The inflammation + protein deficiency cycle

If you're not eating enough protein, your body can become deficient in essential amino acids. Since amino acids are the building blocks of protein, and vital for functions like repairing tissues, making enzymes and hormones, your body will start breaking down its own muscle and tissue to release those amino acids! It sounds like a painful process but it's sneaky—you won't even notice it happening . . . until the signs start showing up:

- **Muscle loss** = slower metabolism = more inflammation and weight gain.
- **Weakened immunity** = more colds, flu, poor healing, and long-term risk of chronic health conditions.
- **Blood-sugar roller coaster** = hormonal imbalances = cravings, fatigue, irritability.
- **Loss of vibrancy** = poor healing, brittle nails, thinning hair, or low energy.

It's a vicious cycle and more common than you think. If you don't fuel yourself properly with enough of the right type of protein, eventually you will pay the price.

How much protein + what types to eat

On average, women should have 90–120g of protein per day, depending on size, height, activity level, and goals. If you're exercising and lifting weights, you'll need more protein than someone who isn't. However, 90g is the minimum I'd recommend to anyone.

A good rule of thumb is 1.6–2.2g of protein per kilogram of bodyweight per day. For example, I weigh around 63kg (139 pounds), which means I should be aiming for 100–140g of protein per day. I do this by breaking it down throughout my meals and snacks:

- Around 30g of protein per meal (breakfast, lunch, and dinner).
- An additional 20–30g across snacks.

Another helpful rule of thumb, outlined by Dr. Gabrielle Lyons (an expert in longevity), is to calculate a daily protein intake of 1g of protein per pound of ideal body weight. For example, if you weigh 180 pounds (82kg) but your ideal weight is 150 pounds (68kg), you should aim for 150g of protein per day, distributing it across three meals with a minimum of 30–50g per meal and one or two snacks (as outlined above) to stimulate muscle health.

Spreading it out like this gives your body consistent fuel throughout the day and stops that horrid 3pm crash-and-burn that we're all too familiar with.

If you're not sure what these amounts look like on a plate, don't worry—this book contains lots of inspiration for perfectly balanced meals, ready for you to cook at home.

Not all protein is equal

Some proteins are complete, meaning they provide all the essential amino acids your body can't make on its own, and others are incomplete, meaning you'll need to pair them together. It's for this reason I love eating an animal-based diet. Animal protein is complete in one serving, however, don't forget the impact of processed vs. unprocessed.

Ultra-processed meat will have a higher omega-6 to omega-3 ratio (see page 51), so when I talk about animal-based, I'm specifically talking about the best quality meat your budget will allow. There's going to be a huge difference in the impact of a takeout burger compared to a homemade burger made with local ground beef. There's a lot of confusion around red meat, too. Over the past two decades, red meat has been increasingly blamed for everything from heart disease to cancer, but red meat is a very nutrient-dense food, full of iron, B vitamins, zinc, and protein that the body can easily absorb.

Best protein sources:

» Red meat
» Free range or organic poultry
» Wild fish
» Pasture-raised/free-range or organic eggs
» Greek yogurt
» Bone broth
» Lentils, quinoa, chickpeas (when combined to provide all amino acids)

Limit or avoid:

» Ultra-processed protein bars
» Fake meats with long ingredient lists
» Soy protein isolates and additives

Plant-based note

If you get most of your protein from plant-based food, you need to be more aware of combining various sources to make sure you cover the nine essential amino acids. Plant-based sources of protein are often higher in carbohydrates than animal protein, so sometimes we can unintentionally eat more carbs than protein, sending our blood sugar on a roller coaster. When assessing your protein sources, look at the total macro split to make sure you're not overshooting your carbs on your mission to increase protein.

The muscle metabolism link

Muscle isn't just for making us look better or leaner, it's a metabolically active tissue, meaning it burns energy even while you're resting. So if you have more lean muscle, you burn more energy and become efficient at regulating blood sugar, which lowers overall inflammation.

As we age, we naturally lose muscle, especially after our thirties, which coincides with when our hormones start to decline. This makes managing inflammation even more important as we head into perimenopause and menopause. That's why eating protein and resistance training (see the Movement Pillar, page 120) are some of the best anti-inflammatory investments you can make.

Simple protein wins:

- » Start your day with a savory high-protein breakfast. There are lots of ideas in this book (see pages 142–169) as well as options for those who prefer a sweet breakfast with a protein punch. A blood-sugar-balancing breakfast sets us up to have more stable energy, consistent mood, and control over our cravings.
- » Add meat, fish, lentils, beans, or tofu to soups, curries, and grain bowls.
- » Choose the best animal sources of protein your budget will allow, like meat, poultry, wild fish, or eggs for a complete protein source AND micronutrients.
- » Use bone broth as a protein-rich base for soups, stews, or sauces.

You don't need to overcomplicate it. The way I think of protein is as the anchor of every meal, and I build my carbs and fats around it. When you prioritize high-quality protein, everything gets better—your energy, your mood, your metabolism, your skin, your cycle. Protein is not optional, it's *essential*.

Carbs: the most misunderstood macro

For years, I thought carbs were the root cause of all my inflammation, mainly because every TV series and magazine said so. (Remember the ad slogan, "*Beat the Bloat and Ban Bread*"!?). This was reinforced when I did the keto and carnivore diets. At first I felt incredible: less bloated, less puffy, and I even had more energy. It was like I had finally cracked the code, and I stayed on this low-carb train (on and off) for over a year.

But then reality hit: my sleep started to suffer, my periods became irregular, my acne and anxiety were spiking, and that buzzlike energy just disappeared. I was freezing cold all the time, my hair felt thinner, and my body was clearly not happy.

After years of research, it's now very obvious to me why. Carbs were never the problem. *Processed* carbs were. I wasn't feeling better because I was only eating meat, I was feeling better because I had unintentionally also cut out UPFs and was focusing on eating good-quality protein. However, without enough good-quality carbs in my diet, the magic of only eating high-quality protein would prove short-lived. Here's why...

Why your hormones need carbs

Carbs give you energy, but they also do so much more. Although carbs don't make hormones in the way that proteins and fats do, the process of building hormones requires energy—and that's where carbs come in. So if you want to optimize your fertility, have steady moods, and support an efficient metabolism, cutting carbs completely isn't the answer.

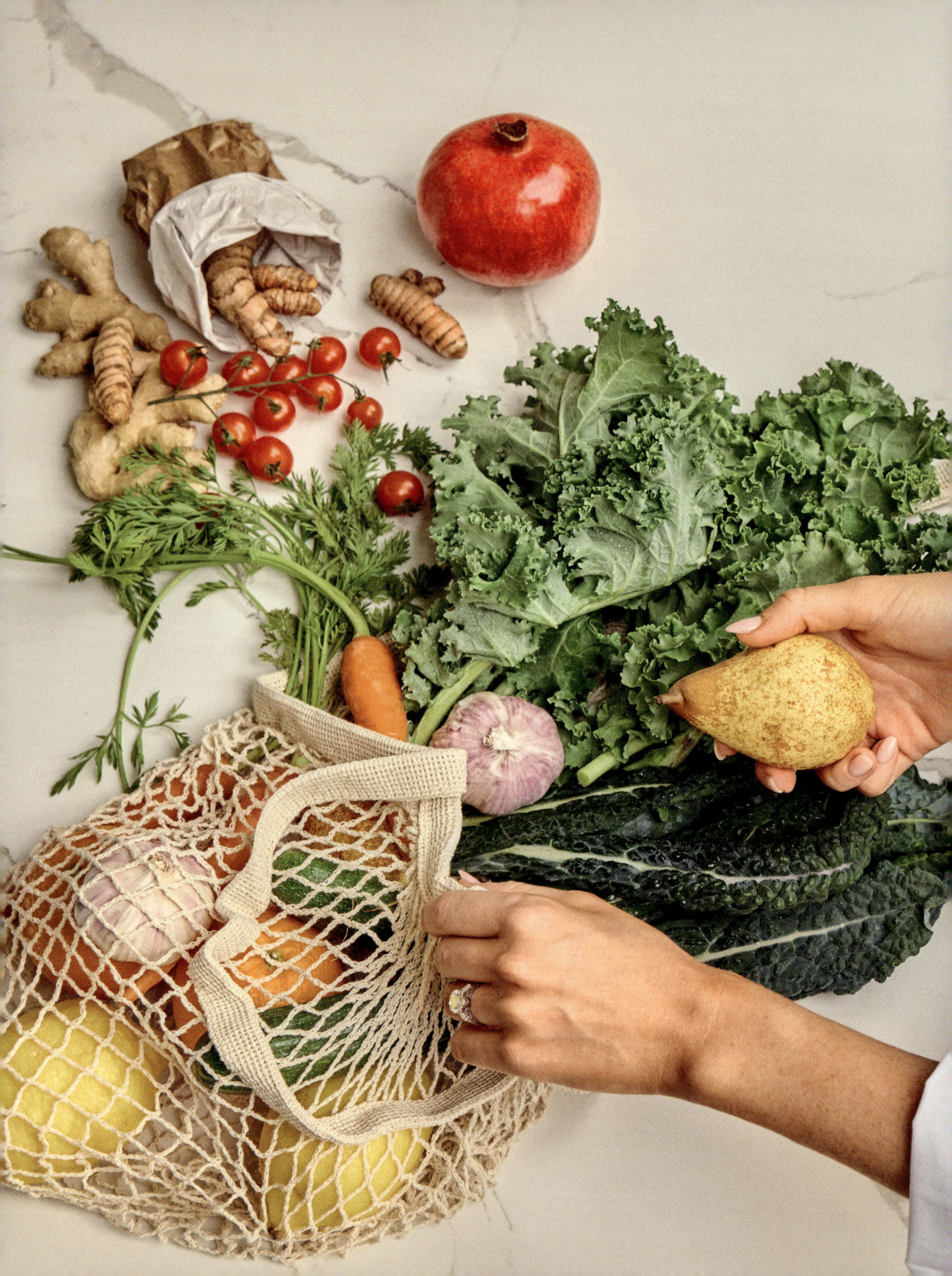

The thyroid–carb connection

Your thyroid is the conductor of your metabolism: it controls how much energy you burn, how warm you feel, and how efficiently your hormones function. But your thyroid needs carbs to produce hormones properly. Without enough carbs, the body down-regulates thyroid hormone production, slowing metabolism and causing:

- » Fatigue that won't go away.
- » Weight gain (or struggling to lose weight no matter what you do).
- » Hair thinning and dry skin.
- » Cold hands and feet.
- » Brain fog and sluggishness.

If you've ever gone low-carb and felt exhausted, anxious, or like your body just wasn't working the way it used to, chances are your thyroid was struggling.

The stress–hormone balancing act

Carbs also help regulate progesterone, your anti-anxiety, pro-sleep, PMS-soothing hormone. When you don't eat enough carbs, your body prioritizes stress hormones (cortisol) over reproductive hormones, because survival will always trump other functions considered "nonessential" under immediate threat. The issue is, many of us constantly feel stressed, resulting in consistently low progesterone.

Long-term low-carb diets can lead to low progesterone, which can cause:

- » Worsened PMS and mood swings.
- » Poor sleep and night sweats.
- » Heightened anxiety and irritability.
- » Shorter or irregular cycles, which also impacts fertility.

This is exactly why women need carbs more than men do. Our bodies are more sensitive to stress, and undereating carbs is a stressor that can throw everything off balance.

Carbs + blood sugar

OK, so we know we want carbs in our diet, but won't carbs spike our blood sugar? Even the best carbs, like sweet potatoes, fruit, quinoa, and lentils, still break down into glucose. If you eat them on their own (Zoe Hindle, functional wellness practitioner, calls this "naked carbs"), they can cause blood-sugar spikes, leading to energy crashes, cravings and, of course, inflammation.

Fear not, we have a solution. **Dress up your naked carbs with . . . protein and fat.** Yes, it's that simple! Not only does this mean you get to enjoy those tasty carbs, but you're ALSO hitting your protein and fat needs. Doing this slows the release of glucose into your bloodstream, keeping blood sugar steady and inflammation in check.

Easy swaps to stabilize blood sugar:

- » Add nut butter to fruit.
- » Pair oats with Greek yogurt, collagen powder, or eggs.
- » Drizzle olive oil over roasted vegetables.
- » Combine quinoa with avocado and grilled chicken.

Notice how I didn't take away anything? In fact I **ADDED** things! Healthy eating is not about restrictions, it's about understanding how food works, and using that to your advantage. When you eat carbs the right way—with "clothes on," i.e., dressed in either protein or fat—they fuel your hormones, support your metabolism, and help you feel full and energized, instead of sending you into an energy crash. And remember: all the wonderful recipes I've shared in this book are balanced, so the thinking has been done for you! You'll find the recipes on pages 142–321.

Fiber: the overlooked carb that's finally having its moment

Fiber is having a real moment in the health world, and for good reason. Fiber, or rather the importance of it, is something I desperately wish I'd understood sooner, as my poor gut health stemmed primarily from avoiding fiber as it bloated me like a balloon.

So, if fiber's that fabulous, why did it make me (and so many other people) bloat so much? And what even is it, anyway?

Fiber is technically a carbohydrate, but unlike other carbs, your body doesn't break it down into glucose. Instead, it passes through your digestive system, playing a key role in blood-sugar balance, gut health and, you guessed it . . . inflammation.

There are two types of fiber, and they are both essential for different reasons:

- » **Soluble fiber:** this dissolves in water, forming a gel-like substance in the gut that slows digestion, balances blood sugar, and feeds good gut bacteria. You'll find it in foods like oats, flaxseeds, psyllium husk, chia seeds, lentils, apples, and carrots.
- » **Insoluble fiber:** doesn't dissolve in water and adds bulk to stool, supporting regular digestion. This comes from whole grains, nuts, seeds, and leafy greens.

When your gut is happy and healthy, fiber is one of the most anti-inflammatory nutrients you can eat. It helps feed beneficial bacteria, stabilizes blood sugar, supports *estrogen* detoxification, and keeps digestion moving so that waste (and excess hormones) don't get stuck and recirculate in your system (see the Gut Health Pillar, page 70). Fiber also slows down how quickly sugar enters your bloodstream, preventing those blood-sugar spikes and crashes that lead to cravings, fatigue, and inflammation. But despite all these benefits, not everyone finds fiber easy to digest.

> *"Fiber and butyrate?"*
>
> *As your gut bacteria break down fiber, they produce short-chain fatty acids like butyrate, which is an incredible compound that helps tighten your gut lining, reduces inflammation, and even improves insulin sensitivity! Think of butyrate like a PT for your gut cells—it keeps them strong and resilient. So fiber absolutely is our friend, and it's time we mended our relationship with it!*

Why some people struggle with fiber and how to fix it

If you've ever eaten a fiber-rich meal like a big bowl of salad and then felt bloated, crampy, or constipated, it's likely not the fiber itself that's the problem, it's your gut health and how it's responding to the fiber. A compromised gut (which we'll dive into in the Gut Health Pillar, page 70) can struggle to break down fiber properly, leading to discomfort instead of the benefits you're supposed to be getting.

The most common culprits? Grains and legumes. While these are fantastic sources of fiber, they also contain compounds like phytic acid and lectins, which can make them harder to digest if your gut isn't in top shape. This doesn't mean you should avoid them altogether (which is the mistake I made for YEARS!)—far from it. It just means that you need to slowly build up your resilience to fiber, while also preparing them properly to make them easier to digest.

Some of the best fiber-rich foods also act as prebiotics (the food your gut bacteria loves to eat!), e.g., leeks, onions, asparagus, and lentils. Including these in your diet helps maintain your microbiome, which supports your digestion, immune system, mood, and hormones . . . without having to buy expensive supplements to do the job.

The recipes later in this book have been carefully designed to include fiber-rich foods that support blood-sugar balance while being gentle on digestion.

Here are a few easy ways to make fiber-rich foods easier to digest:

» **Soak and sprout grains and legumes:** soaking overnight or sprouting helps break down antinutrients that can cause bloating, making them easier for your gut to handle.

» **Prioritize cooked over raw:** steamed, roasted, or blended foods (like soups and smoothies) are gentler on digestion than raw, fibrous vegetables.

» **Start small and increase gradually:** if you're used to a low-fiber diet, suddenly increasing it can overwhelm your gut. Slowly adding fiber-rich foods lets your microbiome adjust.

» **Pair fiber with healthy fats and protein:** this helps slow digestion and reduces bloating while keeping blood sugar stable.

Just like fat, protein, and the traditional "carb," fiber isn't just nice to have, it's essential for blood-sugar stability and for long-term gut health, which is a core metric for inflammation control. So rather than avoiding it, the goal is to build up your resilience to fiber so it helps, not hinders, your health. A great goal for fiber is 25–35g per day. Build up to this slowly, as outlined above.

Micronutrients: more important than you think

Hitting your macros without micronutrients is like plugging your phone in to charge and not switching it on at the plug—you're missing what really matters! Micronutrients (vitamins and minerals) drive every function in the body, and despite only needing a small amount of them (hence the term micro), they're **VERY** powerful. If you're thinking, "Oh no, another thing to track," don't worry! When you're hitting your macros goals with protein, carbs, and fats, by eating real whole foods that aren't ultra-processed, you'll also hit your micronutrients targets, because whole foods naturally contain them. The problem comes when we eat UPFs that technically hit your macros, but are completely stripped of the micronutrients your body needs, so the focus should be on whole foods that satisfy your macro *and* micronutrients!

My all-star micronutrients

Here are the most important vitamins and minerals for reducing inflammation and supporting hormone regulation, and where to get them in real food:

1. *Magnesium: the ultimate anti-stress mineral*

   Why you need it:
   - » *Calms the nervous system (reduces cortisol and stress-induced inflammation).*
   - » *Supports deep sleep (essential for hormone balance and recovery).*
   - » *Helps regulate blood sugar (prevents insulin resistance and cravings).*

   Where to get it:
   - » *Dark leafy greens (spinach, kale, Swiss chard).*
   - » *Nuts and seeds (pumpkin seeds, almonds, cashews).*
   - » *Dark chocolate (yes, really!).*
   - » *Avocados.*

2. *Omega-3 fatty acids: the inflammation fighters*

   Why you need them:
   - » *Reduces inflammation (balances omega-6 intake from processed foods).*
   - » *Supports brain function and mental clarity.*
   - » *Regulates hormones (essential for estrogen and progesterone balance).*

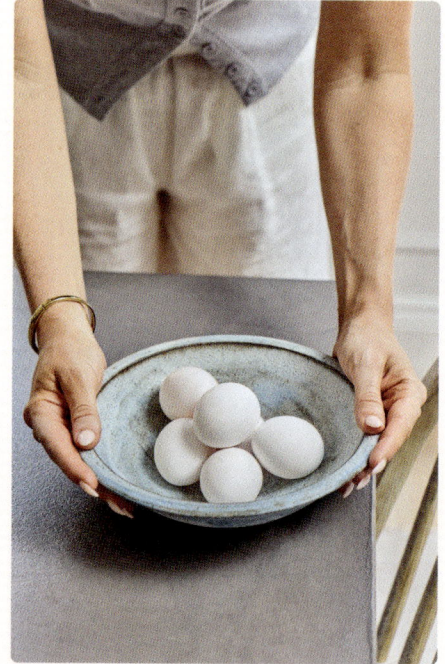

Where to get them:

- » *Wild-caught fish (salmon, sardines, mackerel).*
- » *Chia seeds and flaxseeds.*
- » *Walnuts.*
- » *Algae-based omega-3 supplements.*

3. ***Vitamin D: the mood and immune booster***

   Why you need it:

   - » *Supports immune function (low vit-D linked to autoimmune conditions).*
   - » *Reduces inflammation (especially in e.g., endometriosis and PCOS).*
   - » *Helps with energy and mood (prevents slumps and seasonal depression).*

   Where to get it:

   - » *Sunlight (the best source—aim for 10–20 minutes a day without sunscreen and only available Mar–Oct in the northern hemisphere).*
   - » *Fatty fish (salmon, mackerel, sardines).*
   - » *Egg yolks.*
   - » *Mushrooms (exposed to sunlight).*

4. ***Zinc: the hormone balancer***

   Why you need it:

   - » *Regulates immune function (lowers inflammation, helps fight colds).*
   - » *Supports skin health (reduces acne and inflammation).*
   - » *Essential for hormone balance (supports ovulation and progesterone production).*

   Where to get it:

   - » *Shellfish (oysters, crab, mussels).*
   - » *Beef and lamb.*
   - » *Pumpkin seeds.*
   - » *Chickpeas and lentils.*

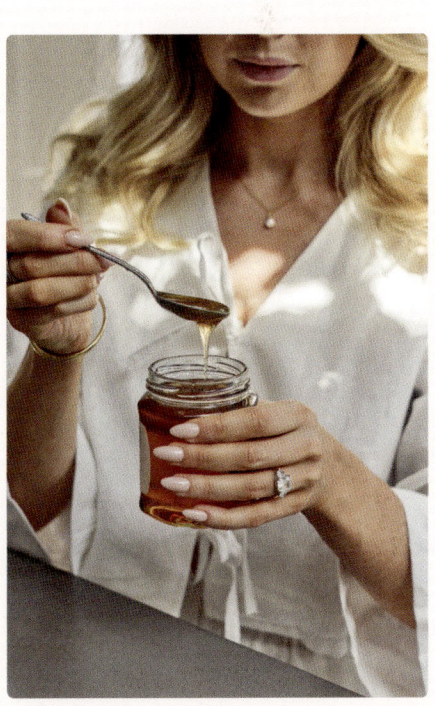

5. *B vitamins: the energy and metabolism boosters*

   Why you need them:

   » Convert food into energy (support metabolism and brain function).
   » Reduce stress and fatigue (especially B_6 and B_{12}).
   » Support liver detox (essential for clearing out excess hormones).

   Where to get them:

   » Red meat (especially liver).
   » Eggs.
   » Leafy greens (spinach, kale, Swiss chard).
   » Nutritional yeast (a great B_{12} source for plant-based eaters).

6. *Iron: the oxygen carrier*

   Why you need it:

   » Prevents fatigue and brain fog (oxygenates your cells).
   » Supports immune function (low iron = getting sick more often).
   » Essential for women's health (especially if you have heavy periods).

   Where to get it:

   » Red meat (beef, liver).
   » Shellfish (clams, oysters, mussels).
   » Spinach (pair with vitamin C for better absorption e.g., citrus foods are full of vitamin C).
   » Legumes (lentils, chickpeas, black beans).

7. *Selenium: the thyroid protector*

   Why you need it:

   » Essential for thyroid health (helps produce thyroid hormones).
   » Lowers inflammation (protects against autoimmune conditions like Hashimoto's).
   » Supports fertility (important for hormone production).

   Where to get it:

   » Brazil nuts (literally one nut a day gives you enough selenium!).
   » Wild-caught fish (salmon, tuna, sardines).
   » Eggs.

And remember, it's not just what you eat but what you absorb! Stress, gut issues, and inflammation can affect nutrient absorption, so looking after your gut is just as important as getting enough vitamins and minerals in the first place.

Supplements

Micronutrients are vital, and if we don't have enough (whether our diet is deficient or because our body is struggling to absorb them), supplementing can be helpful. I want to preface this by saying, as you can see from the previous list, we can naturally supplement with food, which should always be our default. However, with busy lifestyles and compromised immune systems, sometimes extra help is welcome. I always recommend testing (vs. guessing!) to find out what you're deficient in, or else you might end up wasting money on supplements you don't need, or doing more harm than good. If you're dealing with chronic inflammation, I'd always recommend getting a blood test, and if you're interested in functional medicine, get a Dutch test, too. Then you can see what's going on with your body, how you can help it, and IF supplements are the way forward.

> *What's a Dutch test?*
>
> *This is a hormone test that offers a "comprehensive analysis of sex hormones, cortisol levels, and their metabolites. It also includes markers for nutritional deficiencies, oxidative stress, gut health, melatonin, and more." It can be incredibly useful to review someone's hormones over the course of an entire month vs. a snapshot, and goes into more depth than typical blood tests. I'd highly recommend you work with a health-care professional to interpret the results, and because supplements shouldn't be taken lightly—they do have an effect on the body and you want to be sure you take the right ones for you.*

Nature's anti-inflammatory supplements

If you're going to "supplement," here are nature's most powerful ingredients:

» **Ginger and turmeric:** natural inflammation busters that support digestion and reduce pain (see page 309 for my famous ginger and turmeric shot recipe!).

» **Blueberries and pomegranate:** antioxidant powerhouses that protect cells and balance blood sugar.

» **Cruciferous veg (broccoli, kale, Brussels sprouts):** support liver detox, clear excess estrogen, and boost hormone health.

» **Avocado and olive oil:** healthy fats that nourish cells, lower inflammation, and support brain and hormone health.

» **Dark chocolate (min. 70%):** mood-boosting, magnesium-rich treat that supports stress and sleep.

Food intolerances

Food intolerances are not the same as allergies. They don't trigger an immediate immune reaction, but they can make your body struggle to digest or process certain foods. Over time, this can drive inflammation and show up as bloating, skin breakouts, brain fog, headaches, fatigue, and damage to the gut. When the gut is inflamed or imbalanced, foods that are usually well tolerated can suddenly become a trigger, which is why symptoms often seem unpredictable. The most common culprits include gluten and wheat, dairy, and—for some people—eggs, nightshades (tomatoes, peppers, eggplants, chiles), and certain grains.

The tricky part is knowing whether it's the food itself causing inflammation, or poor gut health making you react badly. Stress, lack of sleep, nutrient deficiencies, and other lifestyle factors can all compromise the gut lining, changing how it responds to food. That's why your favorite meal might be fine one day and cause havoc the next.

Because so many of us are living with compromised gut health, what looks like a food intolerance is often a gut issue in disguise. This is why I encourage everyone to try the anti-inflammatory reset in this book. By working through the six pillars (food, gut health, detoxification, stress, sleep, and movement), many people see their symptoms calm without needing to cut out long lists of foods.

However, if symptoms persist, a more targeted approach can be useful. This is where short-term protocols like AIP (Autoimmune Protocol), low FODMAP or low-histamine diets come in. These require short-term restriction and they're not designed for life, as their purpose is to uncover hidden triggers. Personally, AIP changed my life. It helped me identify that chiles, despite their health benefits, are one of my biggest triggers. From the many women who've used my AIP guide, I know I'm not alone in this!

The challenge with elimination diets is knowing what to do after. That's why this book includes anti-inflammatory recipes you can use before, during (adapted to your protocol), and after, so you feel supported at every stage. You can also do the reset alongside the protocols below! I personally believe their effectiveness would be enhanced if used alongside the 30-day reset in this book, as inflammation is driven by all six pillars, so these should be managed alongside food implementations.

If you'd like to explore these protocols further:

» **Low FODMAP:** widely used for IBS, with evidence-based resources online.
» **Low histamine:** can help some people, though results vary depending on genetics and tolerance.
» **AIP (Autoimmune Protocol):** the protocol that made the biggest difference for me. You can find a link to my downloadable AIP guide via my Instagram page **@sophie.richards**.
* *Always discuss elimination diets with a doctor, dietitian, or qualified health practitioner before starting, to ensure you are supported and safe throughout.*

You can also find support at **@found.womenshealth**, where we host talks, courses, and retreats for women exploring these protocols or looking for a more immersive anti-inflammatory lifestyle.

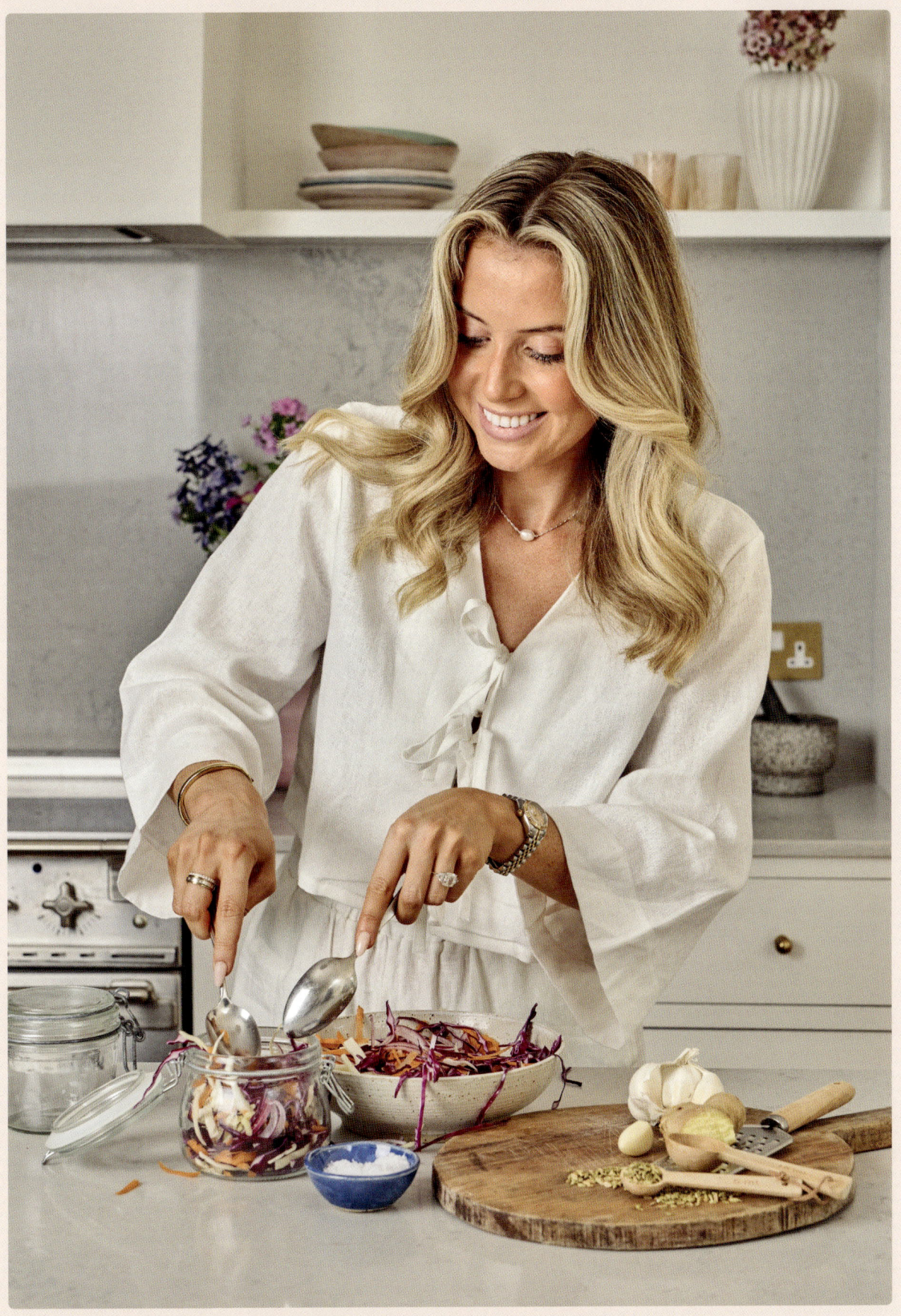

The takeaway here is that food intolerances are real, but they are not always the root cause. By first addressing the six pillars of inflammation, many people find their bodies can tolerate foods again. And if not, a short-term protocol can provide the clarity you need to move forward with confidence.

Actionable steps

Now that you understand what inflammation is, what drives it, and how food can either fight it or fuel it, here are practical steps to get you on your way. This is my go-to checklist that never fails me, and something I refer back to whenever I've lost my way.

1. **Prioritize whole, real foods**

    Build your meals around single ingredient foods you recognize, i.e., fresh vegetables, fruit, high-quality proteins, healthy fats, and whole grains. If it doesn't come with an ingredients label, you're on the right track! I used to get overwhelmed by reading labels until I realized that the best food doesn't have any—easy!

2. **Crowd out, don't cut out**

    This isn't about restriction, it's about filling your plate with all the good stuff, which helpfully crowds out the food that doesn't serve you. So, instead of focusing on what to eliminate, start by adding more nutrient-dense options to your plate. My anti-inflammatory recipes will help with this (see pages 142–321). I found that once I anchored my food with protein and added plenty of healthy fats and fibrous carbs, there wasn't any room for the processed stuff!

3. **Balance your blood sugar at every meal**

    I anchor each meal with 30g of protein at least, and then add healthy fats and good-quality fibrous carbs. This combo keeps blood sugar stable and helps avoid horrid energy crashes that drive you toward coffee and sugar. Increasing protein can feel intimidating at first, so note that my recipes that don't hit this target have helpful advice on how you can "top up" your protein needs in a way that suits you.

    My guide for macronutrient focus is:

    » Protein: 25–30%
    » Fat: 30–35%
    » Carbohydrates: 40–50% (mostly from non-starchy vegetables)

    My personal diet (based on maintaining my weight of 139 pounds), usually looks like:

    » Protein: 100–140g / day
    » Fat: 50–65g / day
    » Carbohydrates: 150–200g / day (or more if I'm exercising)

4. **Focus on quality, not just the macros**

   Sticking with real whole foods from good-quality sources (organic, free range, and local as much as your budget will allow) will get you the micronutrients your body needs instead of UPFs that replace valuable nutrients with chemicals, emulsifiers, and sweeteners. I personally shop 60–70% organic, as that's what my budget allows. The dream would be 100%, but it's not always possible, so whole food over processed is my main focus.

5. **Build your fiber resilience**

   Fiber supports your gut, blood sugar, and inflammation levels. If it makes you bloat, go slowly, and build up gradually. Start with cooked veg, soaked grains, and blended soups . . . the aim is to hit 25–35g per day, but you can do this slowly over time.

6. **Use nature's supplements**

   Daily anti-inflammatory boosters like ginger, turmeric, berries, cruciferous veg, and dark chocolate are nature's gifts to us. A simple ginger and turmeric shot in the morning, or a nibble on dark chocolate at night, is quick, easy, and rewarding, while having a huge positive impact on your body.

7. **Reduce food triggers, don't fear them**

   If you think dairy or gluten are triggering symptoms, try removing them short-term and reintroduce them slowly. It's why the recipes in this book are all GF and DF. Don't label yourself intolerant unless there's a medical reason; it's about healing, not restriction, and both gluten and dairy have their pros, too.

Conclusion

These steps are a guide to help you navigate the anti-inflammatory world. It's never about perfection: I'm living proof that as long as you work on these consistently 80% of the time, you can achieve everything you've wanted (and more!). It's about looking after yourself and making the right decisions as much as possible, so when the 20% creeps in, you get to enjoy it freely without painful symptoms flaring back up.

5 Daily Quick Goals

- ✓ Eat a high-protein breakfast every single day, before 10am.

- ✓ Build every meal with protein, healthy fats, and whole carbs—no naked carbs.

- ✓ Crowd out ultra-processed foods as much as possible with REAL good food. Stick to real, recognizable ingredients that usually don't have a label!

- ✓ Add at least one fiber-rich food to every meal! Cooked veg, lentils, seeds, or whole grains are great, and if you're sensitive to fiber, slowly build up to 30g/day over two or three months.

- ✓ Include one of nature's anti-inflammatory ingredients daily, e.g., ginger, turmeric, berries, or olive oil.

Top 10 Things to Remember About Food!

1. **Food is more than fuel**—it's memories, celebrations, comfort, and culture. It's OK to love it!

2. **Ultra-processed foods** are one of the biggest drivers of inflammation. They mess with your hunger, spike blood sugar, and leave you constantly craving more. The fewer UPFs you eat, the better you'll feel!

3. **You're not broken for craving sugar**—your biology was designed to seek it out and sadly the food companies have taken advantage of this! BUT this ends now—you know how food works and what it does for you vs. falling for the clever packaging and addictive ingredients.

4. **Most extreme diets "work" because they cut out UPFs**... not because they're magical!

5. **Real, whole foods are your foundation!** The more color, fiber, healthy fats, and good-quality protein, the better.

6. **It's not just how much protein, fat, and carbs you eat,** it's the quality that counts. Remember, the more processed, the fewer micronutrients, and they matter just as much as your macronutrients!

7. **Protein is non-negotiable,** especially for women. It fuels your hormones, muscles, skin, mood, and energy, and most of us aren't eating enough.

8. **Fat isn't the enemy,** it's essential for hormone health, brain function, and blood sugar. So stock up on good-quality olive oil, avocados, nuts, and seeds.

9. **Carbs are not the problem**—ultra-processed carbs are. Your body needs natural, whole carbs to support your cycle, thyroid, mood, and more.

10. **Fiber is a game changer!** It supports your gut, balances blood sugar, and helps your body detox excess hormones. Start slowly if you're sensitive, but build up over time.

Pillar 2:
Gut Health

"It's all about **GOOD GUT HEALTH**" suddenly seems to be plastered everywhere you look. On Instagram, TikTok, podcasts, in magazines, and even when you turn on the news . . . people all seem to be talking about the importance of good gut health. But what does this even mean?

There's more and more research coming out linking gut health, or rather poor gut health, with chronic conditions like endometriosis,[1] depression and anxiety,[2] weight gain, and obesity.[3] So when it comes to managing our health, the gut has to be one of the core pillars we approach.

I used to think there was good food (the stuff that didn't bloat me) and bad food (the stuff that did). But now I know that to label food good vs. bad is not helpful. Yes, there are foods that are healthier for us, full of nutrients, and that help us thrive; and there are other foods that are full of sugar and processed ingredients and can cause inflammation (ultra-processed foods). So why did I used to label broccoli, cauliflower, and other healthy foods as "bad"? They're full of nutrients and should therefore clearly go in the "good food" category, right? Well . . . it was because they used to make me feel very bad, very bloated, and caused me quite a bit of pain, along with grains, legumes, and sometimes even nuts and seeds, and I know the same happens to a lot of other people, too.

So what's going on? How can some people eat a big bowl of greens and have a flat stomach, and yet when others do the same they bloat up like a balloon? The answer is all in the gut. It's easy to blame the food itself, but the reality is that food isn't always the problem, it's the state of our gut health, and as a result how our gut is responding to this food. When the gut is compromised, it struggles to digest and absorb nutrients properly, which means we end up with nasty symptoms like painful bloating, discomfort, and inflammation. Thankfully we can repair our gut, so instead of cutting out all these foods that are really great for us (and can in fact nourish our gut), we need to focus on healing and strengthening the gut, building a good foundation so that we can digest these foods that have been causing a problem. Then we can finally enjoy all these veggies, grains, etc. to help supercharge our health for great digestion, which as you'll soon learn is the powerhouse for balanced hormones, a resilient immune system, and, as a result, lower inflammation throughout the body.

So **YES**, there really is a way of getting to the bottom of your bloat, by understanding the gut, and most important how to heal and strengthen it. I'm living proof of this, as someone who can now successfully eat broccoli without blowing up or being painfully gassy.

The gut: where it all begins

When it comes to understanding the gut, Step 1 is to stop thinking of it as just your tummy. Good gut health is achieved via a combination of factors that affect your intricate digestive system, and this actually starts in your mouth.

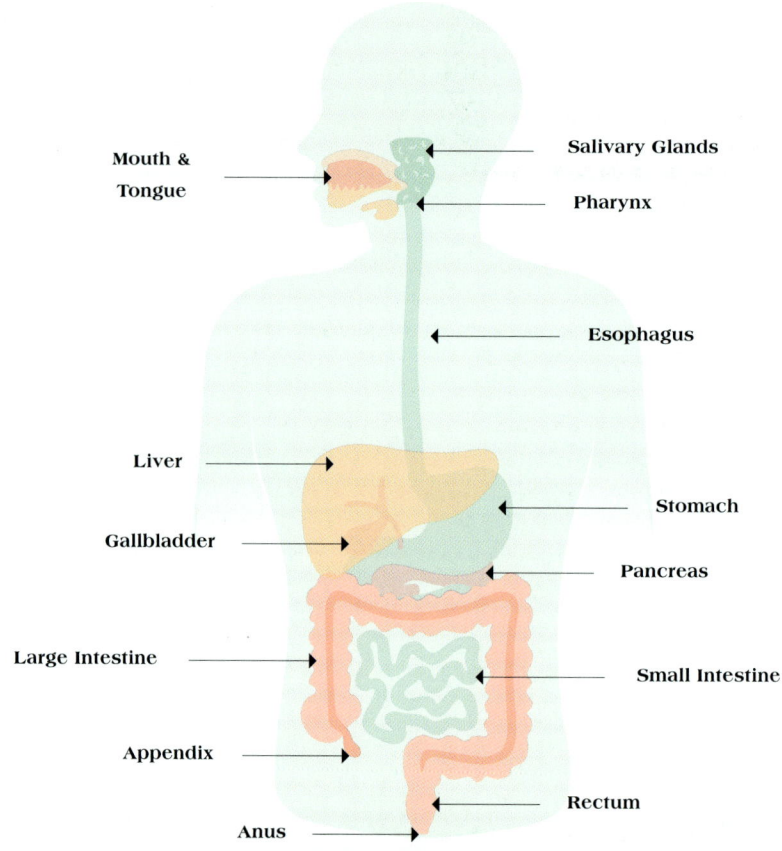

You may have heard people talk about how chewing your food more will help you lose weight and reduce bloating, and this is technically true. The simple act of chewing is one of the most powerful tools for better digestion, which in turn will mean you're less inflamed, carry less water, and, as a result, will feel leaner and lighter. However, the scales aren't the only place where you'll see a difference: it's the impact that properly chewed food has on your gut that is the REAL reward.

Chewing your food breaks it down mechanically and stimulates the release of digestive enzymes in your saliva, making it easier for the stomach and intestines to absorb nutrients. Think of it like this: when you swallow food, your gut needs to receive it in manageable pieces in order to decipher what it is and to absorb it successfully, so that you're getting all the goodness from it. It then shuffles these pieces through your digestive system and later on you'll see them in your toilet.

However, when we rush through meals, eat on the go or while distracted, and usually swallow large bites without chewing properly, this puts unnecessary stress on the rest of the digestive system. Your body struggles to identify what food it's looking at when it's broken down, forcing it to move down the chain without absorbing all the good stuff. The ideal scenario is that you chew your food well (twenty to thirty times per mouthful according to the science), it makes its way into your small intestine to be digested and absorbed, and then it makes one last stop at your large intestine, which is full of bacteria to help with the remaining digestion and absorption . . . and off it goes to your toilet! However, when we wolf down our food, it shoots through the small intestine, missing all the good digestion and absorption pit stops, and then these large bits of food end up fermenting in the large intestine, which if you remember is where all that bacteria is. This absolutely isn't what we want and will leave you feeling gassy, bloated, in pain, and wondering what food caused the issue, when it might have been a simple case of not chewing your food enough or eating your meal when stressed.

Doing this day in, day out, puts more and more pressure on your gut, damaging the lining, triggering an immune response (here come the bodyguards), and the constant fire fight begins.

Interestingly, around 70% of the immune system is housed in the gut, acting as a first line of defense against harmful pathogens and toxins. This proves once again that a strong gut isn't just about digestion, it also helps prevent illness and keeps inflammation in check. So the next time you wonder why your acne is flaring up, your stomach is bloated, or you're feeling under the weather, remember how crucial the gut is, how important it is to feed it the right food and nutrients, and that you also take your time to actually chew. Next time you eat, count your "normal" number of chews and then consciously chew twenty to thirty times on your subsequent bite. Was there a difference? Chances are it took you a lot longer the second time.

What damages the gut?

OK, so what about if you are chewing your food well and you are STILL having problems with your gut?

A healthy gut thrives on balance, and besides not chewing our food, there are other things that can also damage the gut. Modern diets and stressful lifestyles can also have a huge impact not only on the gut, but on our brain and hormones, too. Some of the biggest disruptors include:

» *Ultra-processed foods (UPFs):* these are stripped of nutrients and loaded with additives that alter the gut microbiome. Some are loaded with sugar, which feeds the "bad bacteria," crowding out the good guys.

» *Chronic stress:* when the body is in a constant state of fight-or-flight, digestion slows down, stomach acid production decreases, and gut motility is affected, leading to bloating and discomfort.

- » **Blood-sugar imbalances:** *frequent spikes and crashes in blood sugar can increase stress hormones like cortisol, which signals the body to stop focusing on "nonessential" activities like digestion, which over time damages the gut lining.*
- » **Low-fiber diets:** *good gut bacteria rely on fiber from fruits, vegetables, and whole foods. Without it, these bacteria die off, leading to gut microbiome imbalances and inflammation. These bacteria HELP you, but if you don't feed them fiber, they'll die!*
- » **Toxins and environmental chemicals:** *pesticides, artificial sweeteners, and preservatives can weaken the gut lining, contributing to leaky gut and activating the immune system.*
- » **Poor sleep patterns:** *sleep and gut health are deeply connected. Poor-quality sleep can disrupt the gut microbiome in the same way that stress does. Poor sleep stimulates cortisol to spike blood sugar for energy, which over time increases inflammation, ultimately impacting the gut's ability to digest the food you eat.*

The gut, inflammation, and chronic health conditions

When the gut is in good shape, everything keeps ticking along and inflammation is under control. However, if your gut has been under any of the pressures listed in the previous section that disrupt its day-to-day job of keeping things moving, it can weaken your gut's ability to function properly, and that's when pesky symptoms start popping up! Think of the gut lining like a two-way sieve, filtering all the good nutrients to the right place and keeping out all the bad stuff like harmful bacteria and toxins. When the gut is weakened or damaged, we can't absorb the nutrients properly from our food (making us crave more food because our cells aren't getting the good stuff), and it also starts allowing harmful bacteria and toxins to enter the bloodstream. This is often referred to as "leaky gut." When these unwanted substances slip through the gut, they trigger an immune response. If this was once in a while, no biggy, your body is doing its thing and using inflammation for all the good reasons to clear up the problem. However, if your gut is constantly compromised and therefore activating the immune response day in and day out, it eventually leads to chronic low-grade inflammation, which is linked to conditions like autoimmune diseases, endometriosis flare-ups, skin issues, and metabolic disorders. So looking after your gut is so much more than stopping the bloat, it's about taking care of your overall health, whether that be conditions you're currently struggling with, or future conditions that may develop as a result of this consistent gut damage and inflammation.

For those with chronic health conditions, gut health is even more crucial. Because the immune system is already working in overdrive, you're more likely to struggle with maintaining a strong and resilient gut. This feels unfair, trust me, I know … but always remember that chronic health issues or not, a resilient strong gut is something we ALL need, otherwise ill health is in the cards for everyone. It just means that those of us with chronic conditions need to put some extra effort in to keep things ticking along. The reason being that when gut health declines, it places further strain on the immune system, making it less effective at fighting illness and more reactive to triggers that cause flare-ups. This explains why people with conditions like endometriosis, PCOS, or autoimmune disorders usually experience more symptoms when their gut is struggling. I know this is the case for me because I've always said that when I'm constipated, it's like a snowball effect . . . my acne flares, my endo flares . . . and before you know it, I'm back in bed with crippling period pain, heavy bleeding, and a migraine that won't shift. So healing and supporting gut health isn't just about digestion, it's about keeping the entire body in balance and reducing the intensity of flare-ups and inflammatory responses.

Constipation tip

While my philosophy stands that food should be our primary source of nourishment, and supplements should only be used when really needed . . . magnesium citrate has changed my life when it comes to constipation. It not only helped with the bloating and pressure in my tummy, but supported my hormones, too. That being said, it's definitely possible to have too much magnesium . . . My cousin was once staying with me the night before a big opera performance and struggling to sleep from the excitement. Thinking I could help, I gave her a good dose of my magnesium and she went to sleep soundly. The next day, however, I received a very unimpressed text that she was stuck on the toilet experiencing violent diarrhea! I had slightly overdone her dosage of magnesium, and this was my first lesson in how supplements really work, and how important dosages are. If you are looking for a supplement to help with constipation, getting your gut right is the number one priority, but in the meantime I have loved Magnesium Breakthrough by Bioptimizers, and so does everyone I recommend it to!

The gut–brain connection

When I was younger, I was encouraged rather forcefully to compete in what we call the "Eisteddfod" in Wales. It's where you take the stage and showcase your talents, whether that be singing, reciting poetry, playing the piano . . . or even clog dancing (and yes, I have done all those things . . . to a very below-par standard). Anyway, before getting on stage, I used to get this horrible sicky feeling like my stomach was about to fall out of my ass . . . a feeling people call "butterflies." What I didn't know was that this was all down to something called the gut–brain axis, where your brain speaks to your gut.

How bizarre, right? Even more strange . . . your gut can speak back—it's a two-way thing!

This connection is so strong that scientists now call the gut our "second brain." So, if you're mentally stressed, e.g., me at the age of seven strapping on a pair of wooden clogs and attempting to dance in a full Welsh traditional outfit (top hat and all . . .), your gut feels it, and if your gut is off, it signals distress to the brain. It's a two-way street, which is why gut health is so deeply linked to mood, stress, and overall well-being.

Stress can damage your gut, BUT a damaged gut can bring you stress!

When you're under pressure, your brain releases stress hormones like cortisol, which can slow digestion, decrease stomach acid, and throw off the balance of gut bacteria. This is because your body is in fight-or-flight mode, and digestion is the last thing it wants to have to worry about. This is also why stress often leads to bloating, discomfort, or even IBS-like symptoms such as constipation or diarrhea. On the flip side, if your gut is inflamed or imbalanced, it can send distress signals to the brain, leading to anxiety, brain fog, and low mood. In fact, around 90% of serotonin (your "feel-good" neurotransmitter hormone) is produced in the gut. So if your gut is struggling, it's no surprise that your mood might take a hit, too.

The gut-hormone connection

We've talked a lot about how important your hormone health is, and without it you're guaranteed a world of inflammation. So anything that involves hormonal health is very important to focus on, and that includes your gut. Your gut is a powerful regulator of your hormones, and influences everything from hunger and metabolism to stress and even reproductive health. It produces and interacts with multiple hormones, making it a key player in keeping that hormonal hierarchy in check, and as a result your overall health.

Below are the main hormones that interact with the gut:

Ghrelin and leptin

Your gut helps regulate ghrelin (your hunger hormone) and leptin (your fullness hormone). When the gut is imbalanced, these signals can get confused, which is why so many of us struggle with cravings and overeating and find it impossible to know when we're full. When my tummy was really bad, I remember eating huge meals and just never feeling full. If anything, finishing a big meal was followed by this intense need to eat something sweet . . . so once again I was eating more and more. I wish I'd known that this wasn't me being greedy, but actually a sign that my gut was off and it needed a reset!

Estrogen detoxification

We know how important estrogen is to our bodies: too much or too little, and your body will FEEL it. Mood swings, low libido, intense emotions . . . yep, estrogen is a strong hormone. What you might not know is that your gut actually plays a crucial role in breaking down and eliminating excess estrogen. So if the gut is out of balance, the estrogen that has arrived there to be detoxed ends up getting reabsorbed instead of excreted, which is a huge driver of symptoms like PMS, bloating, heavy periods, and worsening/flaring conditions like endometriosis and PCOS. Remember earlier

I said that whenever I was constipated it was the start of health chaos for me? Well, this explains exactly why. The way your gut detoxifies estrogen is through a set of gut bacteria known as the estrobolome, which helps maintain hormonal balance. When the gut isn't working properly, excess estrogen can fuel inflammation and disrupt the menstrual cycle . . . and we all know how important our menstrual health is not only for the now, but also for perimenopause and menopause.

Thyroid function

Your thyroid is the heart of your metabolism and energy, and even though your thyroid is located in the front of your neck (think Adam's apple!), a large portion of thyroid hormone conversion happens in the gut. If you want to get into the science of it, the inactive thyroid hormone (T4) needs to be converted into its active form (T3) so that your body can actually use it, and your good gut bacteria have a big role to play in this process. If gut health is compromised, thyroid function can slow down, and this can have a huge impact on your life . . . things like fatigue, brain fog, weight gain, and a sluggish metabolism (leading to weight gain).

Cortisol and stress

The gut helps regulate the body's stress response by interacting with cortisol, the primary stress hormone. When gut health is strong, your body is more resilient to stress—brilliant! However, if your gut is inflamed or compromised, cortisol levels can stay higher for longer, which increases inflammation and worsens gut-related symptoms like bloating, discomfort, and irregular digestion. If you're stressed, your gut suffers, and if your gut suffers, you feel stressed!

Keeping the gut healthy allows these hormones to function at their best, meaning you avoid everything from food cravings and low energy to hormonal imbalances and symptoms from inflammation-driven conditions like endometriosis, PCOS, and thyroid disorders.

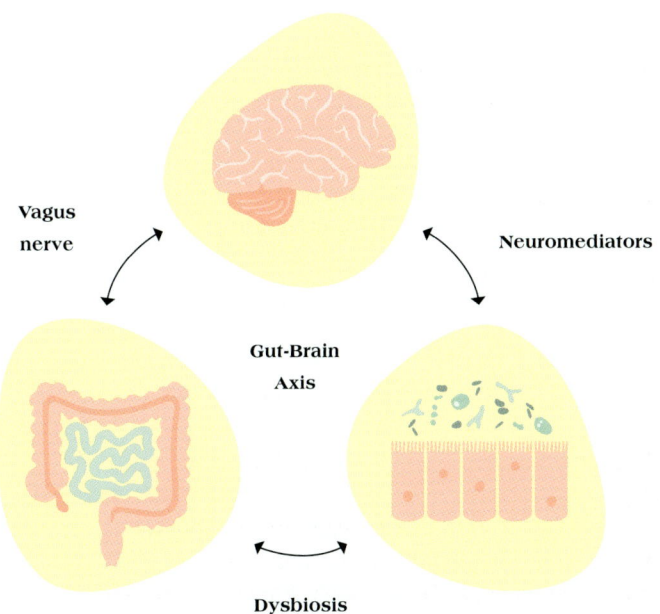

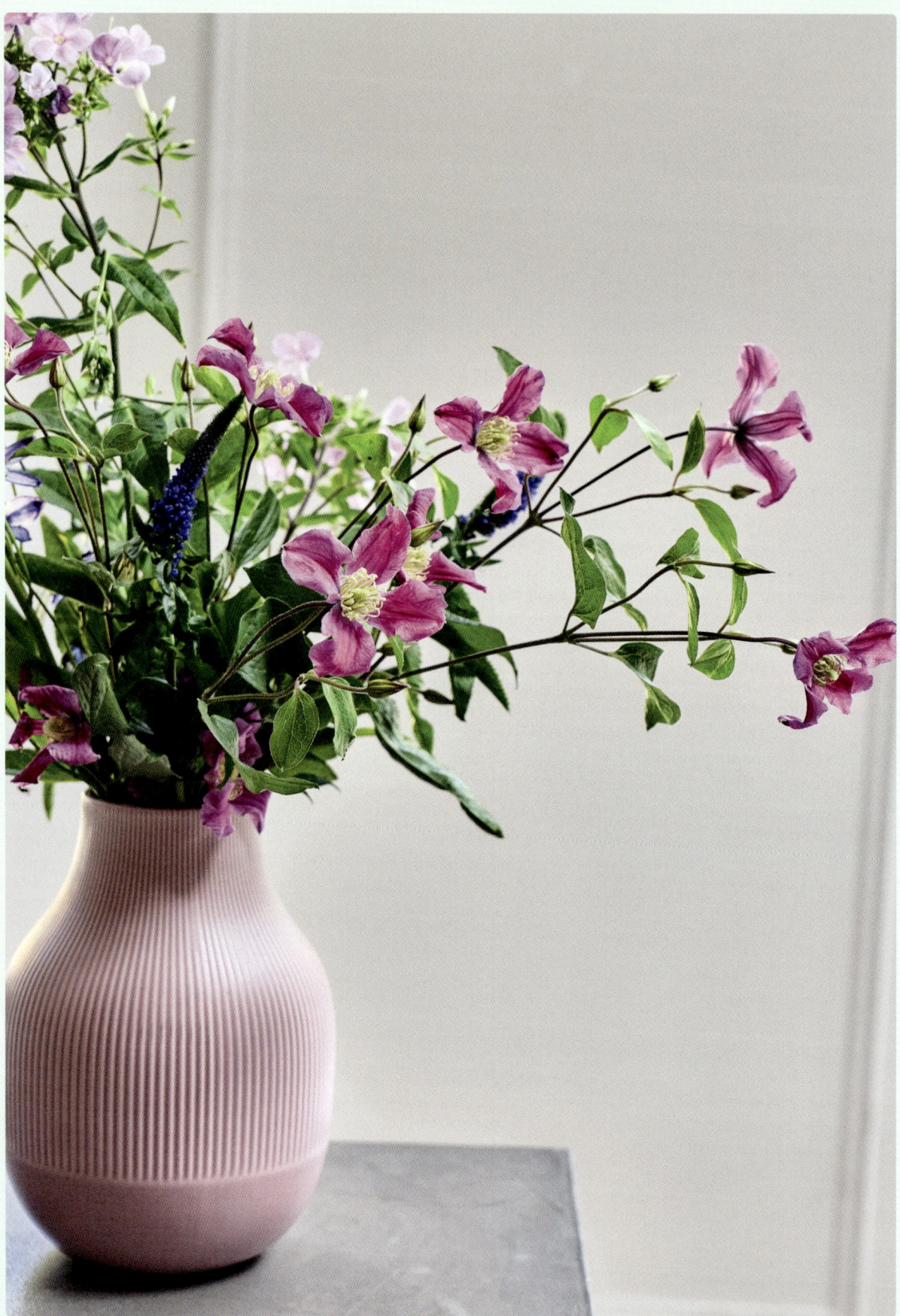

The gut and your menstrual cycle

Just as your cervical mucus changes throughout your cycle, so does your digestion. Some changes are normal; however, when things start to get extreme, like severe constipation or diarrhea, it can be a key indicator that you may have an underlying imbalance that needs your attention.

Follicular phase

During this part of your cycle, estrogen and testosterone are rising and muscle contractions (peristalsis) that move your food and waste along your intestines in a wave-like fashion are doing a good job. You should be experiencing regular bowel movements (once a day, usually in the morning), and they should score a 3–4 on the Bristol stool chart (see page 80).

Ovulation phase

As estrogen rises to its peak, it can start to disrupt the gut, causing some gassiness and lower tummy bloating. This is to a small degree "normal," as our body is responding to fluctuating hormones. However, for people with endometriosis, PCOS, and cystic ovaries, ovulation can be a very painful experience, with extreme bloating, pain, and drastically changing bowel habits. This was definitely something I struggled with until I found an anti-inflammatory way of living, and it is one of the first symptoms to return if I'm less diligent about any of the six pillars explored in this book.

Luteal phase

Progesterone rises, and due to its cool, calm, collected influence on our muscles, it can relax our intestines to the point where bowel movements become less frequent. It's why so many pregnant women struggle with constipation, as progesterone remains high during pregnancy vs. dropping for menstruation. Again, to some degree this is normal, but if you're experiencing extreme constipation pre-period, it can be an indication of underlying hormonal imbalances or conditions that should be investigated.

Menstruation

A few days before your period, progesterone drops and estrogen is at its lowest. Prostaglandins are firing away at your uterine lining, causing muscle contractions, which helps your uterine lining shed. However, your bowels are very close to your uterus, and sometimes these prostaglandins stray and cause contractions to your bowels, too! If you've ever had radiating cramps and "period poos" that will likely be down to prostaglandins. People who are more inflamed tend to have higher numbers of prostaglandins than those who aren't, so this is a key sign to look out for and something that should hopefully subside once you've worked on lowering levels of inflammation.

Bristol stool chart

Type 1		Separate hard lumps, like nuts (hard to pass).
Type 2		Sausage-shaped but lumpy.
Type 3		Like a sausage but with cracks on the surface.
Type 4		Like a sausage or snake, smooth and soft.
Type 5		Soft blobs with clear-cut edges.
Type 6		Fluffy pieces with ragged edges, a mushy stool.
Type 7		Watery, no solid pieces. Entirely liquid.

Our bowel movements can tell us a lot about what's going on in our gut, digestion, and as a result our hormonal health—so don't be a stranger to having a look at what's in your toilet and seeing what's going on.

Fiber: it's supposed to help, so why does it hurt?

Fiber is one of the most powerful tools for improving gut health because it acts as fuel for beneficial gut bacteria, which, as you now know, help with detoxifying hormones and reducing inflammation. Fiber helps bacteria produce short-chain fatty acids (SCFAs), which reduce inflammation, strengthen the gut lining, and support immune function, but that's not all. Fiber also promotes regular bowel movements, which is why if you're struggling with constipation, increasing your fiber is a great way to bulk up your stool and get things moving. However, when I was constipated, adding fiber initially made things worse. For those with a damaged gut lining or a history of low-fiber intake (which is the majority of the population, especially those who have been on a ketogenic or low-carb diet), suddenly adding large amounts of fiber can be overwhelming and can cause bloating, gas, or discomfort. So you need to slowly increase your good bacteria by increasing your fiber intake gradually. Doing this, alongside all the other ways of healing the gut, will mean you'll be eating your recommended daily 30g of fiber in no time!

This low and slow approach gives the gut microbiome time to adapt, building up plenty of good bacteria over time. It also avoids putting unnecessary stress on your gut, while also improving digestion and resilience. As the gut heals, its ability to process fiber naturally improves, making it easier to transition to a fiber-rich diet.

Steps to strengthen and support gut health

The good news is that the gut is incredibly adaptable, and with the right support it can heal and function in all the ways you need it to. Making changes overnight is great in theory, but your body needs time to build and heal, so please bear this in mind and be patient and consistent when you start your journey to better gut health. Here's a reminder of the steps you need to take:

1. **Chew your food.**

    Slow down and chew each bite at least twenty to thirty times. This gets those digestive enzymes working, breaking down your food and readying your system for digestion, ensuring that your food is in smaller particles that don't put pressure on your stomach or intestines AND that your body will recognize the nutrients and be able to easily absorb them.

2. **Balance blood sugar.**

    Eat in the way I outlined in the Food Pillar (page 42), with your carbs, fats, and proteins balanced to avoid blood-sugar spikes, since these put pressure on the gut.

3. **Prioritize whole foods.**

    Focus on minimally processed, nutrient-dense foods such as meat, fish, fresh vegetables, fruits, nuts, seeds, and whole grains. For example, swap refined white bread for a whole grain sourdough, which contains gut-friendly fiber and natural prebiotics.

4. **Stay hydrated**

    I haven't covered this in depth because we all know that drinking at least two liters of water a day is important, but the reason for this is that liquid is essential for all this food to actually move along the digestive tract. So if you're feeling blocked up, it could be because you're not drinking enough water.

5. **Gradually increase fiber intake**

   As we've covered, fiber is fantastic, as it's what feeds those wonderful gut bacteria that HELP your health. However, if you have a damaged gut or haven't been eating much fiber, you need to build up the good bacteria slowly by introducing more and more fiber gradually into your diet. Start by introducing one new fiber-rich food at a time, and gradually build to a total of 30g of fiber per day. A super simple recommendation from Dr. Megan Rossi (@theguthealthdoctor) is to incorporate the "**Super Six**," the essential plant-based food groups that feed the gut microbiome. These are:

   » **Vegetables:** leafy greens, carrots, and bell peppers.
   » **Fruits:** berries, apples, and citrus fruits.
   » **Whole grains:** quinoa, oats, and brown rice.
   » **Legumes:** chickpeas, lentils, and black beans.
   » **Nuts and seeds:** almonds, walnuts, flaxseeds, and chia seeds.
   » **Herbs and spices:** e.g., turmeric, ginger, and cinnamon, which also have anti-inflammatory properties.

6. **Prebiotics and probiotics**

   Prebiotics and probiotics are two key players in gut health, working together to support a strong and diverse microbiome. If you notice bloating after consuming them, gradually introduce them into your diet one by one in small amounts. For best results, combining prebiotics and probiotics is key. Think of prebiotics as the "food" and probiotics as the "workers" that keep the gut running smoothly. Eating a variety of both means you'll have a well-nourished and resilient gut microbiome, and before you know it, these foods will be a staple in your diet and you'll be bloat-free, instead of avoiding them as you might do now.

   » **Prebiotics** are types of fiber that feed the beneficial bacteria in your gut, helping them grow and thrive. They are found in foods like onions, garlic, leeks, asparagus, bananas, and oats. Without enough prebiotics, good bacteria struggle to multiply, making it harder for the gut to maintain balance.
   » **Probiotics** are live beneficial bacteria that help restore gut balance. They are found in fermented foods like kefir, sauerkraut, kimchi, miso, tempeh, and natural yogurt. They help populate the gut with good bacteria, which can be especially useful after antibiotic use or periods of gut distress.

7. **Sleep!**

   Prioritizing sleep is one of the most underrated tools for gut health, as poor sleep can disrupt the balance of your gut microbiome, reduce beneficial bacteria, and increase inflammation and gut permeability (leaky gut). It also affects the gut–brain axis, which as you know by now plays a key role in digestion, immunity, and even mood.

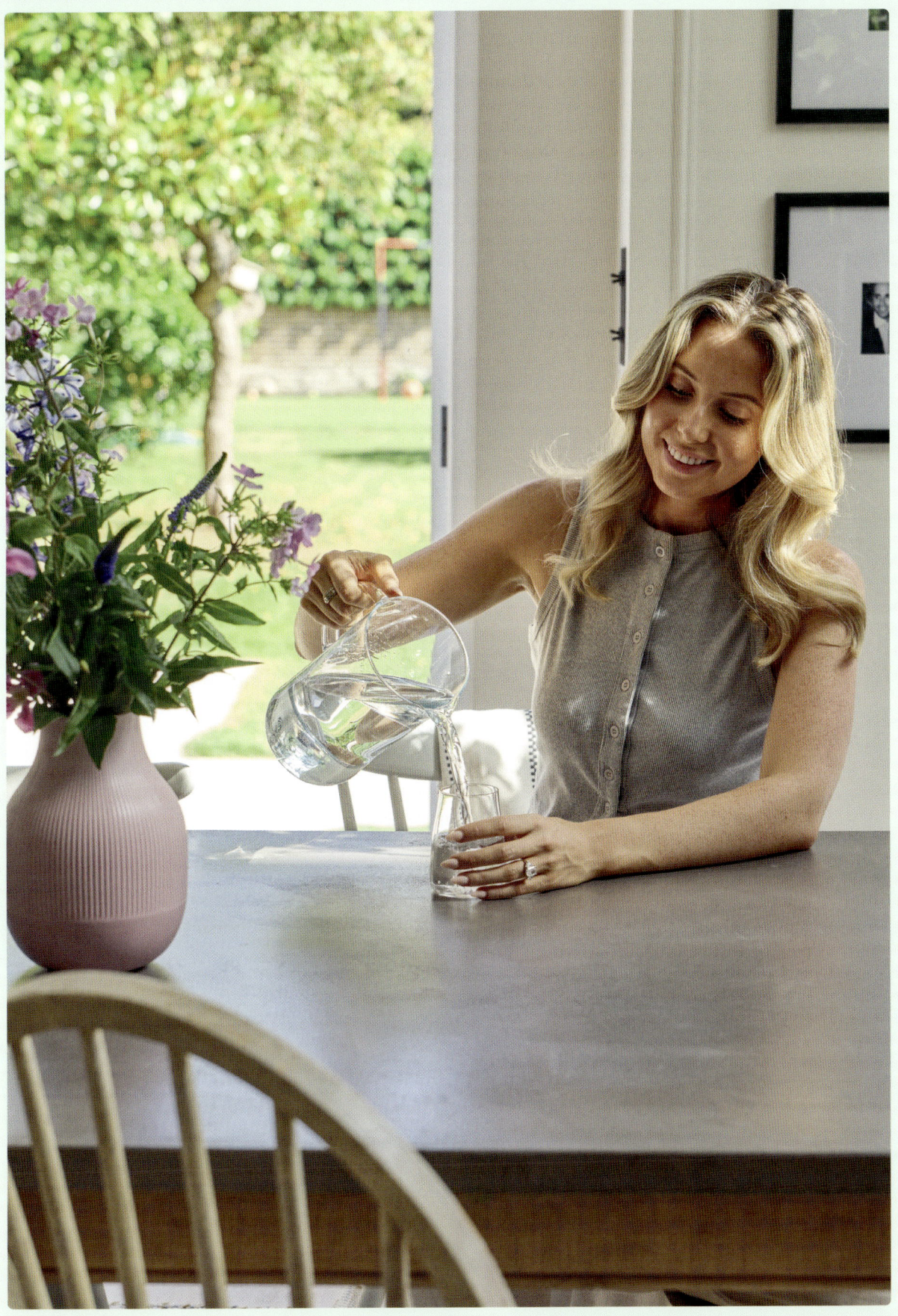

Conclusion

The gut is a complicated system that isn't just in your tummy, but starts in your mouth and impacts your whole body, and as a result, the health of your gut dictates the health of your body. It fights inflammation, keeps hormones balanced, and supports the immune system. By taking small but meaningful steps to prioritize gut health, you'll be laying the foundation for your long-term health.

If you want to dive deeper and learn even more about gut health, there's an episode of the *Finally Found* podcast entirely devoted to the topic, in which I speak to leading gut health expert Dr. Megan Rossi (@theguthealthdoctor).

5 Daily Quick Goals

- ✓ **Chew your food properly—aim for twenty to thirty chews per bite and avoid distracted, rushed meals.**

- ✓ **Drink at least two liters of water a day to keep everything moving.**

- ✓ **Add at least one fiber-rich food to each meal, e.g., cooked veg, chia seeds, oats, or lentils.**

- ✓ **Include prebiotic or probiotic foods like garlic, onions, leeks, kefir, sauerkraut, or miso.**

- ✓ **Prioritize good sleep and reduce stress—both are massive for gut health (more on this in the Sleep and Stress Pillars!)**

Top 10 Things to Remember About Your Gut!

1. **Your gut is more than just your stomach**—it starts in your mouth and plays a role in everything from your mood to your hormones, skin, energy, and immune system.

2. **Bloating doesn't always mean the food is the issue**—it often means your gut is struggling to digest properly.

3. **Chewing your food properly** (twenty to thirty chews per bite) is one of the simplest, most effective ways to help your gut.

4. **70% of your immune system lives in your gut**—so if your gut's inflamed, chances are the rest of your body will be, too!

5. **A damaged gut lining can lead to "leaky gut,"** which lets toxins into the bloodstream and can fuel chronic inflammation.

6. **Your gut talks to your brain,** and your brain talks to your gut. Those butterflies or sicky feeling in your tummy are your gut-brain axis working!

7. **Your gut also helps detox hormones like estrogen,** so if you're constipated or inflamed, you might reabsorb what your body was trying to get rid of and this can lead to hormonal imbalances.

8. **Thyroid function relies on your gut, too,** and a sluggish gut can slow the conversion of thyroid hormones, leaving you tired and foggy.

9. **Fiber feeds your good gut bacteria,** so we need plenty of it! However, if you're struggling with digestion of fiber, start slowly and build up to 30g a day over two or three months.

10. **If you're always hungry or never feel full,** your gut hormones, like leptin and ghrelin, may be out of sync.

Pillar 3: Detoxification

Your body's natural cleansing system

Detoxification is something I used to think we had to force our bodies to do... usually after a heavy night out or a long weekend of eating nothing but fast food! However, despite the clever marketing of fancy juices or teas that claim to "detox" your sins away, your body is naturally detoxing every single day.

Detoxification is your body's natural process for eliminating waste, toxins, and harmful substances that accumulate from food, the environment, and internal metabolic processes. It involves multiple organs, including your liver, kidneys, gut, skin, lungs, and lymphatic system, all of which work together to filter and remove these substances efficiently, if everything is working correctly.

Chronic conditions and the stresses of our modern lifestyles, however, can slow down or overload these detox pathways, making it harder for your body to eliminate waste.

Common signs your body is struggling with detoxification:

- » Fatigue or brain fog.
- » Sensitivity to smells, alcohol, or caffeine.
- » PMS, heavy periods, or breast tenderness.
- » Skin issues (acne, eczema, hives).
- » Gallbladder pain or upper right stomach pain.
- » Strong reaction to medication.

How does your body detox?

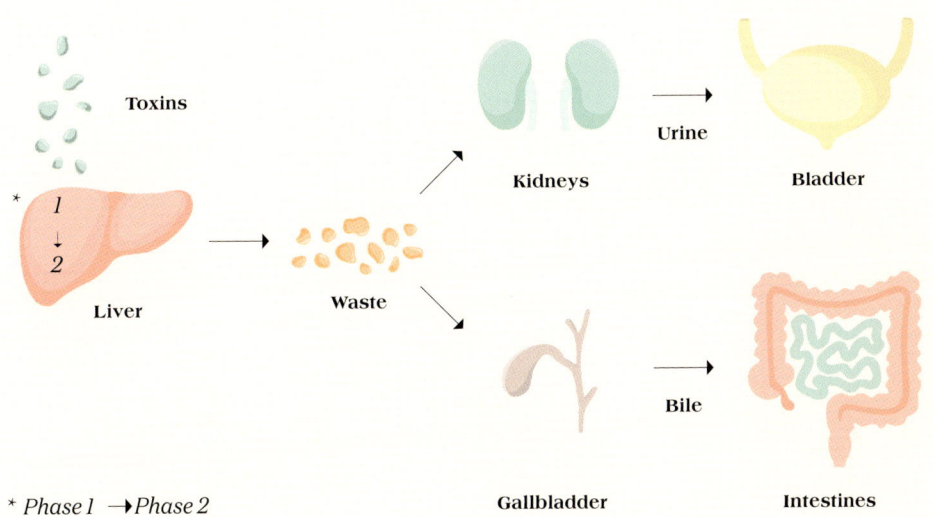

*Phase 1 → Phase 2

I like to visualize the body's detoxification pathways as a road map with lots of turns and junctions. To get from point A to point B, you need to take the right exit at the right time, and hope the roads are clear so you don't get backed up in traffic.

Liver

The liver is your primary detox organ—it's very clever and can even regenerate if it gets into trouble, but we need to look after it. It filters toxins from the blood and breaks them down into forms that can be safely removed. It does this in two phases:

- » **Phase 1:** The toxin is converted into a form that's water soluble; however, this can make the toxin more reactive and potentially more harmful, which is why it's VERY important our pathways are kept clear, so that these toxins can swiftly move to phase 2.[1]
- » **Phase 2:** This is where those toxins are neutralized, by binding them to useful molecules (e.g., glutathione, sulfate, and amino acids) so they can be safely moved on to the next detoxification phase in the gut.

After phases 1 and 2, the by-products are then transported to the gut and kidneys for the final stages of detoxification.

Gallbladder

Your gallbladder works with your liver to store and concentrate bile. When you eat, especially fats, the gallbladder contracts to release concentrated bile into the small intestine to help with digestion. If your liver health isn't optimal, the quality and quantity of bile can suffer, directly impacting your gallbladder. Women are significantly more prone to issues like gallstones than men because of the impact that estrogen and progesterone have on bile production. Estrogen can increase the amount of cholesterol in your bile, making it thicker and more likely to form sludge or stones. Progesterone can slow down the emptying of the gallbladder, leading to bile stagnation. Gallbladder removal is one of the most common surgeries worldwide, with women roughly twice as likely as men to need it due to gallstones.

Gut

Once the liver has neutralized toxins, the gut helps get rid of them for good. This is why a healthy gut is so important; without it, detoxification can't run smoothly.

The liver packages fat-soluble waste products into bile, which is released into the gut. From there, your body clears it out through your stool. Yep . . . having a good poo is one of the main ways we eliminate toxins. But if you're constipated, or not eating enough fiber to keep things moving, those waste products can actually be reabsorbed back into the bloodstream through the gut wall. This is important because even your hormones need to be excreted if there's an excess, but if this process isn't working efficiently, hormones like estrogen can be reabsorbed in the gut contributing to estrogen dominance, which can cause symptoms like PMS, bloating, tender breasts, and more. That's why gut health is such a vital piece of the detoxification process, and why I'm so passionate about everyone having a daily bowel movement!

Kidneys

The kidneys are another major detox organ. After the liver has done its two-step detox process, many of the by-products re-enter the bloodstream in a water-soluble form. From there, the kidneys act like filters, removing these compounds and carrying them out of the body through your urine. This is why hydration matters so much: drinking enough water helps keep blood flowing through the kidneys, supports filtration, and makes sure waste products are flushed out efficiently.

Lungs

The lungs are the body's built-in air filters, constantly working to remove toxins, pollutants, and waste. Every time you exhale, you're helping clear out waste from your cells. Healthy lungs are vital for detoxification, so anything that damages or overloads them should be avoided or limited, e.g., smoking and vaping. They introduce harmful chemicals that irritate and inflame the lungs, meaning they can't do their job as effectively. Keeping your lungs clean and strong is one of the most powerful detox steps you can take.

Skin

The skin is the body's largest organ and acts both as a protective barrier and also a powerful filtration system. Your skin helps eliminate toxins via sweat, which is why movement, exercise, and even sauna sessions help support detoxification. The skin also sheds dead cells, constantly renewing itself to remove impurities and maintain balance. But detoxing through the skin isn't just about what it excretes through sweat, but what we put on it, too. Harsh chemicals in skincare can be absorbed into the body, adding to the "toxic load" (more on this later). When we support our skin, it not only looks better but plays a vital role in keeping the body clean from the inside out.

Lymphatic system

The lymphatic system is like the body's drainage network. The concept is similar to your circulatory system, except there's no pump, and it's why so many of us wake up feeling puffy in the morning, or if we've sat down for too long. The lymphatic system relies on movement (exercising, deep breathing, massage) to remove waste, toxins, and excess fluids. When your lymphatic system is working well, it helps flush out toxins, supports the immune system, and reduces inflammation.

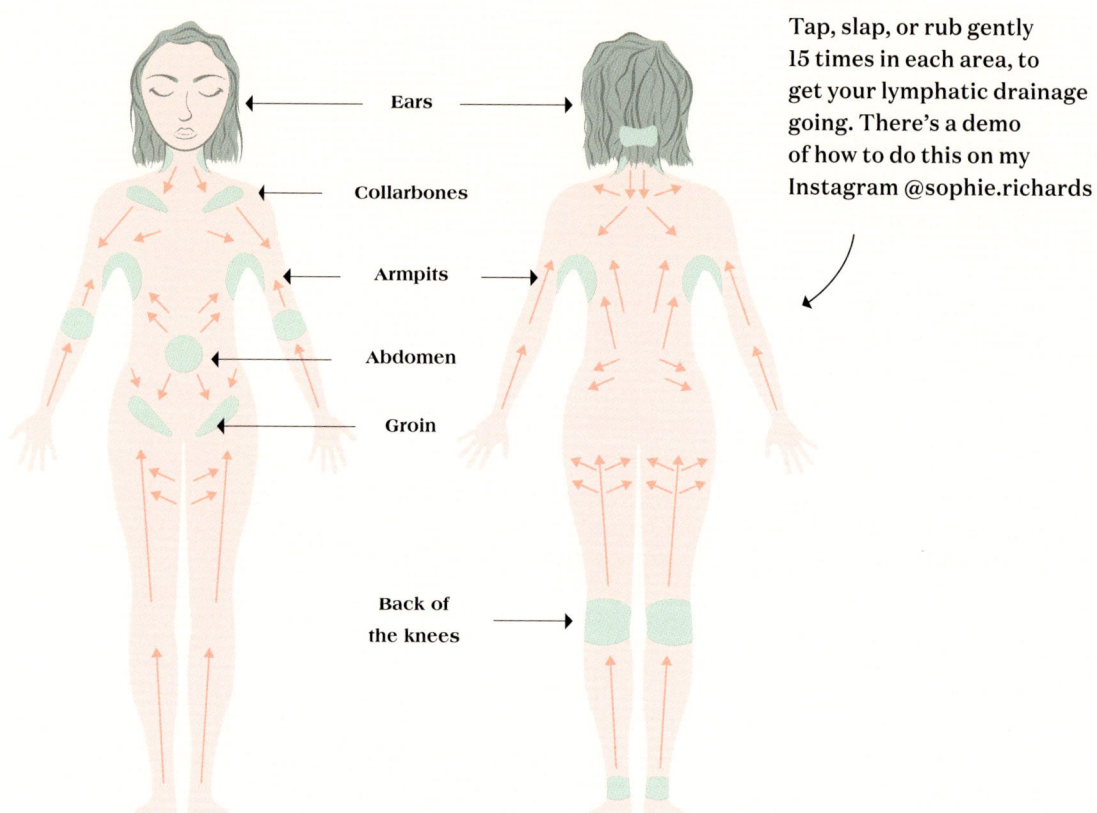

Tap, slap, or rub gently 15 times in each area, to get your lymphatic drainage going. There's a demo of how to do this on my Instagram @sophie.richards

What stops these systems running optimally?

Even though our bodies are **INCREDIBLE** at detoxifying naturally, there are some things that can cause these pathways to get clogged up.

1. **Nutrient deficiencies**

   For your body to work well, your detoxification pathways need a good amount of vitamins, minerals, and antioxidants to support this process. So not only is the Food Pillar important for building hormones, it's also important for supporting your detoxification.

2. **Gut issues**

   Constipation, "leaky gut," and imbalanced gut bacteria can also lead to a buildup of toxins.

3. **Liver overload**

   Our liver is strong, and can even regenerate if damaged (to a degree). However, things like too much alcohol, UPFs, medications, environmental toxins like pesticides, plastics, and heavy metals can be overwhelming for the liver. This is incredibly problematic, as this is where Phase 1 and 2 of detoxification happen. Without a healthy working liver, you can see the domino effect this can have on the rest of the body.

4. **Chronic stress**

   No surprises here, as stress crops up in every pillar. Stress increases cortisol, which can slow down detox pathways and also weaken digestion. This combined effect means that toxins not only move more slowly than you'd like, but they also struggle to be removed due to the impact of stress on your digestion.

5. **Hydration**

   As you know, toxins come out through urine and sweat, both of which NEED water. So without water, both those detoxification systems are impacted. So . . . drink your water, ideally two liters a day!

6. **Lack of movement**

   The lymphatic system is incredible; however, unlike our circulatory system of veins and arteries with our heart pumping all that blood around, the lymph system sadly doesn't have a pump, which means WE need to be our own pump, by moving our body. This could be as simple as jumping up and down on the spot for a few minutes. Massages are also a GREAT way to get the lymph system moving, and a perfect way to help relax and de-stress too—a bonus! It doesn't need to be a full professional massage, just five minutes' good lymphatic self-massage in the morning does the trick, too (see opposite for the steps to a lymphatic drainage self-massage). Exercising also really helps, which is why you might look a little more angular in your face after a run. It's your stagnant lymphatic system moving all that fluid away, giving you your jawline back.

7. **Hormonal imbalances**

   Hormonal imbalances, like estrogen dominance or an underactive thyroid, are very common and unfortunately can slow down the liver's ability to detox properly. When the liver isn't processing hormones and toxins efficiently, it can lead to sluggish bile flow, causing issues with your gallbladder, and making it harder for the body to eliminate waste (as the toxins go from the liver to places like the gut via bile). This buildup can lead to bloating, fatigue, and skin issues and can even worsen hormone-related symptoms—it's a vicious cycle.

So how to support natural detoxification?

You'll be glad to know that strict juice cleanses, detox teas, and any other extreme protocols are not necessary. I'm not going to tell you to trash all your products and cosmetics either. The goal isn't perfection, it's about minimizing your toxic load and supporting your detox pathways so that your body isn't constantly overwhelmed. When your detox systems are functioning well and you're reducing unnecessary exposure, those occasional toxins, e.g., from air pollution or the occasional UPF, won't have a drastic impact on your health. Instead, your body will be resilient and primed to handle them efficiently.

There's more good news! The six steps I am about to recommend for supporting detoxification are also steps you should be taking for overall inflammation management, so they won't only be supporting detoxification, but all six pillars of this book—so know that the effort you're putting in won't just help detoxification, but every process in your body!

Six steps to support detoxification

1. **Support your liver.**

    As our liver is the MVP (most valued player) of the detoxification organs, with two crucial phases occurring here, it's vital we support our liver as much as possible. How?

    » **Increase your intake of cruciferous vegetables**, such as broccoli, cauliflower, and kale, to support liver enzymes. These enzymes help break down and eliminate toxins in Phases 1 and 2 of liver detoxification, which will make it easier for your body to neutralize and remove harmful substances.

    » **Incorporate sulphur-rich foods**, e.g., onions, garlic, eggs, to boost glutathione production. Glutathione is the body's master antioxidant and plays a key role in Phase 2 of liver detoxification by neutralizing toxins, heavy metals, and free radicals, making them safe for elimination. It also reduces oxidative stress, supports immune function, and protects cells, helping your body to efficiently detox and stay resilient.

    » **Prioritize protein** intake, as amino acids like glycine, taurine, and cysteine are crucial for detoxification. As discussed in the Food Pillar (see page 42), protein is very important for balancing blood sugar, and the recipes included in this book are naturally nourished with protein, so you'll be supporting your detoxification pathways AND balancing blood sugar all at the same time.

    » **Minimize alcohol and UPFs**, as they place unnecessary strain on the liver and can slow down detoxification. Alcohol is processed by the liver first, as it sees it as a priority toxin, which means other detox functions (such as hormone metabolism and toxin clearance) get put on hold. Excessive alcohol consumption can also deplete glutathione, increase inflammation, and lead to fatty liver buildup, making detoxification less efficient. Processed foods, especially those high in refined sugars, trans fats, and artificial additives, can contribute to cell damage, gut imbalances, and excess toxin load, forcing the liver to work harder. Reducing the amount of toxins we put in our body allows the liver to focus on eliminating toxins and hormones efficiently, keeping your body in balance and you feeling your best.

2. **Up your gut health!**

You'll be a gut health pro by now, as you've already read up on the gut in Pillar 2. However, I find it incredibly motivating to focus on my gut health when it helps not only with hormone health and inflammation, but also with detoxification. Here are some quick tips on how to boost your gut health:

» **Eat fiber-rich foods**, such as vegetables, flaxseeds, and chia seeds (there are loads of recipes in this book that include these!), as they support that daily bowel movement we all want, which is one of the ways we can excrete those toxins.

» **Drink plenty of water**, to help with moving along the food in your colon, once again helping with that bowel movement.

» **Support your gut bacteria**, with fermented foods like kimchi, sauerkraut, and kefir. Getting plenty of good bacteria will help with your digestion and inflammation, which in turn will help with your bowel movements and ability to get rid of those toxins vs. reabsorbing them.

3. **Sweat**

Another way to remove toxins is by sweating, so do whatever you need to and get that sweat dripping! There are a couple of ways of doing this:

» **Exercise:** There are no rules here, just whatever gets you nice and sweaty. Sometimes a quick power walk can do the job.

» **Sauna:** a great way to get your body sweating. If you don't have access to one, a really hot bath with some Epsom salts can also do the trick.

4. **Reduce toxin exposure**

Your detox pathways don't just need support, they also need fewer obstacles. So reducing your toxin exposure can also help free up those detox pathways. Ways to do this include:

» **Choosing organic produce** where possible, to limit pesticide intake. Going organic also helps with the omega-3 to omega-6 ratio, which we covered in Pillar 1, so this has multiple benefits.

» **Wash your fruit and veg.** I know going organic isn't always realistic, depending on budget and availability. So a simple way to reduce exposure to chemicals is to wash produce in a baking soda solution.

Fill a bowl or sink with water, add one teaspoon of baking soda for every two cups of water and let produce soak for 10–15 minutes before rinsing well. It's an easy way to lower toxic load without breaking the bank.

» **Limit or avoid plastics** and nonstick cookware. BPA and other endocrine disruptors are very common in plastic, especially when they're exposed to heat. Some chemicals act like hormones in our bodies, so when it comes to balancing hormones the last thing we want is to be adding additional ones to the mix! Water bottles, plastic containers, takeout coffee cups, etc., should be limited or avoided, and glass or stainless steel should be used instead. I know this isn't always possible, but if you can buy reusable containers, not only will you be helping your body, but you'll also be helping the planet.

» **Filter your drinking water** to remove heavy metals and contaminants. I used to think this was a conspiracy, until I looked into my water supply. There are a wide variety of affordable easy-to-fit water filters you can add to sinks and showers, and I would highly recommend doing this.

» **Pads and tampons.** These are essential for managing our period, so you'd assume they're harmless, right? However, you'll be shocked to know that your favorite brands are often riddled with chemicals, and on top of that, the insertion and removal of tampons can often cause tears and open our vaginal microbiome up to unwanted bacteria! I've since switched mainly to period pants (they're incredible, and yes, you can get period thongs, too!), as well as organic pads when needed.

5. **Prioritize sleep and stress reduction**

Rest and relaxation are just as important for detoxification as food and movement. We will cover sleep and stress in more depth in upcoming pillars, but for some quick tips on detoxification:

» **Aim for seven to nine hours of quality sleep**, as this is when your body does its deepest detox work.

» **Manage stress** through meditation, deep breathing, or time in nature, as chronic stress slows digestion and therefore slows one of our key detox pathways.

6. **Move your lymphatic system**

Your lymphatic system is like the body's drainage network, but it needs **YOU** to keep it flowing. Social media can imply you need special tools, oils, and fancy routines, but in reality you don't. These methods work perfectly well:

» Rebounding through jumping up and down on the spot as well as skipping, running, or even jumping on a trampoline.

» Self massage is a great free way to help your lymph system. Check out my Instagram (@sophie.richards) for a tutorial of the "six-step lymphatic drainage method" I use every day, devised by Dr. Perry Nickelston.

» Stay hydrated, as lymph fluid relies on water to transport waste efficiently.

Detox? Done!

I hope you're starting to realize that our bodies already know exactly what they need to do to keep us fit and healthy, and that it's just about supporting them from the inside and out.

When we support one pillar, we often support the others, too. When we're detoxing properly, everything moves through our system as it should, reducing stress on the body and inflammation. Sounds good, doesn't it?

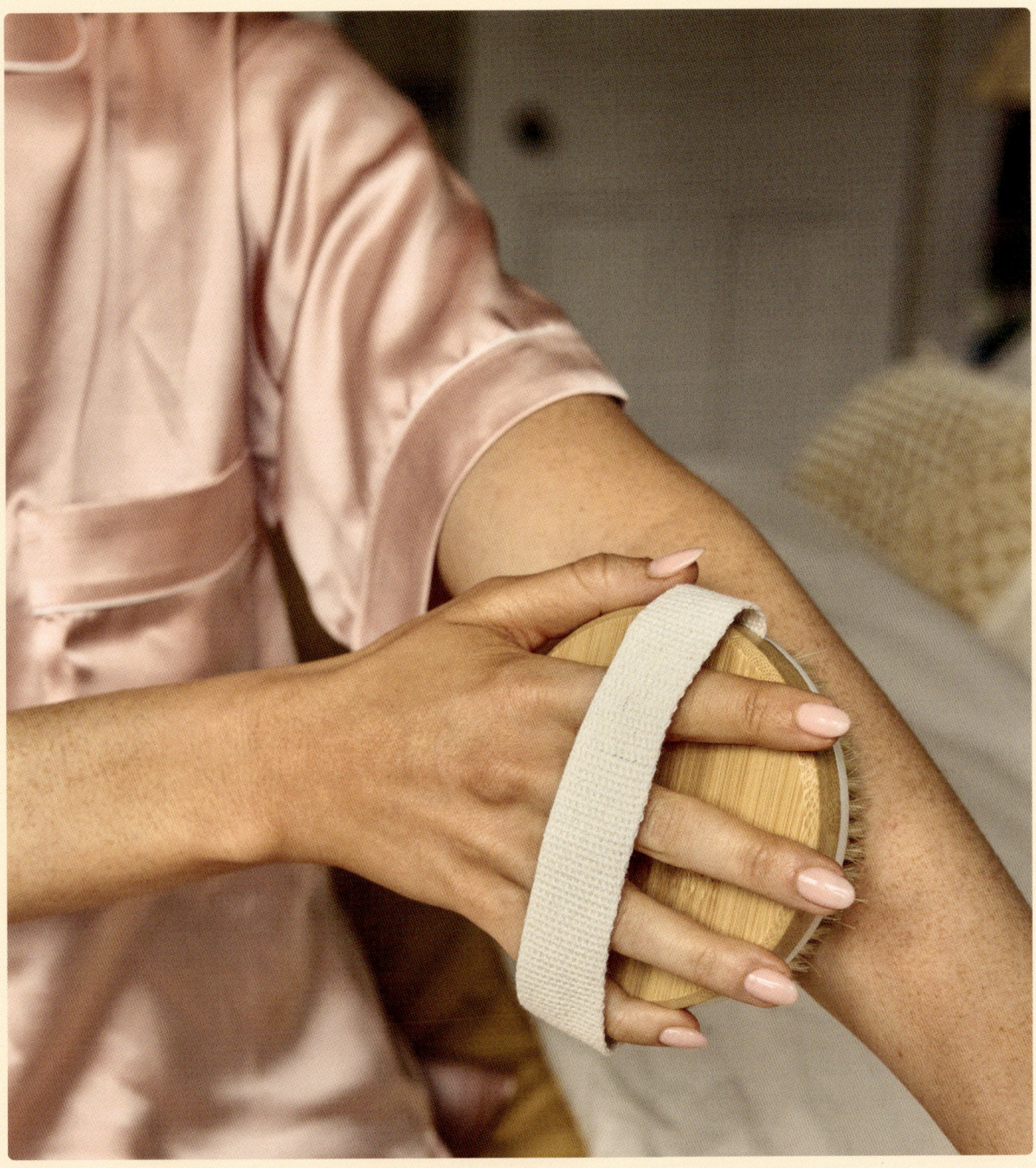

Conclusion

5 Daily Quick Goals

- ✓ Eat cruciferous veg like broccoli, kale, or cabbage every day to support liver detox pathways.

- ✓ Drink two liters or more of water to support kidneys, bowel movements, and lymph flow.

- ✓ Sweat daily through exercise, sauna, a hot bath, or even cleaning the house!

- ✓ Reduce toxic load by cutting back on alcohol and UPFs, washing fruit and veg, switching cookware and swapping out plastic bottles—perfection is not the aim, it's about doing better where we can.

- ✓ Do one thing daily to support lymph, e.g., a walk, a two-minute bounce up and down, or five minutes of self-massage such as the lymphatic drainage protocol.

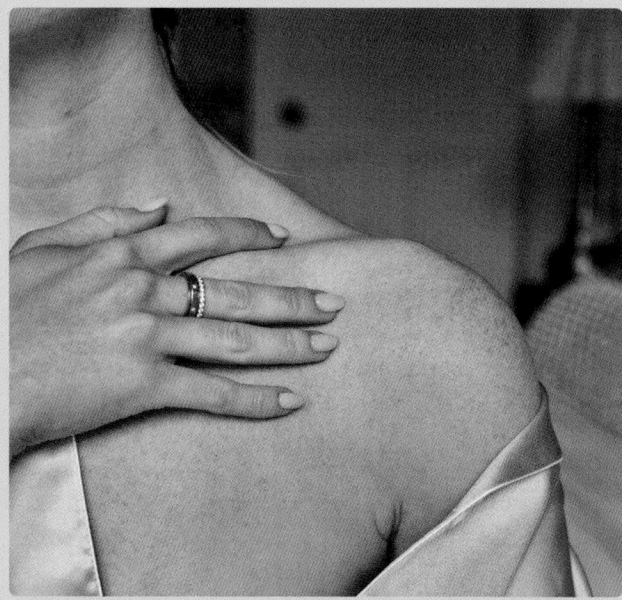

Top 10 Things to Remember About Detoxification!

1. **Your body detoxes itself every single day,** through your liver, gut, kidneys, lungs, skin, and lymphatic system.

2. **The liver is your main detox organ.** It works in two phases to neutralize toxins and send them to the gut and kidneys to be removed.

3. **Your gut is ESSENTIAL for detoxing,** and so are your bowel movements! You need to be having a proper daily poo to remove toxins. If you're constipated, they can be reabsorbed and cause havoc.

4. **The kidneys filter out water-soluble toxins** through your urine. Hydration is key to keeping this process running smoothly—so get those liters in!

5. **Your lungs are detox organs, too!** Every breath helps eliminate toxins, which is why fresh air, breathwork, and avoiding pollutants (like vapes) really matters.

6. **Your skin detoxes through sweat,** so you can support it with movement, saunas, dry brushing, and clean skincare that's not filled with chemicals.

7. **Your lymphatic system doesn't have a pump,** so it relies on YOU to move it. You can do this by moving your body (jumping, walking, exercise) as well as by massages.

8. **You don't just need to support detox organs . . .** you need to reduce the toxic load, too. This means less alcohol and fewer UPFs and endocrine disruptors (chemicals like pesticides and ingredients in personal care and period products).

9. **Nutrient deficiencies** (like low B vitamins, zinc, amino acids) can slow detox pathways, so food quality and protein intake are essential. When you eat real whole foods, you're doing it all!

10. **Detoxification affects all your other systems**—hormones, skin, energy, immune health, and inflammation. When it's working well, you'll feel the difference in every part of your body.

Pillar 4: Sleep

Growing up on a farm, with very hard-working parents, meant not only that sleep was **NOT** a priority, but that it was borderline shameful to be well rested. Going to sleep after 11pm and waking at 5am was "normal" in my household, so if you **DARED** to still be in bed past 7am, you were in trouble. Not only was there a lot of work to do, but there was also a culture (which exists not only in farming, but everywhere) that sleep is a luxury, and those who work hard don't need it!

For years, I bragged about how I only needed five hours of sleep. I convinced myself I was still laser focused and somehow "built different" to my friends who casually slept ten hours on the weekend. Sadly, I was not. That wired, buzzing feeling I thought was productivity? Just cortisol spikes from chronic sleep deprivation. No wonder my so-called laser focus was always followed by depressive crashes, zero energy, and an uncontrollable need for sugar and caffeine. My blood sugar was all over the place, fueling the cycle even more. The pillars are all connected—which is a **GOOD** and a **BAD** thing. Sacrifice one, and you'll likely see a domino effect on the others. However, the same is true when you start fixing one pillar: the positive domino effect will occur, which is exactly what you'll see once you start implementing the changes in this book.

It's easy to think that sleep is just about feeling rested, but that's the least of it. It's the foundation for everything. When sleep is not prioritized, it has a knock-on effect on the entire body. Poor sleep disrupts blood sugar, which triggers inflammation, which throws hormones out of balance, which then makes it even harder to sleep . . . sound familiar? It's a vicious cycle that leaves so many of us exhausted, bloated, irritable, and constantly reaching for caffeine or sugar to compensate.

For years, I thought my health was dictated by what I ate, but now I know that sleep is just as important. And once you understand why, you'll never take it for granted again.

Why sleep is the foundation of your health

I always like to imagine sleep as your body shutting up shop for the day, and cleaners coming in for the night shift. Every night, if you allow it, your body hits the reset button, letting you wake up fresh in the morning. Your hormones regulate, your brain detoxifies, your metabolism stabilizes, and inflammation lowers. But when we don't sleep? Those processes are cut short, the clean-up crew clock off early, and you're left with the mess from yesterday.

A single night of poor sleep can have several immediate effects on the body:

» Increasing inflammation markers, which can worsen pain and bloating.

» Elevating cortisol levels, leading to higher anxiety and less stress tolerance. When cortisol is high throughout the day, it can impact your sleep at night, causing that annoying "tired but wired" feeling.

» Impairing insulin sensitivity, which results in blood-sugar fluctuations and energy crashes.[1] Starting the day on the blood-sugar roller coaster means you'll be more likely to seek out sugar and caffeine, which then messes up your mood and sleep and keeps you stuck on this hamster wheel.

» Increasing appetite, particularly for refined carbohydrates and sugars.[2]

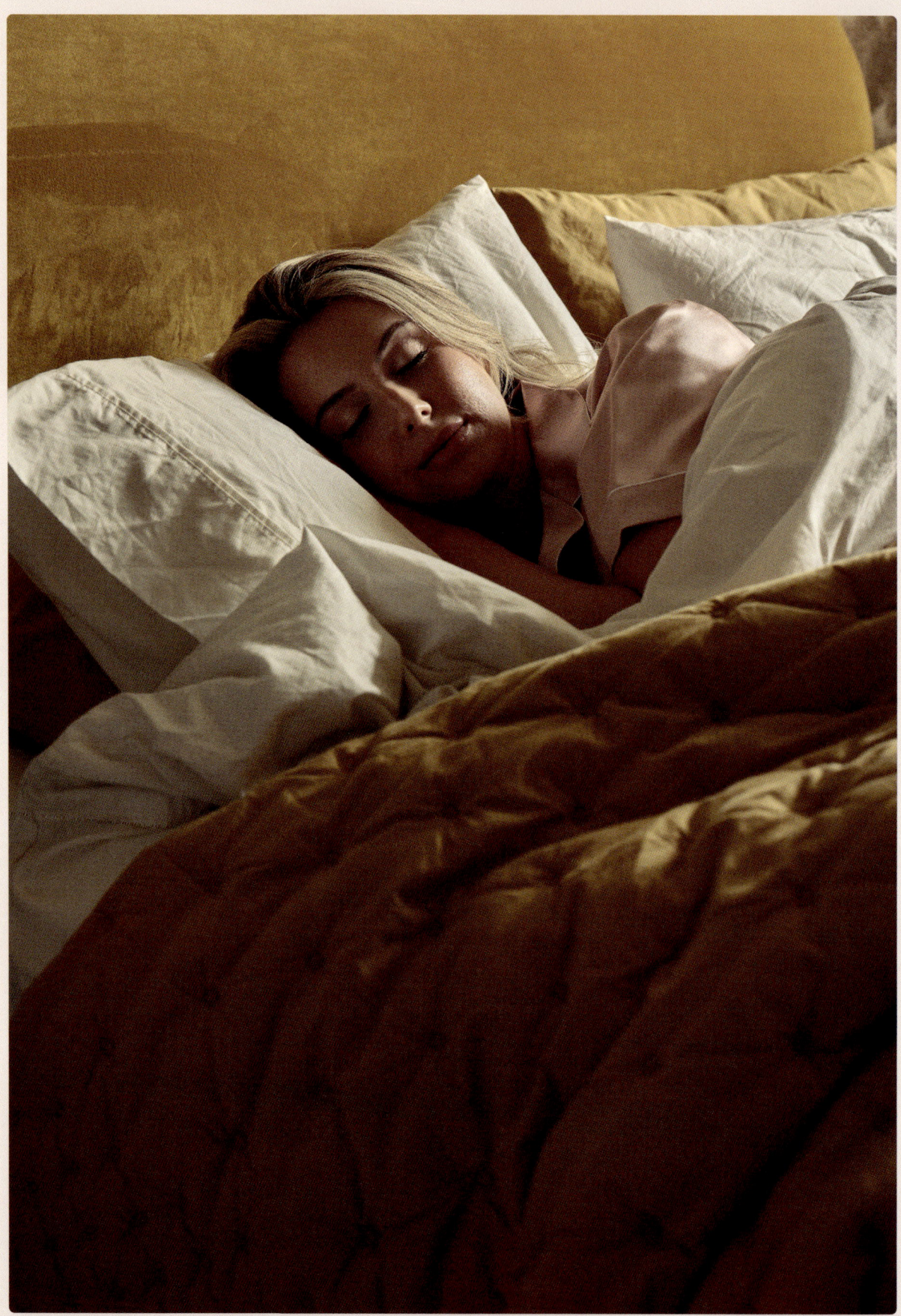

Look, one bad night's sleep here and there isn't a big deal; your body is adaptable and it's also unavoidable—life happens! It's also important not to become obsessive—sometimes a late night is worth it for a celebration, a fun trip, or just having a great time with people you love. Writing this book, for example, has been the most exciting project I've ever worked on, and sometimes it's taken me through the night because I just can't stop typing! Dr. Sophie Bostock recently joined me on my *Finally Found* podcast, where we discussed the ins and outs of sleep, and she shares exactly the same view about sacrificing sleep when the time is right, because life is worth living, after all!

However, when sleep deprivation becomes a long-term pattern, that's when the real problems start. Dr. Bostock advises that it becomes a notable problem when you've been struggling with sleep for over three months. Poor sleep fuels inflammation, throws hormones off balance, and sets off a domino effect in the body. For women, this is even more impactful. As you know, when cortisol and insulin are disrupted, the impact isn't isolated to stress and blood-sugar crashes; they also interfere with key hormones that regulate the menstrual cycle and impact transition through perimenopause and menopause. That alone is a reason to prioritize sleep . . . but for those with conditions like endometriosis and PCOS, it's even more important. Hormonal fluctuations can make sleep more difficult for some, and when we don't prioritize sleep it can make symptoms worse, recovery harder, and falling asleep even harder because we are running on stress hormone, which makes us more prone to that tired but wired feeling. If we don't prioritize sleep, we're fighting an uphill battle every single day.

The circadian rhythm = your body's master clock

At the heart of your sleep is your circadian rhythm, which is the twenty-four-hour internal clock that regulates your sleep–wake cycle, digestion, metabolism, and even your immune function. It's what makes you feel awake in the morning and sleepy at night, mainly down to a hormone called melatonin.

Melatonin is your body's natural sleep hormone, with anti-inflammatory and antioxidant properties. It is produced by the pineal gland (a small pea-shaped gland deep in the center of your brain) in response to darkness and acts like a signal to your brain that it's time to wind down. This process starts in the evening when light naturally drops, helping lower your brain activity, body temperature, and alertness so you can fall asleep more easily. This process was seamless back in the day when TVs, phones, and fluorescent lights didn't exist . . . but when was the last time you just sat in darkness as the sun set? Thankfully we don't have to, we just need to adapt our surroundings to mimic this experience as much as possible. Bright lights and screen exposure can be a nightmare when it comes to our melatonin production and therefore our sleep. But not to worry, by the end of this pillar, you'll know exactly how to master your sleep.

Just like a clock, you need to set your body's circadian rhythm, which is primarily done by three things:

- » Light exposure
- » Movement
- » Food timing

This is why getting morning daylight, keeping a consistent sleep schedule, and eating meals at the right times all impact your ability to sleep well.

When this rhythm is thrown off, it can throw everything off. The effects include:

- **Cortisol spikes** at the wrong times, making you feel wired at night and groggy in the morning.
- **Melatonin gets suppressed**, making it harder to fall and stay asleep.
- **Metabolism slows down**, making weight management harder.
- **Inflammation increases**, which can trigger bloating, skin issues, and joint pain and keep you in a vicious loop of discomfort.
- **Hormonal balance is disrupted**, potentially reducing progesterone and increasing estrogen, affecting menstrual cycles.

Your body is highly adaptable, so if a restful sleep feels like a beautiful dream for you right now, just know that there are small steps we can all take to improve our sleep. Just like you can reset a clock, you can reset your circadian rhythm, and when you do, your short and long-term health will thank you.

The science of sleep:
what else happens when we don't get enough?

If you're still thinking, "I can get by on little sleep," here's what the research says about sleep deprivation:

- **Increases inflammation and immune response.** Sleep deprivation has been shown to negatively impact genes related to the management of immune and inflammation-related processes.[3]
- **Menstrual cycle changes.** For women, fluctuating hormones mean sleep can be disrupted regardless. However, when hormones are unbalanced, e.g., by poor sleep (i.e., higher or lower than the usual cycle fluctuations), this further drives the poor sleep cycle as cortisol and insulin send the hormonal hierarchy into a spiral, causing worsened menstrual cycle pain, as well as harsher perimenopause and menopause symptoms.
- **Mental health** is also impacted. Studies have shown that lack of sleep can change activity in the brain, negatively affecting our decision-making and problem-solving, our ability to control our behaviors and emotions and how easily we cope with change.

Now imagine months or years of poor sleep? It's no wonder so many of us struggle with inflammation, hormone imbalances, and stubborn weight gain. But now that you know exactly why sleep is important, and how it might be a major contributor to why you're feeling the way you are . . . it also means you can change it!

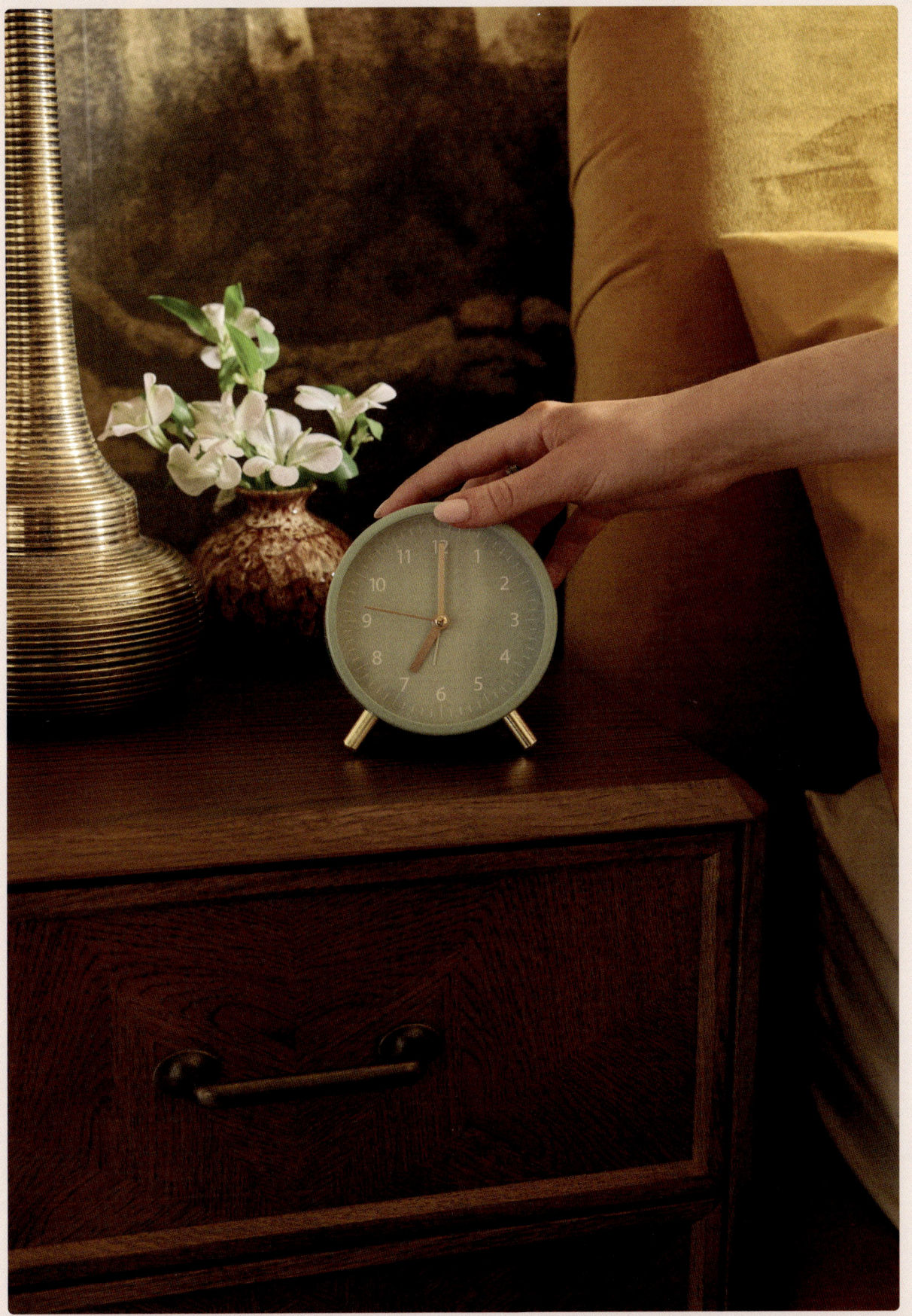

How to fix your sleep for optimal health

If you want better sleep, better energy, and better health, then listening to the sleep king himself—Dr. Andrew Huberman, professor of neuroscience at Stanford University—is the best place to start. I found Dr. Huberman's work in 2023, and it was one of those A-HA! moments when I finally realized that following an evidence-based, systematic approach to a problem I was having was the way forward.

Below are some of Dr. Huberman's favorite tools,[4] combined with insights from my menstrual health training and from sleep expert Dr. Sophie Bostock's work, designed to get your sleep schedule SOLID.

1. **Get morning daylight.**

    Exposing your eyes to natural daylight within an hour of waking helps regulate your circadian rhythm and tells your body it's time to wake up. This is down to the morning daylight exposure reducing melatonin and triggering the natural release of cortisol, which helps you feel alert and energized. Ideally you'd get thirty to sixty minutes of daylight in the morning, but even just ten minutes on a clear day can help your body wake up.

2. **Keep a consistent sleep schedule.**

    Going to bed and waking up at the same time every day trains your body to sleep deeply and wake up naturally. Once you're in the habit of waking up and sleeping at the same times, your body will be doing it in a seamless rhythm, and the early wake-up call you used to dread will naturally happen with ease. The amount of sleep that is required varies from person to person, but research shows that on average we need anywhere from seven to nine hours per night.

3. **No caffeine after 2pm.**

    Dr. Sophie Bostock shocked me when she said caffeine stays in your system for almost nine hours after consuming it. Meaning that even an afternoon coffee can disrupt your sleep. If you struggle to fall asleep, cutting caffeine earlier in the day can make a huge difference.

4. **Reduce screen time at night.**

    Blue light from screens suppresses melatonin, making it harder to fall asleep. Try dimming lights after sunset, wearing blue-light-blocking glasses, or switching screens to night mode.

5. **Balance blood sugar before bed.**

Large spikes in blood sugar at night can cause energy crashes and wake you up in the middle of the night. Following the principles from the Food Pillar (page 42) will massively help with sleep, so focus on balanced carbs, fats, and proteins, and don't eat too late before bed. No later than two or three hours before bed is ideal, to give your body time to digest and space to wind down in preparation for sleep.

6. **Create a wind-down routine.**

We work well when we have routines or rituals to follow. Just as waking up and going to bed at the same time will help create a sleep routine, so will a "wind-down" routine that helps prepare you for sleep.

> » My personal wind-down routine includes listening to Dr. Huberman's 10 minute NSDR audio—it's free on YouTube and is a non-sleep deep-rest protocol that you can use at any point in the day.

7. **Sleep in a cold and dark room.**

I am a lover of warmth and cannot stand a chilly room; however, when I met my partner, Dillon, he was obsessive about having a cold room for sleep. I tend to be more agreeable at the start of a relationship (which Dillon reports didn't last long . . .), so I agreed to having a colder room to sleep in. I couldn't believe the difference not only in how quickly I fell asleep, but also in how deep that sleep was. And there's a reason for this. Dr. Huberman states: "Your body needs to drop in temperature by 1–3 degrees to fall and stay asleep effectively. Body temperature increases are one reason you wake up."[5] Therefore keeping your room cool and as dark as possible is the best way forward for a good night's sleep.

Conclusion

Dr. Huberman's philosophy has always been that sleep is the cornerstone of both mental and physical well-being and influences how we function in every part of life. Skipping a night of good rest or missing morning light once in a while won't cause major issues, but we will start to suffer if we neglect these behaviors for too long. My life notably changed when I started focusing on my sleep, and when I started slipping back into old habits, the impacts were very obvious. My recovery crashed, and so did my energy. No matter what your lifestyle or ambitions are, master your sleep. Your body and mind will thank you!

5 Daily Quick Goals

- ✓ Get ten-plus minutes of morning daylight within an hour of waking. Ideally, go for a walk outdoors—this maximizes light exposure and also supports movement, digestion, and lymphatic drainage. If a walk isn't possible, standing outside in your garden is still very effective. And if you can't get outdoors, sitting next to an open window will provide some benefit.

- ✓ Keep a consistent sleep and wake time every day—even on weekends! Set your alarm to go off seven days a week, and before you know it, you'll have the ideal sleep/wake routine that feels effortless (no more fighting the snooze button!).

- ✓ Avoid caffeine after 2pm to help your body wind down properly.

- ✓ Reduce screen time and dim lights after sunset to support melatonin production.

- ✓ Create a calming wind-down routine to signal to your body that it's time to sleep, e.g., gratitude practice, journaling, light reading (nothing too stimulating), or NSDR meditation (see page 105), to prepare your body to drift off and have a restful sleep!

Top 10 Things to Remember About Sleep!

1. **Sleep isn't a luxury**—it's the foundation of your health, hormones, and energy. Poor sleep creates a domino effect that impacts blood sugar, cravings, mood, and inflammation.

2. **You're not built differently!** Running on five hours' sleep a night might feel productive, but it's just cortisol keeping you wired. That "buzz" will always be followed by a crash.

3. **One bad night won't ruin your health,** but consistent sleep deprivation over time WILL impact your immune system, hormone balance, and how you feel every day.

4. **Your body repairs, detoxes, and rebalances while you sleep.** If you're not sleeping well, these essential overnight jobs get skipped or cut short.

5. **Your circadian rhythm is your internal body clock.** It regulates your sleep-wake cycle and is controlled by light exposure, food timing, and movement. When you work with it, you're supporting melatonin production, which we want plenty of as it's an anti-inflammatory hormone.

6. **Morning daylight helps set your circadian rhythm** by lowering melatonin and triggering a healthy cortisol spike, helping you feel fired up in the morning and sleepy at night.

7. **A consistent sleep schedule** (yes, even on weekends) trains your body to fall asleep faster and wake up more naturally.

8. **Blue light from screens suppresses melatonin,** your sleep hormone. Reducing screen time and dimming lights in the evening can switch on those sleep cues and get you falling asleep in no time!

9. **Caffeine can stay active in your system** for almost nine hours after your last sip. Cutting it after 2pm can help improve sleep quality drastically (yes, switching to decaf is better, but that still has some caffeine in it!).

10. **Blood sugar affects sleep, too.** Balanced meals and not eating too late can help you get to sleep, and STAY asleep, too!

Pillar 5: Stress

Stress: the silent driver of inflammation

Just like lack of sleep was worn as a badge of honor in my household when I was growing up, so was stress. If you weren't stressed, the assumption was you mustn't be working hard enough!

I spent my teens and early twenties stressed, striving for my top exam results, first-class degree, and shiny graduate job. My dreams had come true... right? **WRONG!**

My symptoms started during my A-levels, and even though this was also when I started my period, knowing what I do now about stress, there is no doubt that my compulsive stressing made matters much worse and unsurprisingly landed me on an operating table. The same wired, buzzing feeling that I used to have from lack of sleep was the same feeling I had when I was stressed. Something I mistook for productivity, energy, and drive was actually my cortisol levels spiking, only to burn me to the ground later in the day... on repeat, for over ten years. The afternoons when I was crashing, ravenous for sugar, as well as suffering from bloating, pain, and horrific endometriosis symptoms, were all partly driven by stress. My poor body was trapped in a state of constant inflammation that was fueling itself daily.

Is stress always bad for us?

Just like inflammation is good for us in small doses, so is stress. Short, controlled bursts of stress can help keep us sharp and fuel us with motivation in times that are challenging. However, when stress becomes chronic, problems arise.

> *Quick test: Are you stressed?*
>
> *Answer yes or no to the following questions:*
>
> - *Do you wake up feeling tired, even after a full night's sleep?*
> - *Do you find yourself craving sugar, caffeine, or carbs throughout the day?*
> - *Is your mind constantly racing, making it hard to switch off or relax?*
> - *Do you often feel bloated, experience digestive issues, or get unexplained headaches?*
> - *Do small things (like emails, traffic, or last-minute changes) easily irritate or overwhelm you?*
>
> *If you said yes to more than one of these scenarios, your body is likely in a state of chronic stress... whether you realize it or not. But the good news is that now that you're aware of it, you can start making simple changes to break the cycle.*

Like every pillar explored in this book, stress doesn't work in isolation. It's tied to everything. Poor diet spikes blood sugar, which triggers stress. Gut issues disrupt the gut–brain connection, making us feel anxious. Lack of sleep fuels our stress hormone cortisol, which makes getting a deep and restorative night's sleep even harder. Even overexercising can stress out the body. That's why managing stress isn't just about meditating or "thinking good thoughts" . . . it's about addressing all the moving parts.

By the end of this pillar, you'll know EXACTLY how to better manage when stressful events crop up and how to reduce the stress that's within your control—because the goal is to remove the cause, not just treat the symptom. As always, once you learn the "why," the "how" makes so much more sense. So let's get into the science and break down what stress actually is, how it shows up in your life, and why it's one of the biggest drivers of inflammation, hormonal chaos, and poor health.

What is stress?
(and why it's not always bad)

Stress is your body's built-in alarm system. It's an evolutionary response designed to keep you alive. There's a famous example often cited, which is to imagine you're being chased by a lion . . . clearly your body needs to react fast. Your brain floods your system with stress hormones (mainly cortisol and adrenaline), which then increases your heart rate. This is for a very important reason: it gets you hyper-focused, and pulls sugar into your blood for easy access to energy, making you ready to **RUN**.

The issue is, this stress response isn't just reserved for life and death situations. It can be triggered by anything you find stressful. In this day and age, constant access to information, and to other people, means we're constantly on. Always expected to respond, with no off switch. The emails build up, the WhatsApps tumble, Instagram notifications are pinging away, negative self-talk gets louder . . . your boss is asking you to "quickly" respond to a client . . . all at the same time, on repeat, every day. THAT feeling, although logically it shouldn't be the same as a lion chasing you, has the same effect. It's overwhelming and stressful and your body responds by trying to help, with cortisol and adrenaline coming to the rescue. To your nervous system, a passive-aggressive email triggers the same fight-or-flight response as running from a lion. And if you don't actively reset your stress response, you stay stuck in that heightened state, resulting in chronic inflammation. It's wild to think that something as harmless as opening WhatsApp can feel like stepping onto a battlefield.

Last year, I made an executive decision to simply do my best with my phone—to reply to only as many people as I reasonably can, rather than every single message. That might seem selfish to some, but for me, it had become a genuine problem. I was constantly filled with dread and guilt for not replying to people. But as the group chats multiplied and I (rookie error) started giving work contacts my personal number, that little red "99+" bubble started to feel like a personal attack.

It hit me one day that we're living in a world of constant access—always on, always available—which just didn't exist a few decades ago. Back then, you'd write a letter, post it, and wait a week for a reply. That, I could have kept up with.

So I waved the white flag and I told my friends I'm hopeless on my phone, and that if there's ever a fire, just call me. And honestly? It's been a game changer. I don't feel guilty any more for the unread messages. And that fear of letting people down? Turns out it was just that—a fear. No one actually cares, and if anything they're also fighting the same WhatsApp battle!

Being a good friend isn't about replying to every micro-message in real time, it's about showing up when it matters, in the big moments, the tough moments, and everything in between. Prioritizing your health (mental included!) isn't selfish . . . it's essential!

The science: stress, blood sugar, and inflammation

When you're stressed, your body releases cortisol, one of the key stress hormones and—as you now know—one of your two CEO hormones. Cortisol's job is to get you a quick injection of energy, so it raises blood-sugar levels by signaling to the liver to release stored glucose into the bloodstream. This gives you an instant burst of fuel since the sugar is now easily accessible—super-useful if you're running from danger, less so if you've been triggered by something unpleasant while doom-scrolling on your phone. However, chronically elevated cortisol can lead to insulin resistance over time, as constantly high blood sugar forces the body to produce more insulin to clear it. This cycle can lead to energy crashes, sugar cravings, and inflammation. Can you see the similarity between when we eat too many UPFs or refined sugars, or don't balance our blood sugar? The same response happens, proving once again that no single pillar is the sole cause of inflammation—they *all* have an impact! The more inflammation, the more your body stays in a state of stress, creating a vicious cycle that fuels:

» **Hormonal imbalances:** Cortisol and insulin are your CEO/dominant hormones in the hierarchy. If they're out of balance as a result of stress, so will your other hormones that play a key role in your menstrual cycle, perimenopause, and menopause.

» **Blood-sugar dysregulation:** Stress makes us crave sugar and carbs, leading to spikes, crashes, and consequently more stress. Insulin goes on a roller coaster that feels impossible to get off.

» **Gut issues:** The gut and brain are directly connected. Chronic stress can alter gut bacteria, trigger bloating, and even cause IBS-like symptoms. So your "bad tummy" that you blamed on dairy might actually be from stress having impacted the gut that's now responding poorly to various foods.

» **Weakened immune function:** Stress diverts resources away from healing and repair, making the body more susceptible to illness and inflammation. This was one I struggled with during A-levels, my degree, and basically every corporate role I worked in: I was constantly catching any bug that was flying around and it just felt like I couldn't catch a break.

» **Poor sleep:** Stress makes it harder to fall asleep, which means you don't get that deep restorative sleep we talked about in the previous chapter . . . which has a huge knock-on effect on the body, and of course the less you sleep, the more stressed you feel . . . another vicious cycle.

Stress works in mysterious ways

> *Years ago, I went to a healer who suggested that pain in the body could be a physical manifestation of our mental thoughts. While I don't fully agree with that idea, one of her examples stayed with me. She explained constipation as the body physically "holding on" to waste—and asked whether I also tended to hold on to rumination and negative thoughts, i.e., mental waste that didn't serve me. At the time it sounded a little woo-woo, but what I later learned was that science actually backs this up in a different way: the gut-brain axis communicates stress directly to the gut, and stress is a well-known trigger for constipation. So what first seemed like a purely holistic interpretation actually does have a physiological explanation, too.*
>
> *My cousin had a similar experience just before her wedding, when she suddenly lost her voice. The holistic practitioner she saw asked her: "Is there something you're not saying, even to yourself?" Holistically, the idea was that she was suppressing her true feelings—she couldn't voice the fact that she didn't want to marry her partner of over ten years. Her body, in turn, expressed this by literally taking away her ability to speak. Now, this sounds very woo-woo to me, but stay with me. Because sometimes the woo-woo is backed by science. So let's get into it.*

What happened to my cousin might sound insane, I know, but if we put aside the "spiritual" element of it, there's actually a really physical reason behind it. It's all down to something called the vagus nerve, which is a long nerve that runs from your brain all the way down your body, connecting to most of your major organs along the way (heart, lungs, gut, vocal cords, and more!). It's part of your parasympathetic nervous system, which is responsible for keeping you calm, digesting your food properly, and helping your body feel safe. When it's working well, your heart-rate drops, your digestion improves, your mood lifts. When it's not . . . you stay stuck in fight-or-flight.

This is why stress isn't just a feeling, it's a full body experience. If your vagus nerve isn't firing properly, your digestion slows, your breath shortens, your body tenses, your voice might even go (like hers did!). You feel like you're on edge all the time . . . even when there's no real danger.

So how do we help our vagus nerve?! Well, there's a whole host of simple but powerful ways to help it. Things like deep breathing, cold showers, humming, even singing or gargling can all help stimulate it and bring your body back into a calm, rested state. It sounds small, but these little practices send a signal to your body that you're safe now, and when your body feels safe, it can finally begin to heal. The lymphatic drainage routine (page 90) also helps do this, as it's a slow, mindful process using self-touch, which reassures your body that you're safe and helps you come out of fight-or-flight and into rest-and-digest. It's why I love doing it first thing in the morning with intentional breathwork at the same time.

Causes of stress

I used to think stress would creep up when I was either overworked or feeling like someone was being passive-aggressive (my biggest pet peeve and it puts me on edge!). Although both are valid, there's so much more to it than that, and stress can sneak up on all of us in different ways. Here's a few common ones:

» **Emotional stress:** Work pressure, difficult relationships, social media, self-doubt, or unresolved trauma can all take a toll on your emotions, even if you think your mind has put it all in a box... your body knows better.

» **Blood-sugar stress:** Skipping meals (e.g., fasting), eating lots of refined carbs and UPFs or relying on caffeine can throw your blood sugar off and signal to your body that something's wrong, creating a stress response.

» **Gut stress:** Poor digestion, food intolerances, and gut imbalances don't just affect your stomach. Remember that gut–brain connection? It can increase anxiety and stress, too.

» **Overexercising:** Music to my ears, because I don't like exercising too much anyway. However, in all seriousness, intense workouts without proper recovery and adequate fueling can spike cortisol and stress the body even more... it's why female athletes and bodybuilders often "lose" their periods during competition seasons!

» **Toxic load:** From alcohol to UPFs and environmental toxins, the liver can become overwhelmed, which keeps your stress response switched on.

» **Lack of sleep:** As you now know from the last chapter, lack of sleep or poor-quality sleep increases cortisol and makes it harder to cope with everyday challenges, leading to that snappy, on-edge feeling no one enjoys.

» **Negative self-talk:** Your thoughts alone can trigger a physical stress response. I personally love manifesting, and the concept of your thoughts becoming reality. However, even if you don't believe in the "woo-woo" magic of manifesting, on a real biological level mental stress can trigger a physical stress response, so that inner critic isn't just annoying to have, but it's triggering inflammation, too.

So do you still think of stress as just a "mental" thing that "some" people are good at dealing with and others aren't? Or do you see it for what it is? A full body response that, when left unchecked, will show up in your cravings, your cycle, your skin, your energy levels, your digestion... everything!

How to reduce stress and lower inflammation

Stress can feel both trivial and monumental at the same time (for me, anyway). My mindset used to be torn between the fact that on the one hand stress is "normal" and just a part of life, so I should just get on with it . . . and on the other hand, I was so crippled by stress from all the angles above that it felt impossible to escape, so what was the point? If you're reading this and thinking SNAP, then I want you to remember three things:

1. You only get one life, and you deserve to enjoy it! Stress really is the thief of joy, and it's quietly stealing your energy, mood, and peace.
2. Stress directly fuels inflammation, the very thing you're trying to reduce, so if you REALLY want to feel better, lowering your stress is a non-negotiable.
3. The goal isn't to eliminate all stress (because some stress is out of our control and some stress is GOOD!). The goal is to reduce what's in your control and support your body to respond better to the rest.

You know **WHY** stress can cause havoc on your body, you know **WHERE** stress comes from . . . and now it's time to learn **HOW** to reduce and manage your stress to live a healthier and happier life.

Balance your blood sugar

Bored with hearing this? GOOD! Balancing blood sugar keeps coming up because it's one of the most crucial ways of managing inflammation across all the pillars. A quick reminder of key ways to balance blood sugar:

» Start your day with protein and healthy fats, not just caffeine!
» Don't skip meals, especially if you're already feeling stressed. If you don't think you have the time to make food, meal prepping is a great option. This book is full of meal-prep-friendly recipes (see pages 142–321).
» Avoid big sugar spikes, especially late at night. Swapping my evening coffee and custard creams for chamomile tea really helped with this, and it has some powerful extra benefits, too. Chamomile contains a powerful antioxidant called apigenin that binds to receptors on the brain, helping to promote sleepiness, and even reduced symptoms of depression in a study with postpartum women. Chamomile tea has also been found to improve insulin sensitivity and blood-sugar regulation,[1] which goes to show the power of natural remedies. So an evening chamomile tea should be on everyone's menu!

Get morning daylight + restorative movement

Setting our circadian rhythm, which we covered in the previous pillar, is not only vital for sleep, but also for the impact it has on stress! Pairing your morning light exposure with a little walk outside will also mean you're making the most of that morning cortisol spike, helping regulate cortisol for the rest of the day, and as a result the rest of your hormones in that hierarchy. As well as walking, you can do yoga, pilates, strength training (or any form of movement you enjoy)—whatever helps get you moving without causing additional stress. Exercise should energize you, not exhaust you . . . and the extra endorphins will help set you up for the day, while the movement will also help with digestion—but more on this in the next pillar.

Cut down on caffeine

Caffeine can raise cortisol, especially when you're already in fight-or-flight mode. I used to go through five or six cups a day . . . and now have one (occasionally two) after my breakfast and before lunch, then switch to herbal teas from there on. When it comes to coffee, you don't need to go cold turkey, just have your morning brew after your breakfast, and no more after 2pm (gold stars if you stop by noon!).

Chamomile[2] and rooibos are my go-to teas, as not only do they taste amazing, but they also help calm the nervous system.

Support your nervous system

Breathwork is often overlooked, but is VERY powerful! Even just for five minutes a day it can help calm the body and reset your stress response. A simple but powerful technique is **"Box Breathing."** It helps calm your nervous system by activating the parasympathetic "rest and digest" mode. Just a few rounds can lower stress, steady your mind, and leave you feeling more centered. Give it a go now—and come back to it any time you need a reset.

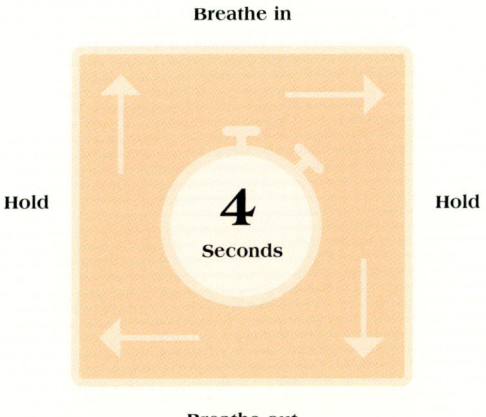

I also really enjoy the **4-2-6 Breath Technique**, where you take one long inhale for four beats, pause for two, then slowly exhale for six. Andrew Huberman does this in his NSDR videos and the extended exhale vs. inhale helps calm your nervous system down almost immediately! Give it a try and repeat three times—you'll be floating in no time.

Cold exposure (ice baths or even a cold shower) can also help calm the body and mind and help you relax. However, a quick note on this! There's more research emerging that for some people, cold water exposure can have the opposite effect on the body, i.e., causing more stress than reducing it. This is a good example of where some science can contradict itself and proves how we are all individuals and have different needs. So what to do? We listen to our bodies! For me, jumping into the ice bath after being in a hot sauna makes my body switch off in all the best ways. I feel calm and relaxed, my muscles feel like they've had some much-needed TLC, and I sleep better for it. My friend Rebecca, on the other hand, has the total opposite reaction. She feels stressed, anxious, and worse than before she got in. Find out what works for **YOU** and **YOUR** body, and apply this to all the advice you receive. Just because a study says that you have a 99.9% chance of feeling better when you do certain activities or take certain supplements, it doesn't mean it's going to work for you! Listen to your body and how it's responding—that's what really matters.

Set boundaries and protect your peace

1. Doom-scrolling on social media feels "good" at the time, as it's a distraction; however, it can also be a major source of low-grade constant stress. Videos are designed to **HOOK** you in and keep you watching, and they often use stress tactics to do this—so put your phone away and focus on being in the present moment rather than losing an hour of your life to TikTok.

2. Creating buffers between work and home life is a great way not to "bring work home." Creating physical buffers like changing your clothes when you get home, or even if you're working from home, can signal to your brain that work is now complete, and "normal life" resumes. I like to go for a long walk at the end of the day and pack my laptop away before I leave, **(a)** to avoid jumping on emails when I get back in and **(b)** because having a clear space absent of my laptop or work-related visuals helps me mentally switch from work to personal life.

3. Make time for joy! As much as spontaneous fun is wonderful, unless we actively plan it, adult life can get in the way and we experience less and less of what makes life so good. Don't underestimate spending time with friends, family, loved ones, and being in nature! These are all stress-reducers and a great form of natural medicine. If you still think making time for "joy" sounds like nonsense, well, I'm about to change your mind! Studies show that positive social connections boost levels of oxytocin, which has been dubbed the "love hormone" as it's been shown to reduce cortisol, inflammation, and even promote wound healing! How cool, right? One study also found that higher levels of oxytocin were directly linked to lower blood pressure and stress during social bonding moments.[1] So go and grab a friend and give them a big *cwtch* (a Welsh hug!); your hormones will thank you for it!

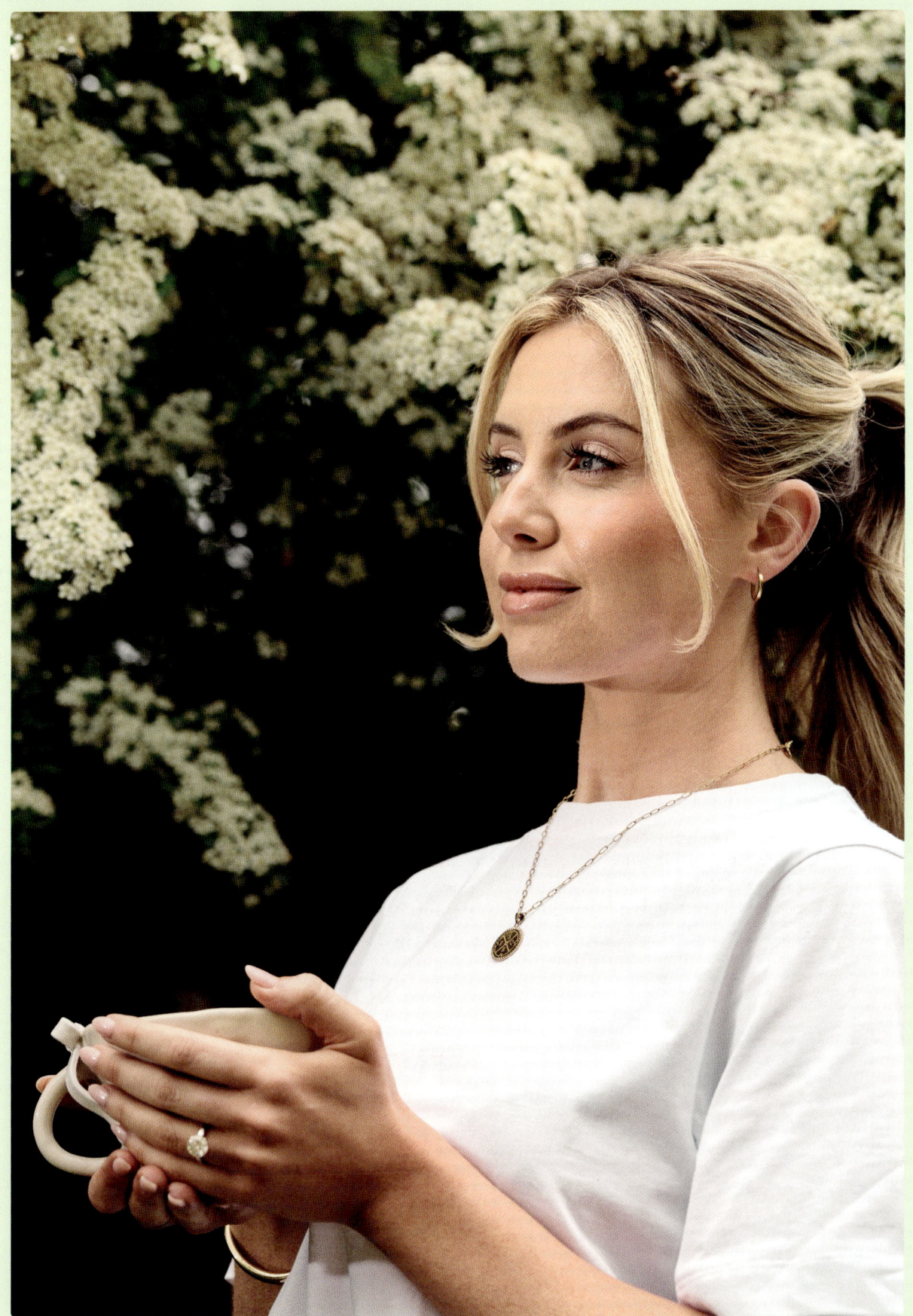

Conclusion

For so long, I thought stress was just a mindset thing. That if I could just "get a grip" or think positively, it would go away. But stress shows up in your body whether you realize it or not. If you're constantly tired, craving sugar, snapping at people, bloated, or just not feeling like yourself... stress is likely playing a much bigger role than you think.

Managing stress isn't about being perfect. It's about giving your body and mind the tools to feel safe again, and when you do, everything changes. Because when your body stops fighting itself, it finally gets to heal, and that's what this book is all about.

If you want to learn more about stress, listen to my episode of the *Finally Found* podcast with psychotherapist Anna Mathur, where we discuss stress we've personally experienced and ways of overcoming it. It's a great conversation and another reminder of how important managing stress is for a healthy, happy life.

5 Daily Quick Goals

- ✓ **Start your day with a protein-rich breakfast to keep blood sugar balanced and cortisol in check.**

- ✓ **Get outside in the morning for ten-plus minutes of natural light and gentle movement.**

- ✓ **Do one calming practice like NSDR (page 105), breathwork, or a short meditation—even a few minutes can have a big impact.**

- ✓ **Limit caffeine to one or two cups before midday, then swap to herbal teas such as chamomile or rooibos.**

- ✓ **Take one hour away from screens and messages and do something joyful or grounding—a walk, a bath, a chat, a stretch, or just silence—this will help take you out of any stressful work context, and ground you back into your life!**

Top 10 Things to Remember About Stress!

1. **Stress is not just a mental state**—it affects your whole body. Chronic stress can drive symptoms in every system, so it's something we should absolutely focus on reducing!

2. **Not all stress is bad.** Short bursts can be helpful, but long-term, low-grade stress keeps cortisol high and takes its toll on your body, lowering your stress resilience and weakening your immune system.

3. **Cortisol raises blood sugar** to give you a quick energy boost . . . useful if you're running from danger, not so much when you're just dealing with emails or traffic!

4. **Your body can react to everyday stress** in the same way it would to a life or death situation. Over time, this creates chronic inflammation.

5. **Stress and blood sugar are linked.** Cortisol spikes = sugar cravings, crashes, fatigue, and more inflammation.

6. **Stress can come from so many angles**—poor sleep, overexercising, processed foods, emotional strain, and even your own negative self-talk!

7. **Your nervous system needs support to regulate.** Breathwork, NSDR (page 105), morning walks, and gentle movement all help reset your stress response.

8. **You don't need to fix everything at once.** The goal is to reduce what's in your control and support your body to handle the rest better.

9. **Social connection is just as powerful as medicine.** Human touch, hugs, laughter, and quality time with loved ones releases oxytocin, which helps lower cortisol and, in turn, inflammation.

10. **You're not weak, broken, or dramatic if stress is affecting you.** It's biological, not personal. And once you learn how to manage it, your whole body starts to feel safer . . . and better.

Pillar 6: Movement

Movement: the misunderstood magic pill

When we think of movement or exercise, we often tend to picture aggressive HIIT classes, sweaty, painful running, flushed cheeks, lack of breath . . . and ultimately an unpleasant experience. At least that's what my immediate feelings were when someone told me that "movement" was important to my health.

I **HATED** all kinds of "movement" in that sense. Growing up, like many others I was launched into the realm of exercise by a humiliating "bleep" test at school, because apparently it was "healthy competition" to push us to our max. If you don't know what a bleep test is, count yourself lucky. It's essentially running lengths of an old school hall with loud bleeps that get faster and faster until eventually you don't make it to the other end before the bleep. At that point, you're eliminated. Anyway, my first bleep test was so beyond humiliating that I made the executive decision, at the age of twelve, that exercise was not, and would never be, for me. A decision I battled with every summer, as I tried to get a "bikini body" in two weeks, which of course never happened. I always **WISHED** I loved exercise purely for the sake of looking "better," which was probably why I never committed to it. It was a superficial goal that was only on my mind during the summer months, and considering everyone around me was usually complaining about their weight, too, I'd just decide that I was struggling, so was everyone else, and that it probably wasn't that important.

So the movement or exercise message back then was very simple: exercise = weight loss.

No one thought to tell us that exercise was **SO** much more than how we looked . . . that it could be one of the most powerful anti-inflammatory tools, that it could boost mood, support our hormones, protect our bones, and give us that injection of energy that overall would improve how we feel day-to-day. Not only that, but also the fact that this physical commitment could psychologically trigger other healthier habits, too, like prioritizing what we eat, because we all know by now that how we fuel ourselves determines how well we perform.

If someone had told me all of **THAT** . . . I might have started moving my body a lot sooner than I did. I only really committed to exercising in a positive way recently . . . and honestly, it's changed my life. So if you're sitting there thinking I **HATE** the gym, I'll never like running, and I just can't be bothered . . . I hear you, I was you, but I promise that everyone can love movement, it's just about finding the right routine that works for **YOU** . . . not the six-minute six-pack routine you found on YouTube that you swore you'd do every morning and then hated every minute of.

So hopefully we're all on the same page when it comes to movement being about so much more than your figure . . . it's about your future! But what does this mean? Should you be jumping into the gym seven days a week, running every morning, and buying a standing desk so you can multitask your meetings with a walking at-home treadmill?

No.

Just as with all the pillars, it all needs to balance, and too much exercise can cause inflammation, too. It's why a lot of people hit a wall when they're bloated, frustrated that they're putting all this effort into exercising loads—and yet feel worse than ever! I had this when I was following an aggressive weight-training plan four days a week, focusing only on adding weight each week (progressive overload, for you gym lovers), with absolutely **ZERO** consideration for my cycle. In my gut I knew that a session would go badly in the run-up to my period, because my energy would be lower and my body would feel weaker, but still I'd try and add more plates to the bar because that inspirational quote on Pinterest said, "Follow the plan, not your mood."

Well, although this is true in some instances, I'm here to tell you that the answer to your movement problems may be just that. You're following the plan rather than listening to what your body truly needs in that moment of time, because with fluctuating cycles, phases, and hormones—not one day is the same.

Too much exercise can cause as much harm as too little, especially if you're already dealing with inflammation, hormonal imbalances, or burnout. So in this pillar my goal is to help you reframe the way you think about movement. To show you what it actually does in your body, why it matters so much (especially for women), and how to find a rhythm that feels good throughout every stage of life, whether you're in your menstrual years, perimenopause, or beyond.

What is movement and why does it matter?

Movement doesn't have to mean crazy gym workouts; it just means moving your body. This could be any of the below—they all count:

- » Walking
- » Dancing
- » Cleaning
- » Gardening
- » Chasing after your kids
- » Yoga
- » Pilates
- » . . . and yes, going to the gym!

Of course, movement can change how we look, we all know that. But honestly? What it does underneath the surface is where the REAL magic happens!

Movement has the underrated power to completely shift how we feel, how we function, and how we show up in life. Just turn the page to look at what's going on inside your body every time you move.

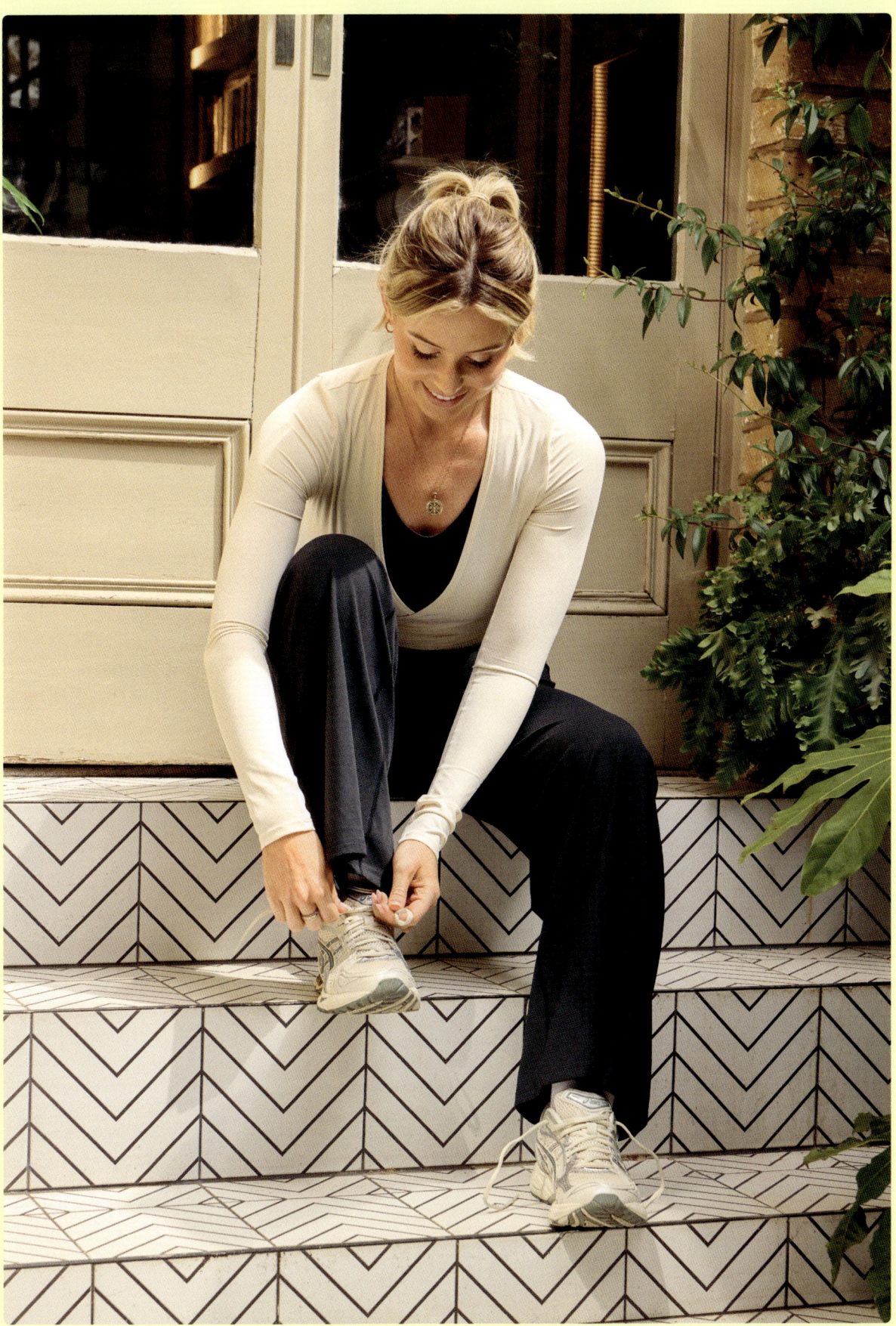

1. **Movement lowers inflammation markers.**[1]

    Regular exercise has been associated with reduced levels of anti-inflammatory markers (such as C-reactive protein and interlekin-6), meaning exercise can help reduce inflammation. But the key word in the study this came from is "regular"... meaning consistency is KEY. But don't worry, that will be you by the time you've finished working through this book.

2. **It supports your lymphatic drainage (natural detox!).**[2]

    Your lymphatic system is a central part of your immune system. Exercise helps get the lymph system going by promoting muscle contractions that help move the fluid around your lymph system, which, as you know from the Detoxification Pillar, helps clear toxins and reduce inflammation.

3. **Movement balances blood sugar (fewer crashes, cravings, and "hangry" episodes).**[3]

    Movement (in any form you like) helps improve insulin sensitivity and lower blood glucose levels, which will help balance blood sugars and keep those CEO hormones (cortisol and insulin) in check. Once again, you can see how balancing blood sugar isn't just managed by food... it's all the pillars working together!

4. **It boosts your mood with feel-good endorphins.**[4]

    Have you ever felt that "high" after doing exercise? That's because movement stimulates the release of endorphins (which are natural chemicals in the brain that help increase your mood). So not only does exercise improve your inflammatory markers, but it also makes you feel happier!

5. **Movement improves your sleep.**

    Once again, working on one aspect of health (in this instance exercise) helps another pillar, too. Exercise has been proven to improve quality of sleep and sleeping patterns,[5] which as you know has drastic effects on your health.

6. **It strengthens your bones and muscles.**[6]

    It's widely recognized that movement can strengthen muscles—after all, that's what we're doing it for, right? However, it blew my mind to learn that it also helps our bones! As we age, our bone density decreases. I think of it as the walls of our house getting weaker... so what do we do? Put scaffolding up and repair it! Muscle is like the scaffolding of a house; it helps support the structure and keep it strong. For those going through perimenopause and menopause, muscle (and building it) is even **MORE** important. This is also why I encourage everyone to exercise, no matter your age, because it will always help you in the present, and even more so in the future. To build muscle, resistance training is needed. This could be using body weight in Pilates, or picking up weights at home or in the gym. You don't need to aggressively lift twice your body weight—there are plenty of at-home workouts with moderate dumbbells that for just thirty minutes, three or four times a week, would make the world of difference!

7. **It supports metabolism and protects against age-related decline.**

   As we age, our metabolism naturally starts to slow down, and a big reason for that is the gradual loss of muscle mass, a process called sarcopenia. From around age thirty, we can lose up to 3–8% of our muscle mass per decade, and this loss speeds up significantly after the age of sixty.[7] Muscle is metabolically active tissue, which means it burns energy even at rest. So the more muscle you have, the more calories required to sustain it . . . which means more food (always a win in my eyes!). However, this also means if you have less muscle = lower metabolic rate = fewer calories burned.[8] This can then spiral into weight gain, fatigue, and generally feeling sluggish . . . sound familiar? If so, don't worry.

   Resistance training and regular physical activity will maintain muscle and BUILD it, too, even as we age. Strength training just a couple of times per week has been shown to increase muscle mass and help prevent metabolic decline.[9]

   So movement isn't just for weight loss. It helps reduce inflammation, revs up our metabolism, and helps us have a smoother transition through perimenopause and menopause. It can help regulate hormones, support energy, and protect against insulin resistance, weight gain, bone loss, and even mood swings.

Finding that sweet spot

I hope you're feeling excited about moving your body more and ready to reap all of these benefits. But first I do want to remind you that there is such a thing as overexercising as well as underexercising. For me, all the results came when I found the sweet spot in between.

As with everything else in this book, it all comes back to balance. We need movement for all the reasons I've covered here, but **MORE** doesn't always mean better! This is especially important if you're already dealing with inflammation, hormonal issues, or burnout.

Too little movement

You know that sluggish, "can't be bothered to do anything" feeling? It could be because you aren't moving enough. Lack of movement can lead to a sluggish lymphatic system (which means poor detoxification), reduced circulation, increased insulin resistance, higher levels of inflammation, and that "puffy" look we all think is excess fat but for many of us is just water weight! Over time, too little movement also impacts our mood and energy, which is why we can feel a bit flat, puffy, and low. This was something I used to struggle with all the time and would mistake for either mild depression, or just part and parcel of having endometriosis!

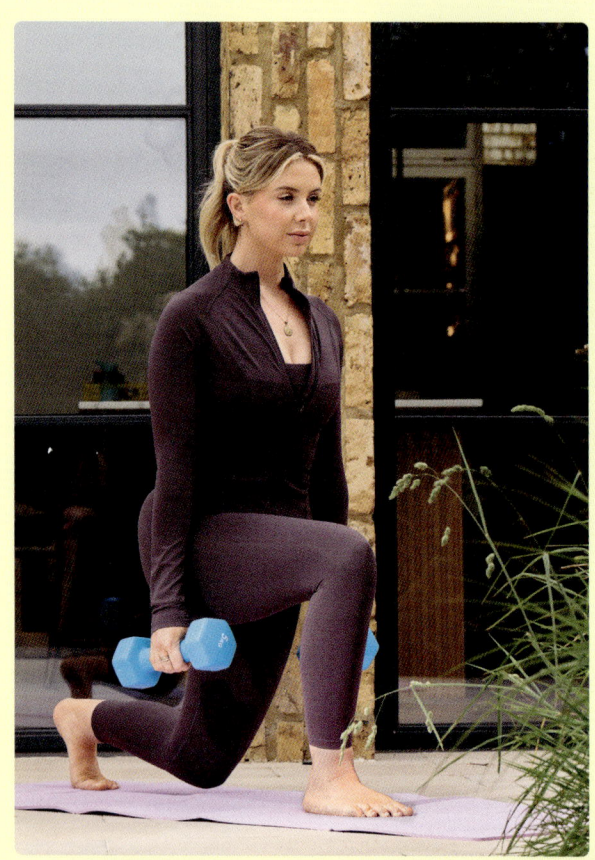
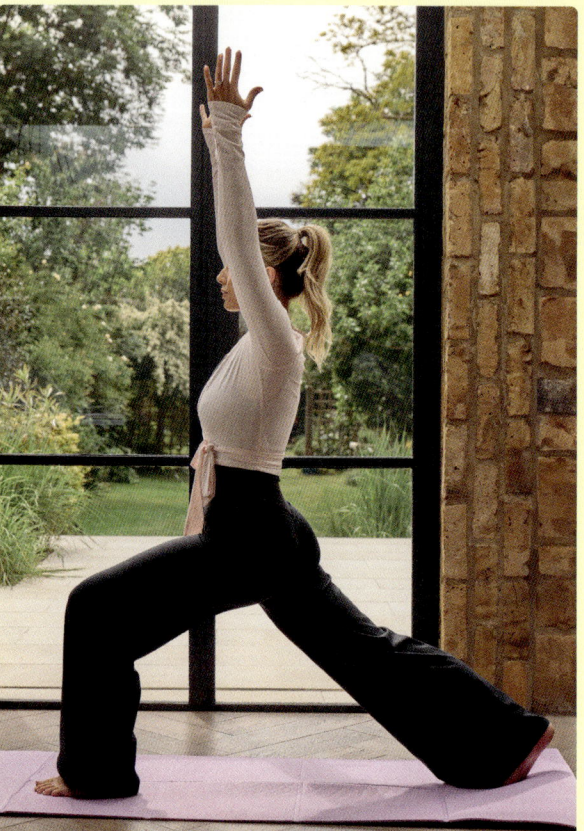

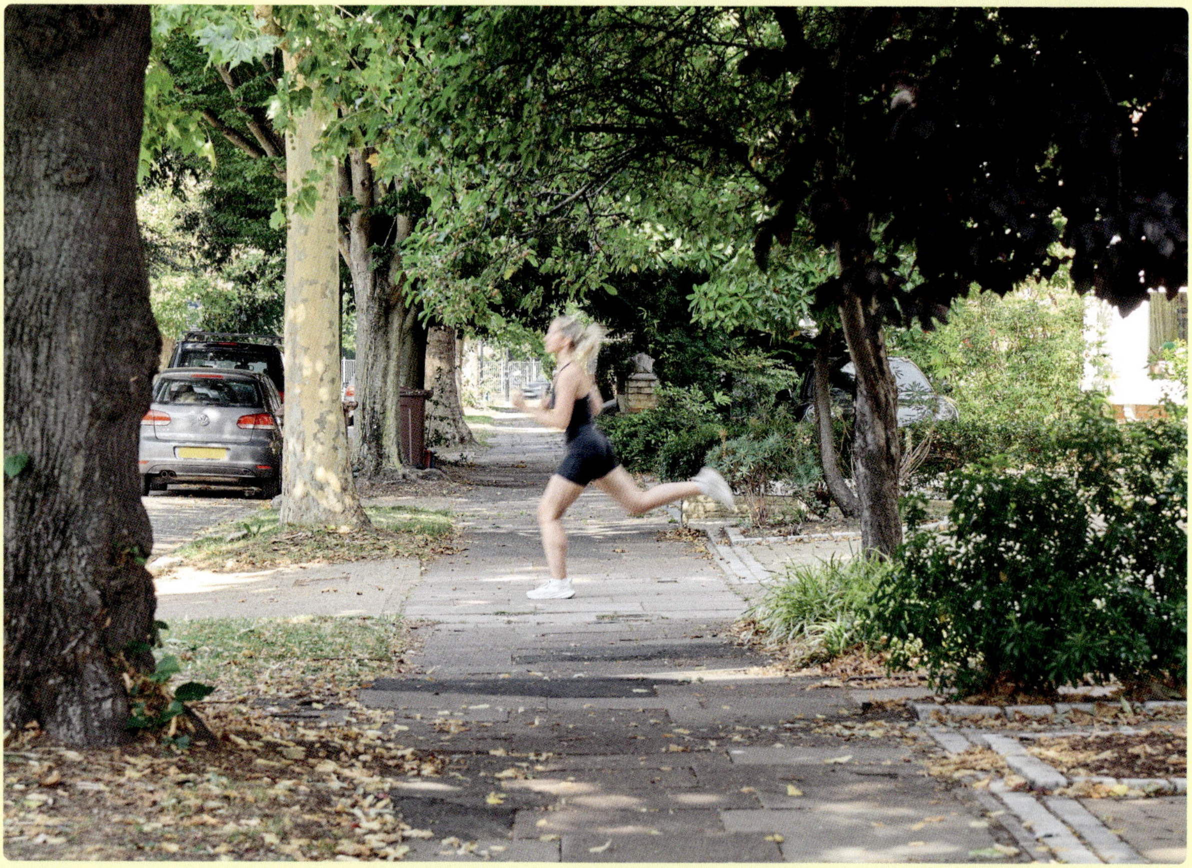

Too much movement

Instagram has glamorized overexercising, celebrating the latest workout craze, whether that's Crossfit, Hyrox, marathons. When I realized the impact of exercising, I went all in and started hammering HIIT workouts every day, with lots of heavy lifting and basically no recovery days. This level of stress on the body can spike your cortisol . . . and, well, you know the rest by now! Inflammation, bloating, weird cycles, and a rocky transition through perimenopause and menopause if it goes on for too long.

So if you've been going 100 miles an hour in the hopes of becoming healthier but are struggling with burnout as a result, OR you're on the other end of the spectrum, where you feel like you should be doing the gym seven days a week but because it's too much there's "no point," and you end up doing nothing at all . . . hopefully it comes as good news that the sweet spot in the middle is where we should all be aiming!

Movement and your cycle . . . sync, don't force

You might have heard the term "cycle syncing," which refers to living life in tune with our menstrual cycle. Earlier in this book, we covered the four phases and I outlined how you can use each phase to your advantage. This awareness of our cycle and pairing complementary tasks and activities is what we call cycle syncing. More and more women are cycle syncing their workouts now, too! I never used to believe in this, as there's limited evidence that it "actually" works. However, with the general lack of female-funded research, are we surprised that there's been little research in this area? No. However, I want to state that what I'm about to discuss is more anecdotal than data-driven. I have, however, spoken to hundreds of women who claim their life, health, and attitude toward exercising has completely transformed since syncing their workouts with their cycle, an experience I myself can personally attest to as well. Here's a quick guide:

» **Menstrual phase (your period):** This is traditionally your low energy time, as it corresponds to when your hormones are at their lowest. Focus on more restorative movements like gentle walks, stretching, or maybe yoga.

» **Follicular phase (after your period):** Hormones are rising, energy is building, and so this is a great time to try new workouts, strength training, or movement that feels a bit more adventurous.

» **Ovulation:** You'll likely feel your strongest and most energized if your cycle is working for you, as estrogen and testosterone (our more competitive hormones) are at their highest. A perfect time for more intense workouts, lifting heavier weights, or smashing a sweaty session.

» **Luteal phase (before your period):** This is when progesterone rises, which is your calming hormone, so you might feel more tired, bloated, or off (I know I do!). Focus on slow strength work, walking, yoga, and rest. Some movement is always good, especially during this phase, as progesterone can bring on constipation, and movement can quite literally help "move" things along.

There are a few things to be mindful of when cycle syncing. First, it's not a rule book, and becoming obsessive about where you are in your cycle defeats the purpose. If you're feeling full of energy and fancy a sprint session while on your period—go for it. However, if you are struggling with hormonal imbalances, inflammation, and stress, then accepting that you need slower periods of time may help you. Additionally, the ovulation phase is "supposed" to be our full of energy phase, but for people with endometriosis, PCOS, and cystic ovaries this can be a challenging time if your hormones are struggling or if you have PMDD (premenstrual dysphoric disorder) and are more sensitive to the rise of hormones.

I personally love cycle syncing and use it as a guide to help me decide whether I want to push more or rest at different points in my cycle. But I don't let it rule my life, and I don't feel I have to stick to certain workouts just because of where I am in my cycle. For example, I enjoy strength training throughout the whole month, but in my luteal phase and at the start of menstruation, I tend to use lighter weights because I know my body doesn't respond well to pushing hard in those phases. Everyone is different, and I encourage you to explore your own cycle, notice how you feel in each phase, and ultimately honor your body—whether that means pushing, resting, or finding a happy medium on that day. Of course, there are also times when a random flare-up will occur, and when that happens, I always listen to my body regardless of where I am in my cycle. I encourage you to do the same. It's about working with your body, not against it—and that's when you'll see the results you're looking for.

Also, I know a lot of people may be on contraception or have no cycle, in which case it's even more about listening to what your body needs, and honoring that. If you do have a cycle, there are apps you can use to keep track of it and identify each phase.

So that's cycle syncing, but what about life after your cycle?

Perimenopause, menopause, and movement

There's so much fear around transitioning through menopause, and confusion about whether you should or shouldn't be exercising, as it's a big change for your body. However, movement can be your superpower during this transition. As estrogen starts to drop, we become more vulnerable to things like bone loss, mood swings, weight gain, and insulin resistance. However, exercise (in particular, building muscle through resistance training) can help with all of that. So I encourage everyone, regardless of where you are in your life cycle, to embrace some movement, because it can be one of the best ways to support your hormones and your body.

Strength training + menopause

Strength training is not just helpful at this stage of your life, it's essential! Here are the reasons why:

» It supports bone health (reducing the risk of osteoporosis).
» It maintains muscle mass (which supports metabolism).

- » It improves insulin sensitivity (which helps balance hormones, cravings, and inflammation).
- » It boosts confidence, brain function, and mental clarity.

That said, recovery is just as important when going through perimenopause and menopause, so once again it comes back to finding the right balance. You might find you don't bounce back from high-intensity workouts like you used to, and that is absolutely not a weakness, it's just physiology. Less can be more during this phase, and slowly building yourself up week by week is a great way of slowly introducing yourself to a new way of living, where movement is part of your routine, not a chore, and a gradual habit change that stays with you for a lifetime. Walking, resistance training with bands or weights, bodyweight exercises, mobility, Pilates, or even a slow yoga flow: they all count as strength training. Remember that rest is also important, and so if some days you're not feeling it? That's okay! Consistency and balance are the way to win.

Building your anti-inflammatory movement routine

You don't need an expensive gym membership or a seven-day workout plan to get the benefits you're looking for. You just need to move in a way that supports your body consistently, intuitively, and in a way that you ENJOY!

Here's a really simple structure that I follow, in case you need some inspiration. However, I encourage you **RIGHT NOW** to make a list of the type of movement you've enjoyed in the past, and start integrating that into your day where it fits best.

- » **Daily walks**—Aim for twenty to thirty minutes a day, ideally in the morning, because you're also ticking that box for a happy circadian rhythm while also helping with kickstarting your lymphatic drainage. Ideally you'd be getting a nice long forty-five-minute walk in, but remember this is about lifelong changes, so start small and build up!
- » **Strength training two or three times a week**—This can be bodyweight, resistance bands, or dumbbells. Explore what you enjoy, whether that's at-home workouts or at the gym.
- » **Mobility or stretching**—If you don't feel like working out, even a few minutes of this a day will keep your joints happy and support your circulation. Remember, something is better than nothing.
- » **Something joyful**—Dancing in your kitchen, gardening, playing with your dog, doing a YouTube Pilates class. If it makes you smile, it counts! I go through phases of quitting the gym and doing completely at-home workouts inspired by @zoeantonio on Instagram, and her results speak for themselves.
- » **Rest days**—Essential. This is when your body actually heals and gets stronger. There's no point pushing yourself to the breaking point— it gets you nowhere and does more harm than good.

Conclusion

Movement is one of the most powerful tools we have to reduce inflammation, support our hormones, clear our minds, and reconnect with ourselves. It's a privilege, **NOT** a punishment, and helps with inflammation directly AND indirectly through helping to strengthen all the other pillars, too. Movement truly is a gift, and once you stop seeing it as something you have to do, and start seeing it as something you **GET** to do, that helps you feel your best. It gets a whole lot easier to keep showing up for yourself and to find the anti-inflammatory benefits you've been searching for!

If you'd like more guidance on how to move your body, whether that's Pilates, weight training, or a mix of both, I've created a fitness guide to help you through it step by step. It's designed to give you structure and confidence and to find a routine that actually works for your body. It can be found via my Instagram **@sophie.richards** and **@found.womenshealth**.

5 Daily Quick Goals

- ✓ **Walk for twenty to thirty minutes a day** (ideally in the morning to support circadian rhythm at the same time!). Or even after a meal can be helpful to support blood sugar regulation.

- ✓ **Strength train two or three times a week**, using body weight, resistance bands, or dumbbells.

- ✓ **Move in a way you ENJOY!** Dance, garden, play with pets or kids, do a class you love—whatever gets you moving in a way you enjoy, do it!

- ✓ **Honor your energy**—rest when you need it and don't push through exhaustion. This journey is about helping and healing, not pushing through pain and giving up because it's not sustainable. Consistent, enjoyable movement is key.

- ✓ **Cycle sync your workouts** if you feel this helps. It can be a great way to ensure you're varying your workouts, while honoring where your hormones and energy levels are at, too!

Top 10 Things to Remember About Movement!

1. **Movement isn't just about fitness or weight loss,** it's one of the most powerful anti-inflammatory tools we have, so it's not optional, it's ESSENTIAL!

2. **Your body was designed to move daily.** Walking, stretching, cleaning, dancing... it all counts, but it doesn't need to be a stressful gym environment—just move in a way that feels good, and resistance is key!

3. **Overexercising can be just as harmful as not moving at all.** More is not always better.

4. **Strength training isn't just for aesthetics**—it supports your bones, hormones, metabolism, and mood.

5. **Movement supports your lymphatic system,** helps your body detox, and keeps inflammation in check.

6. **You don't need to train hard every day.** Consistency beats intensity when it comes to results.

7. **Cycle syncing your workouts** can help support your hormones and energy. Rest days are not lazy, they're essential.

8. **Walking is underrated!** Daily walks are powerful for hormone health, weight management, and stress.

9. **Moving your body helps balance blood sugar,** reduce cravings, and regulate your mood.

10. **You may not love all your workouts,** but they're essential to supporting your health. With time, you can find ways of moving that work for you, that you look forward to, and that make you feel good.

Your 30-Day Reset Plan

Before we start, let's check in

It's time to put everything you've learned into action. Before you embark on this reset, I'd like you to check in on yourself using the below questions to see where you're currently at. Your answers are a helpful indicator not only of how you're feeling now, so that you can compare afterward, but also of which plan level is best for you.

After you've completed your 30-day reset, please revisit this check-in. Thirty days is the minimum amount of time needed to start seeing real benefits, and one of the most rewarding parts of the reset is reflecting on the progress you've made. I think you'll be pleasantly surprised by how differently you answer these questions afterward.

1. **How energized do you feel when you wake up in the morning?**
   (1 = Exhausted and groggy, 10 = Refreshed and full of energy)

   •-----•-----•-----•-----•-----•-----•-----•-----•-----•

2. **How steady is your energy throughout the day?**
   (1 = I crash constantly, 10 = I feel stable and strong)

   •-----•-----•-----•-----•-----•-----•-----•-----•-----•

3. **How well are you sleeping at night?**
   (1 = Tossing and turning, 10 = Deep and restful)

   •-----•-----•-----•-----•-----•-----•-----•-----•-----•

4. **How balanced do your moods feel day-to-day?**
   (1 = All over the place, 10 = Emotionally stable and calm)

   •-----•-----•-----•-----•-----•-----•-----•-----•-----•

5. **How often are you bloated or experiencing digestive discomfort?**
   (1 = Every day, 10 = Rarely or never)

   •-----•-----•-----•-----•-----•-----•-----•-----•-----•

6. **How would you rate your skin right now?**
   (1 = Breakouts, dryness, irritation, 10 = Clear and glowing)

   •-----•-----•-----•-----•-----•-----•-----•-----•-----•

7. **How sharp and focused do you feel mentally?**
   (1 = Foggy and distracted, 10 = Clear and productive)

   •-----•-----•-----•-----•-----•-----•-----•-----•-----•

8. **How connected do you feel to your body and cycle?**
   (1 = No clue what's going on, 10 = Totally in sync)

   •-----•-----•-----•-----•-----•-----•-----•-----•-----•

9. **How much joy and ease do you feel in your daily routine?**
   (1 = Chaos and overwhelm, 10 = Calm, grounded, and happy)

   •-----•-----•-----•-----•-----•-----•-----•-----•-----•

10. **How confident do you feel that your current habits support your health, e.g., food you're eating, movement, stress levels, etc.?**
    (1 = Not at all, 10 = 100% aligned)

    •-----•-----•-----•-----•-----•-----•-----•-----•-----•

Ready to reset? LET'S GO!

Making real change comes down to two things: first, having the right knowledge, and second, putting it into action.

You've already nailed the first step—you've read about my journey and seen how I've improved my health even from the trenches of inflammation; you've learned how inflammation works, the vital role hormones play, and the six pillars of health that can transform your body and mind. Now it's time for step two: taking action. No matter where you are in your journey—whether you're just starting out or have already made progress—a 30-day reset can give you the structure and momentum to create real, lasting change. This is your chance to put everything into practice and feel the difference for yourself.

Your 30-day reset is where your life can really shift. One meaningful check box at a time, making better and more informed choices day by day . . . and finally fulfilling your promise to yourself, that this time you're going to show up for **YOU**!

This isn't to say you haven't been trying. Far from it—I'm sure you have. Before I started my anti-inflammatory journey, I had been taking action for two years . . . just in all the wrong places. If I'd had the information in this book all those years ago, I would have been living my best life **SO MUCH SOONER!** However, I hope that reading about my journey will help you direct your efforts in a way that creates real change.

So, here's the reset you've been looking for! With small, powerful habits that transform your mind and body, the next thirty days can change everything. Why? Because you're not just following a plan. You're learning how to honor your body, support your hormones, calm inflammation, and boost energy in a way that finally lasts.

Something we often overlook is that it's not just the steps we take or the habits we change, but it's all down to our beliefs, too. Research shows that belief and intention activate the same pathways in the brain as action. That means every time you visualize success, every time you remind yourself why this matters, you make it easier to stick with. Your brain is listening, so speak to it with purpose!

You don't need permission . . . you don't need perfection . . . you just need to START!

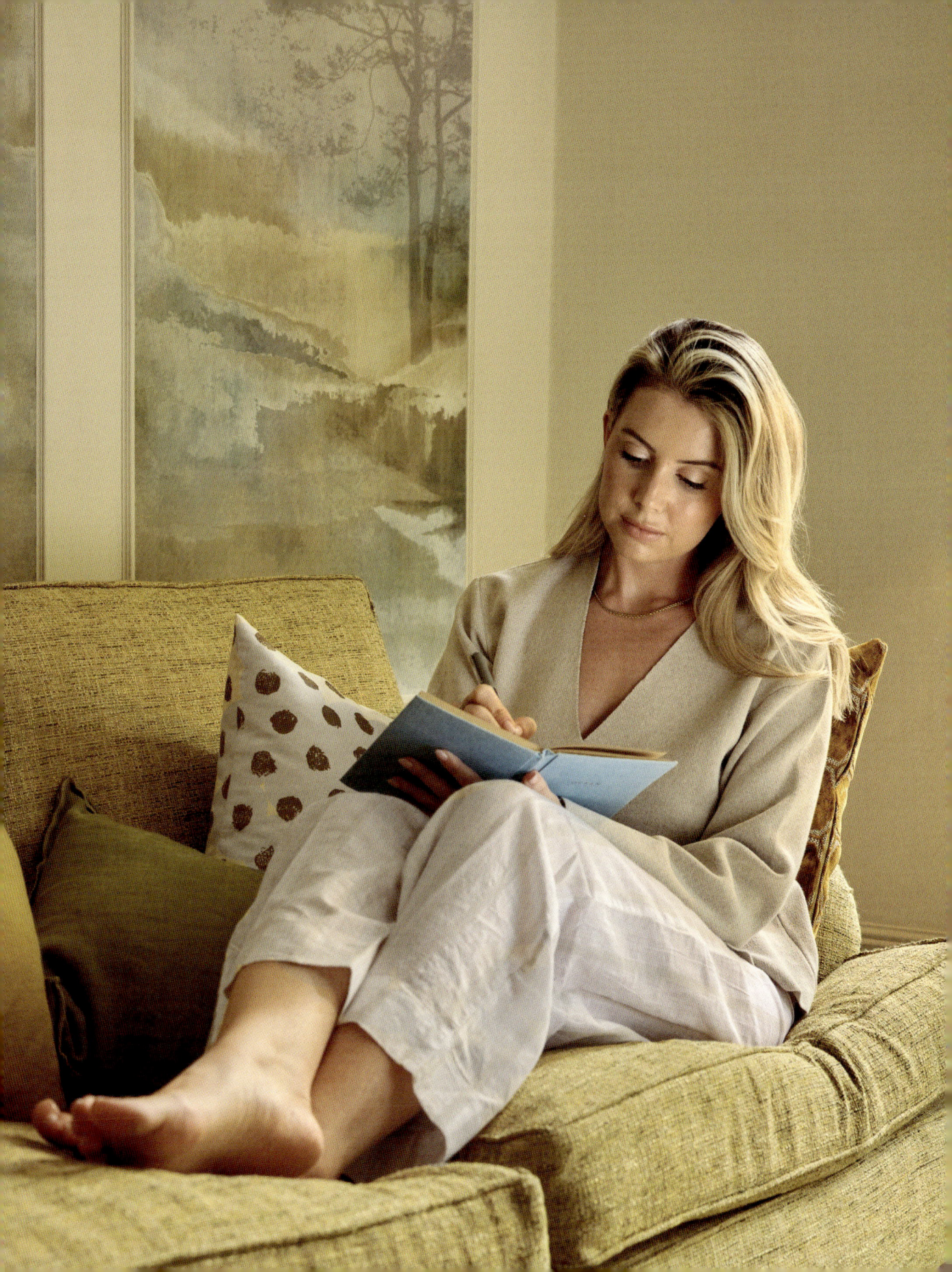

Your Reset Promise

For the best chance of success with your reset, make sure to complete the steps below. There are multiple studies to support the fact that finding the deeper meaning behind your goals, and the act of writing them down, will give you a greater chance of achieving them. It will also help ingrain the principles more deeply into your memory, so that you're reminded daily of the healthy habits you're committing to.

Step 1: What's your WHY? Write it down!

Why are you doing this reset? What aspects of your life do you hope to change? Is it to have more energy? Better digestion? Balanced hormones? Clearer skin? Really think about WHY you're doing this. Then write it down.

E.g., because I want to feel full of energy, have stable moods, suffer from less bloating, and finally start living the life I was meant to live!

_____

_____

Step 2: The commitment

The next step is to commit yourself. Creating a a simple self-contract is a powerful way to do this—when you put your commitment in writing, you're far more likely to follow through and stay accountable. Use the template below, or adapt it to create your own.

I, _____, **am committing to myself for the next 30 days.**

Over the next thirty days, I will:

- » Nourish my body with food that supports healing
- » Move in ways that feels good and energizing
- » Honor my need for rest, recovery, and calm
- » Tune into my body's signals—not ignore them
- » Gently shift habits that no longer serve me
- » And prove to myself what's possible when I put myself first

Because I deserve to feel good. Because the life I want starts with the choices I make today. Because showing up for myself is the most powerful act of self-respect.

This is my commitment to the 30-day reset, and a life of feeling good in my body.

Signed: _____

Date: _____

Accountability tools to keep you going

> » *Morning affirmation (printed or written on a Post-it note) displayed somewhere you'll see it every day e.g., "I make choices aligned with my healthiest self."*
> » *Journal entry each day to remind yourself why you're doing the reset, what you're proud of, and your goals.*
> » *Check off your five daily habits, e.g., write them on your fridge, in your bedroom, or bathroom ... wherever you'll see it!*
> » *Set phone alarms to remind you of key habits (e.g., "Protein breakfast," "Evening wind down")*
> » *Tell someone close to you what you're doing, both for accountability, but also as a check-in.*
> » *Post about your journey and tag* **#30DAYRESET** *to find others in the community who are doing the same.*

Pick your plan!

On the next page, there are three structured resets for you to pick from, each designed to meet you where you're at in your anti-inflammatory journey. Only you can decide which reset is appropriate for you. Think about your answers to the check-in questions, read through all three reset plans, and see which level of commitment you feel able to give over the next thirty days.

It should **NOT** feel like an impossible "challenge" that you dread daily. That is exactly what we want to avoid. The reset is for your health and your journey alone, so pick the plan that feels achievable, motivating, and will get you closer to your end goal. If you're unsure, you could opt for the Gentle Reset first and later move upward ... or customize a reset plan of your own from all the tips you can find at the end of each pillar.

The reset framework

Each plan is built on six simple foundations that help lower inflammation by supporting your hormones and overall well-being:

1. **Morning daylight**— sets your body clock, boosts mood and energy.
2. **Lymphatic drainage**—supports detoxification and reduces bloating.
3. **Food**—balances blood sugar and lowers inflammation.
4. **Mindful moment**—calms the nervous system and lowers stress.
5. **Movement**—improves circulation, hormone balance, and lowers inflammation.
6. **Sleep**—restores the body, supports repair, and reduces stress hormones.

The Gentle Reset

A soft launch that works to remove key triggers, add nourishment, and help you build consistency without overwhelm. This path is for you if...

- » You're feeling burnt out, anxious, or new to anti-inflammatory living.
- » You want to ease in slowly and gently.
- » This is the first time you've considered changing your lifestyle.

1. Morning daylight

10 minutes each morning, even just standing outside with a cup of tea. If you can add a short walk, even better.
Why it helps: regulates circadian rhythm and boosts morning energy.

2. Lymphatic drainage

2 minutes of rebounding (jumping up and down on the spot) or dry-brushing in the morning.
Why it helps: kick-starts drainage and helps reduce fluid retention.

3. Food

Eat a whole-food breakfast with protein and fiber (try my recipes). Avoid ultra-processed foods at this meal.
Why it helps: balances blood sugar and supports digestion.

4. Mindful moment

5–10 minutes daily, e.g., journaling, breathwork, meditation, or NSDR (see page 105).
Why it helps: shifts the body from "fight-or-flight" toward "rest and digest."

5. Movement

20–30 minutes daily, e.g., walking, light yoga, Pilates, or simple weights.
Why it helps: aids circulation, digestion, and muscle support.

6. Sleep

No screens for at least 15 minutes before bed and lights out at the same time each night.
Why it helps: encourages deep, restorative sleep cycles and resets circadian rhythm.

Reset Plan 1

The Core Reset

A balanced, flexible approach that's realistic, effective, and designed to reduce inflammation, without being too intense. This path is for you if...

- » You're ready for change but want flexibility.
- » You want to feel results without it feeling overwhelming.
- » You've got some momentum and want to build on it.

1. Morning daylight

20–30 minutes, ideally combined with a walk to support digestion.
Why it helps: regulates circadian rhythm and boosts morning energy.

2. Lymphatic drainage

Full six-step lymphatic massage routine (page 90), plus 2 minutes of rebounding.
Why it helps: kick-starts drainage and helps reduce fluid retention.

3. Food

Breakfast and lunch to focus on whole foods, protein, and fiber (use my recipes!). Limit ultra-processed foods for the rest of the day where possible.
Why it helps: balances blood sugar and supports digestion.

4. Mindful moment

10–15 minutes daily, e.g., journaling, breathwork, guided meditation, or NSDR (see page 105).
Why it helps: shifts the body from "fight-or-flight" toward "rest and digest."

5. Movement

30–45 minutes daily, with at least two strength-based sessions each week. E.g., brisk walk, yoga, Pilates, at-home bodyweight session, or gym workout.
Why it helps: aids circulation, digestion, and muscle support.

6. Sleep

30 minutes of screen-free wind-down with a consistent bedtime.
Why it helps: encourages deep, restorative sleep cycles and resets circadian rhythm.

Reset Plan 2

The All-In Reset

A powerful, energizing, intentional approach that aligns with how the body functions best. While it may feel like a bigger shift than the other reset plans, this is the lifestyle many of us thrive on when we give it a chance. This path is for you if . . .

- » You've done resets before and are ready to level up.
- » You've tried building habits before but you're now ready to commit to a lifestyle change because you know WHY these habits will help you.
- » You're the kind of person who gets the best results when they go "all in."

1. Morning daylight

30–45 minutes every morning, always combined with a walk.
Why it helps: regulates circadian rhythm and boosts morning energy.

2. Lymphatic drainage

Full six-step lymphatic massage routine (page 90), plus 2 minutes of rebounding.
Why it helps: kick-starts drainage and helps reduce fluid retention.

3. Food

All meals and snacks focused on whole foods, protein, and fiber, every day (use my recipes!). Limit ultra-processed foods as much as possible.
Why it helps: balances blood sugar and supports digestion.

4. Mindful moment

10–20 minutes daily, e.g., journaling, breathwork, guided meditation, or NSDR (see page 105). All at once or 5–10 minutes in the morning and the evening.
Why it helps: shifts the body from "fight-or-flight" toward "rest and digest."

5. Movement

45 minutes daily, with at least three strength-based sessions weekly. Can be brisk walking, Pilates, gym, or yoga, as long as resistance training is included.
Why it helps: aids circulation, digestion, and muscle support.

6. Sleep

1-hour screen-free digital detox before bed. Lights out at the same time each night.
Why it helps: encourages deep, restorative sleep cycles and resets circadian rhythm.

Reset Plan 3

After the thirty days

First, congratulate yourself: you did it! Whichever plan you followed, you should be so proud. You've taken the most important step on any health journey, which is to **START**!

The next step is to review the check-in questions. How do you feel now compared to beforehand—physically, mentally, emotionally? Did you see any shifts (big or small)? Use your answers to guide what you do next. If you started with the Gentle Reset, but want stronger results, you could now try the Core or All-In Reset. If you went All-In and found it too hard, scale back and try a gentler one. Ultimately, it's about finding a rhythm you enjoy, that's sustainable, and makes you feel like **YOU** again. There's no right or wrong, there's just your journey, your body and what feels best for you.

For me? I went All-In, and over time the habits and lifestyle changes became my new norm. Occasionally I do have situations where avoiding UPFs entirely is impossible, usually while traveling or at social occasions. But I prep the best I can and trust that my body is now so strong that some deviation won't cause issues.

These resets are here to help you build habits you can stick to. Whichever level you choose, my only ask is that you commit to it for 30 days to see how good you can feel. The plans aren't restrictive—they're designed with flexibility because it is about creating a lifestyle change, about committing to yourself, and adopting the 80/20 framework. When you show up for yourself consistently (rather than perfectly!) that's when you'll see your energy return, your balance restored, and a freedom to actually enjoy life again.

So, if long-term health is what you're looking for, the reset habits should remain a part of life as much as possible, and as such this doesn't "end" like most fad diets or challenges do. This isn't thirty days, done and dusted—it is just the start of a lifetime of feeling healthier every day. It's not about perfection, but about learning what tools help you thrive. Adapt until you find the right fit; this is your journey!

As for the recipes? I hope they will become lifelong staples. Keep this book on your kitchen counter as a reminder of how good healthy can taste!

This may be the end of your "reset," but it's the start of something even better: your new normal of feeling better every single day.

Note: The following recipes were developed, tested, and originally written using metric measures (including grams, milliliters, and centimeters, with teaspoons and tablespoons, tested at Celsius cooking temperatures). All nutritional information was calculated from the metric measures provided. The imperial measures offered are an approximated equivalent.

Brea

kfast

This is a perfect hearty brunch idea, a little twist on the traditional cooked breakfast. To speed up the process, you can use cooked potatoes left over from the night before. This dish uses bacon and gluten-free sausages, but you can add your own protein choice. It also works really well with fish, gammon (pork), or even marinated tofu if you want to be more plant-based.

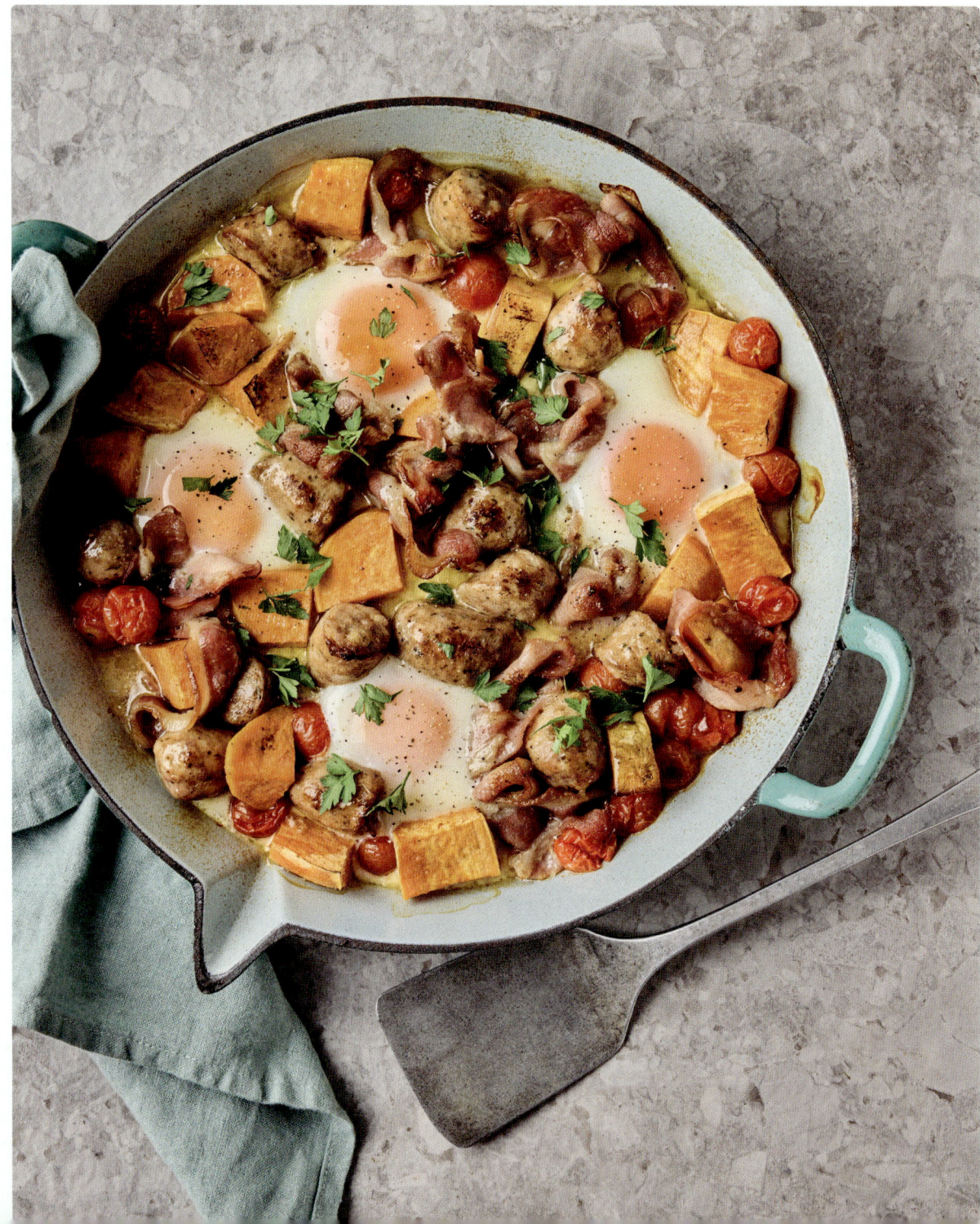

One-Pot Brunch

SERVES 2 ○ HIGH PROTEIN

INGREDIENTS

- 1 sweet potato (175g), peeled and diced
- 1 tbsp olive oil
- 6 strips of nitrate-free thick back bacon, cut into large strips
- 4 nitrate-free, gluten-free, good-quality sausages, cut into ¾-inch pieces
- ⅔ cup/100g cherry tomatoes
- sea salt and freshly ground black pepper, to taste
- 4 eggs

To garnish
chopped flat-leaf parsley

Preheat the oven to 400°F (fan).

Place the sweet potato on a baking sheet and drizzle with olive oil. Add the bacon, sausages, and cherry tomatoes and mix to make sure they are evenly covered in oil. Season to taste.

Bake for 20 minutes, then remove from the oven. Make 4 small areas for adding your eggs, and crack the eggs into the dish. Put back into the oven for 8–10 minutes, until the egg whites are firm, but the yolks are still soft.

Serve immediately. Garnish with parsley and more black pepper.

NUTRITIONAL INFORMATION *(Per Serving)*

Calories 725Kcals ○ Net carbohydrates 21.5g ○ Fiber 3.2g ○ Fat 51.7g ○ Protein 58g

Ultimate Omega Breakfast Toast

SERVES 1 ◦ RICH IN OMEGA-3, HIGH PROTEIN, GRAIN-FREE

INGREDIENTS

2 slices of my Grain-Free Seeded Bread (page 258)
1 small avocado, halved and roughly mashed
sea salt and freshly ground black pepper, to taste
one 4.23oz/120g can of sardines, drained
a squeeze of lemon juice
a sprinkle of chile flakes

Toast the seeded bread lightly.

While this is toasting, mash the avocado and season to taste.

Top the toast generously with the mashed avocado, then add the sardines.

Finish with a squeeze of lemon and a sprinkle of chile flakes. Enjoy!

SERVING OPTIONS

I serve the sardines cold, as they are already cooked, but if you want to warm them through, you can do so very lightly in a pan—be careful, though, as they can be quite delicate. You can also place the can of sardines (unopened), in a bowl of boiling water to warm them through for a few minutes.

You can top the toast with smoked mackerel, canned tuna, or salmon.

For added protein, serve with a poached egg on top.

NUTRITIONAL INFORMATION *(Per Serving)*

Calories 895Kcals ◦ Net carbohydrates 6g ◦ Fiber 17.5g ◦ Fat 82.5g ◦ Protein 46.5g

Omega-3 is your anti-inflammatory best friend, so this simple, quick, and easy breakfast is the perfect way to start your day. It's an incredible blend of nutrients and can double up as a snack on the go.

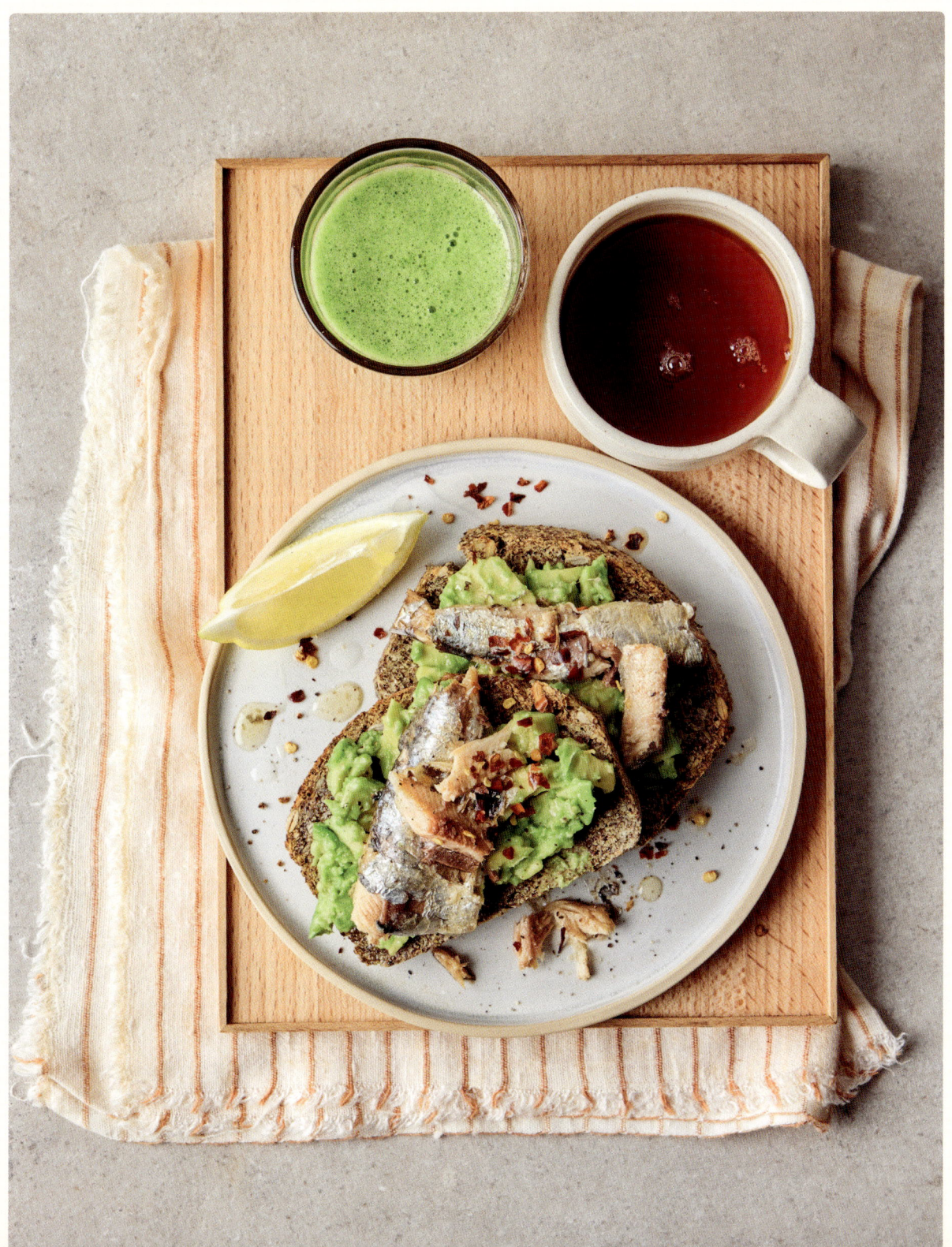

Who doesn't love a shakshuka? It's a classic Middle Eastern dish of poached eggs in a rich spiced tomato and pepper sauce that's full of flavor. High in protein, fiber, and healthy fats, this meal is both delicious and perfectly balanced. It'll keep you full for longer, so it's the ideal breakfast dish—and don't get put off by the preparation time! You can prep ahead by doubling up the base and storing it in the fridge (or freezer) for when you need it— it takes minutes to reheat and just add your eggs for a speedy breakfast.

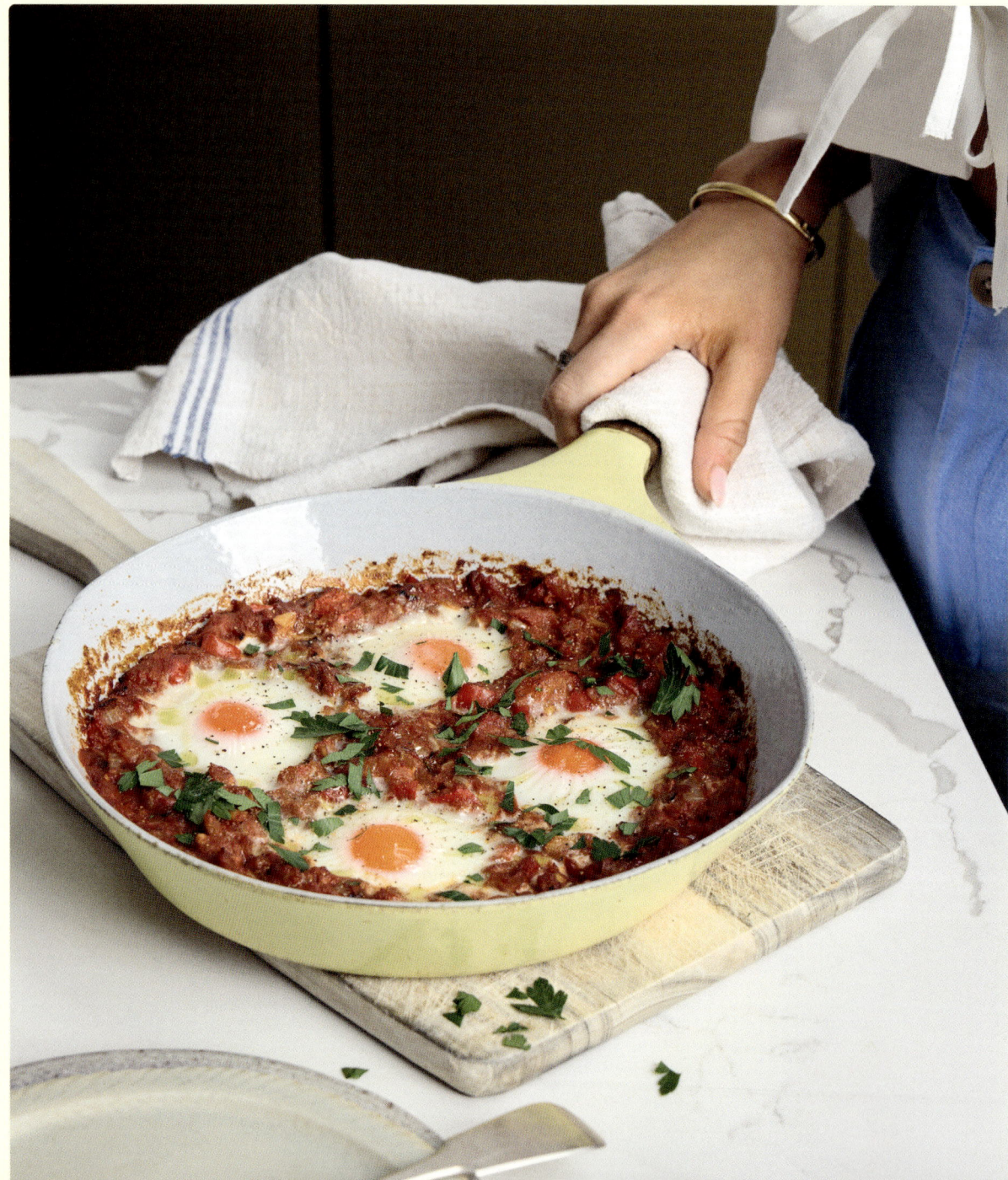

Classic Shakshuka

SERVES 2   ○   VEGETARIAN, HIGH PROTEIN

INGREDIENTS

- 1 tbsp olive oil
- 1 small onion, finely chopped
- 1 red pepper, diced
- 2 cloves of garlic, minced
- 1 tsp ground cumin
- 1 tsp smoked paprika
- ½ tsp ground coriander
- ½ tsp chile flakes
- One 14oz/400g can of chopped tomatoes
- 2 tbsp tomato purée
- sea salt and freshly ground black pepper, to taste
- 4 medium eggs

To garnish
cilantro or flat-leaf parsley, finely chopped

Heat the olive oil in a large frying pan over a medium heat.

Add the onion and red pepper, and sauté for 5 minutes until softened.

Stir in the garlic, cumin, paprika, coriander, and chile flakes, and cook for another minute until fragrant.

Add the chopped tomatoes and tomato purée, and season with salt and black pepper. Let the sauce simmer for 10–15 minutes, stirring occasionally, until it thickens.

Make small wells in the sauce and gently crack in the eggs. Cover the pan and cook for 5–7 minutes, or until the egg whites are set but the yolks remain runny.

Sprinkle with cilantro or parsley before serving, and enjoy hot!

TOP TIPS

Double the base recipe and store in the fridge or freezer, ready to make this delicious breakfast whenever you like. Heat gently before adding the eggs.

PROTEIN BOOSTERS

Increasing the eggs per serving from 2 to 3 will add 7g of protein.

1 tbsp of hemp seeds sprinkled on each serving will add 3g of protein.

1¾ oz/50g of smoked salmon per serving will add 11g of protein.

3 strips of nitrate-free bacon per serving will add 17g of protein.

2⅓ oz/65g of smoked mackerel per serving will add 13g of protein.

2⅔ oz/75g of organic tempeh per serving will add 16.5g of protein.

2⅔ oz/75g of smoked tofu per serving will add 12g of protein.

SERVING OPTIONS

For added fiber, stir in a generous handful of baby-leaf spinach a couple of minutes before adding the eggs.

NUTRITIONAL INFORMATION *(Per Serving)*

Calories 284Kcals   ○   Net carbohydrates 17.2g   ○   Fiber 4.9g   ○   Fat 16.8g   ○   Protein 17.1g

Baked Apple, Cinnamon & Pecan Oats

SERVES 2   ○   HIGH PROTEIN, FAMILY-FRIENDLY, VEGETARIAN

INGREDIENTS

- ½ cup/45g gluten-free porridge oats
- 1 heaped tsp baking powder
- 1 tsp ground cinnamon
- 1 tbsp honey or maple syrup, or to taste
- 2 medium eggs
- 1 tsp vanilla extract
- 2 tbsp plant-based yogurt
- a pinch of sea salt
- ½ an apple, cored and finely chopped
- 2 tbsp/20g chopped pecans

Preheat the oven to 350°F (fan). Grease a small ovenproof dish.

Place the oats in a bowl, and add the baking powder and cinnamon.

In a jug, mix the honey, eggs, vanilla, and yogurt. Add a pinch of sea salt to enhance the flavors.

Pour the egg mixture over the oats. Add the chopped apple and pecans and combine well.

Transfer to your ovenproof dish and bake for 15–20 minutes, until golden, and the top springs back when pressed.

Serve immediately, or enjoy cold from the fridge for a grab-and-go option.

TOP TIPS

Can be stored in the fridge for 3–4 days, or can be frozen for up to 2 months. Simply reheat in the oven at 300°F for 10 minutes.

For a smoother, muffin-like texture, blend the oats before mixing.

FLAVOR VARIATIONS

Chocolate, Banana & Hazelnut
Swap the apple and pecans for 1 small mashed banana and 2 tbsp/15g of chopped hazelnuts. Add 1 tbsp of cocoa powder to the dry mix and a few dark chocolate chips.

Lemon & Blueberry
Omit the apple and cinnamon. Add the zest of 1 lemon, the juice of ½ a lemon, and ½ cup/80g of blueberries.

Coconut, Raspberry & Vanilla
Omit the pecans and cinnamon. Replace the apple with 1 tbsp of desiccated coconut and ½ cup/80g of raspberries. Keep the vanilla and honey/maple the same.

NUTRITIONAL INFORMATION *(Per Serving)*

Calories 227Kcals   ○   Net carbohydrates 29g   ○   Fiber 3.8g   ○   Fat 10.1g   ○   Protein 5.4g

This cozy baked oats recipe is my go-to quick and easy breakfast that's also simple to make in batches for busy mornings. The cinnamon adds a little spice and also helps with balancing blood sugar! It's full of protein and fiber, and the combo of apple, cinnamon, and toasted pecans gives it an "apple pie" vibe that's full of goodness. Enjoy it as a slice of cake, an on-the-go breakfast, or a mid-morning snack!

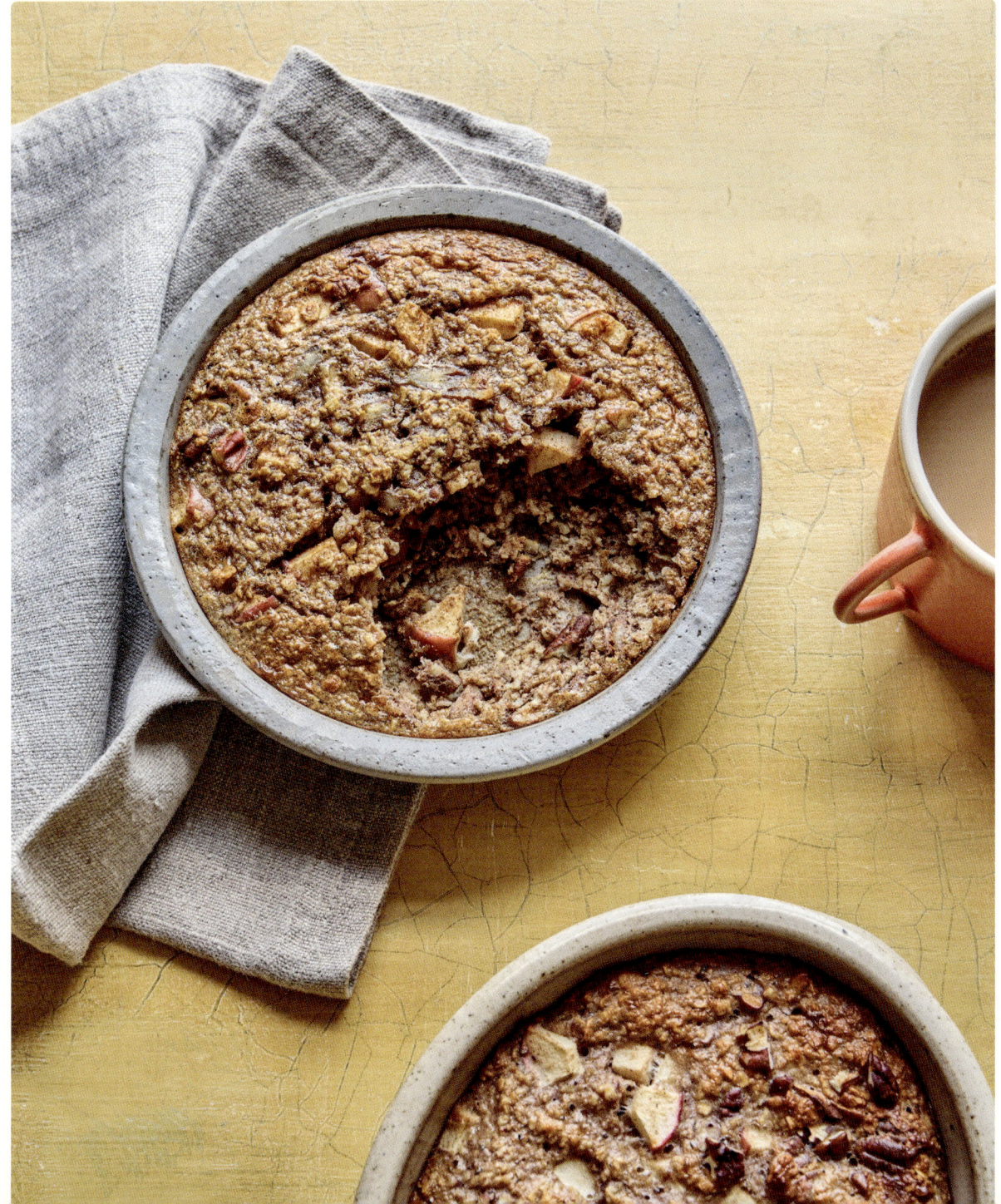

These make a perfect, light start to your day but also give you a healthy balance of protein and fats to keep your blood sugar in check. The spiralized zucchini act as a base, making the nest for your eggs, which will cook perfectly in the oven. If you're feeling hungry, or want an extra hit of protein, add smoked salmon, nitrate-free bacon, or tempeh. I love adding some avocado for extra fats.

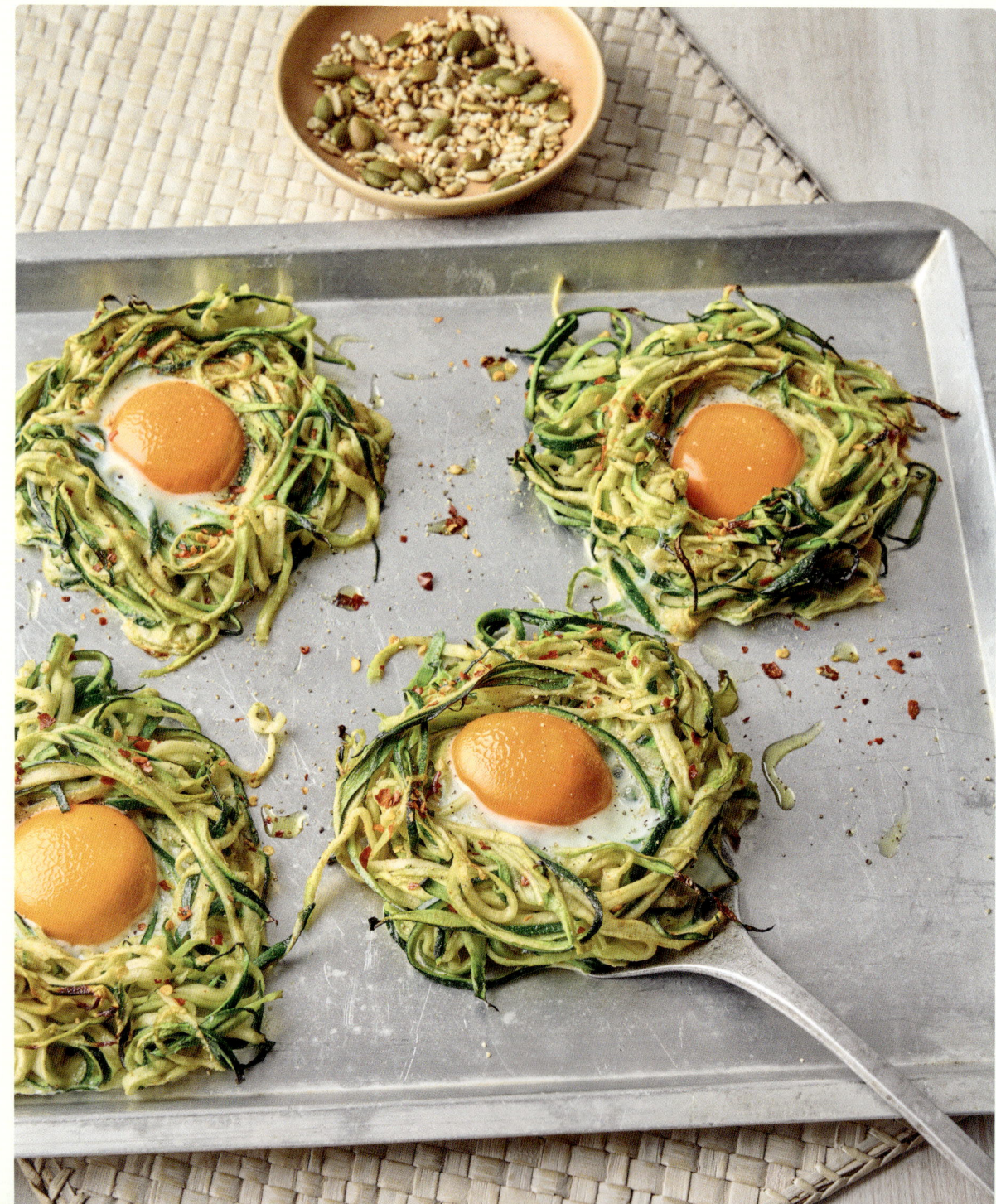

Breakfast Nests

SERVES 2 ○ PERFECTLY BALANCED, VEGETARIAN, GRAIN-FREE

INGREDIENTS

- 3 zucchini
- 1 tsp sea salt
- 1 tsp olive oil
- a pinch of chile flakes
- ½ tsp smoked paprika
- 4 eggs
- freshly ground black pepper, to taste
- 1 tsp toasted mixed seeds

Preheat your oven to 350°F (fan) and line a baking sheet with parchment paper.

Spiralize the zucchini or ribbon them using a julienne peeler. Sprinkle with the salt and allow to sit in a colander for 10 minutes to help remove excess water.

Toss the spiralized zucchini in the olive oil, and season with chile flakes and paprika.

Place the zucchini on your lined sheet and form into 4 rounds. Press down in the center of each round to form little nests, leaving enough space for your eggs.

Crack an egg into each nest before placing the sheet in the oven.

Bake for 10–15 minutes, or until the eggs are cooked to your liking.

Remove from the baking sheet season to taste and sprinkle with the toasted mixed seeds.

Serve on its own or use one of the serving suggestions below.

TOP TIP

Moving the zucchini nests onto your plate can sometimes be tricky, so I recommend you add extra individual pieces of parchment paper under each portion, bigger than the nest, so you can lift them out and slide each nest onto a plate when cooked.

PROTEIN BOOSTERS

1¾ oz/50g of smoked salmon in each serving will add 11g of protein.

3 strips of nitrate-free bacon in each serving will add 17g of protein.

2⅓ oz/65g of smoked mackerel in each serving will add 13g of protein.

2⅔ oz/75g of organic tempeh in each serving will add 16.5g of protein.

2⅔ oz/75g of smoked tofu in each serving will add 12g of protein.

NUTRITIONAL INFORMATION *(Per Serving)*

Calories 277Kcals ○ Net carbohydrates 7.3g ○ Fiber 2.9g ○ Fat 18.6g ○ Protein 19.2g

Morning Zinger Green Smoothie

SERVES 1   ◦   FULL OF ANTIOXIDANTS, ANTI-INFLAMMATORY, VEGAN, GRAIN-FREE

INGREDIENTS

- 1 small (about 1-inch) piece of fresh ginger, peeled and roughly chopped
- One ¾-inch piece of fresh turmeric root, peeled and roughly chopped
- zest of ½ a lemon
- 1 Granny Smith apple, cored, cut into pieces
- ½ tsp ground cinnamon
- ½ tsp maca powder (optional)
- 1 cup/30g fresh baby-leaf spinach
- ⅔ cup/150ml unsweetened almond milk
- ½ cup/100ml coconut water
- a pinch of freshly ground black pepper
- a pinch of sea salt
- 1–1½ tsp maple syrup (optional)

Place all the ingredients in your blender and blend until smooth and creamy. Adjust the liquid as needed.

Drink within 20 minutes, to ensure you get the full nutritional benefits.

PROTEIN BOOSTERS

1 scoop (20g) of collagen or protein powder will add 20g of protein.

1 tbsp of hemp seeds will add 3g of protein.

NUTRITIONAL INFORMATION *(Per Serving)*

Calories 149Kcals   ◦   Net carbohydrates 23.9g   ◦   Fiber 6.4g   ◦   Fat 4.3g   ◦   Protein 4.4g

This refreshing, zesty smoothie is the ideal way to kickstart your morning with an anti-inflammatory, energy-boosting blend of ginger, turmeric, and citrus. The apple adds natural sweetness, while the spinach delivers essential nutrients and fiber. The creamy texture comes from the almond milk, and a pinch of sea salt and black pepper enhances the bioavailability of the turmeric—clever, right? Packed with antioxidants, healthy fats, and gut-friendly ingredients, this smoothie really is the perfect start to your day!

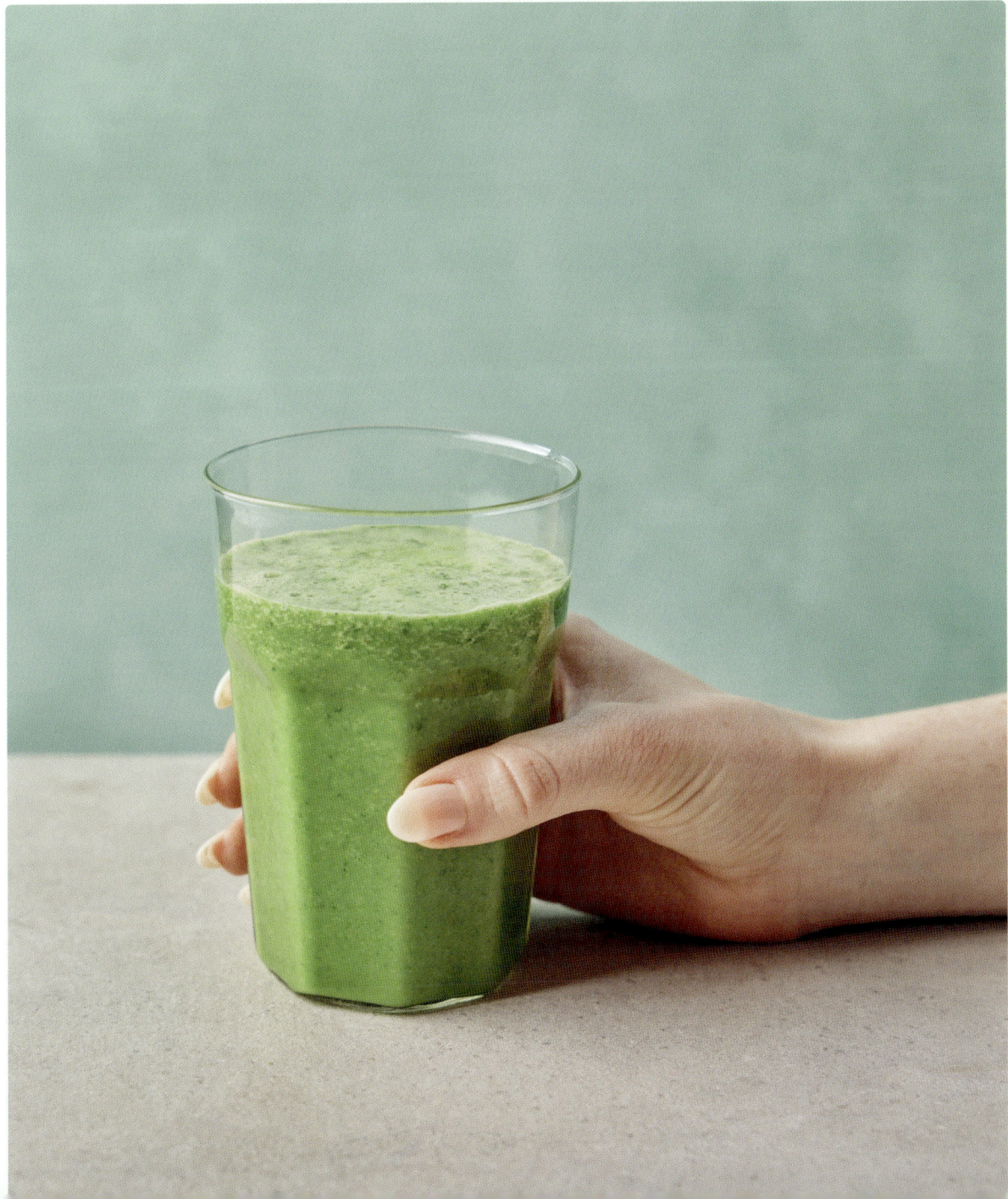

This silky, protein-packed breakfast or brunch dish, with whipped tahini, poached eggs, and a drizzle of warm chili oil, is a delicious combination of Eastern flavors while also providing you with a perfectly balanced meal. It's my go-to lazy weekend breakfast, full of healthy fats and proteins to power you up for the rest of your day.

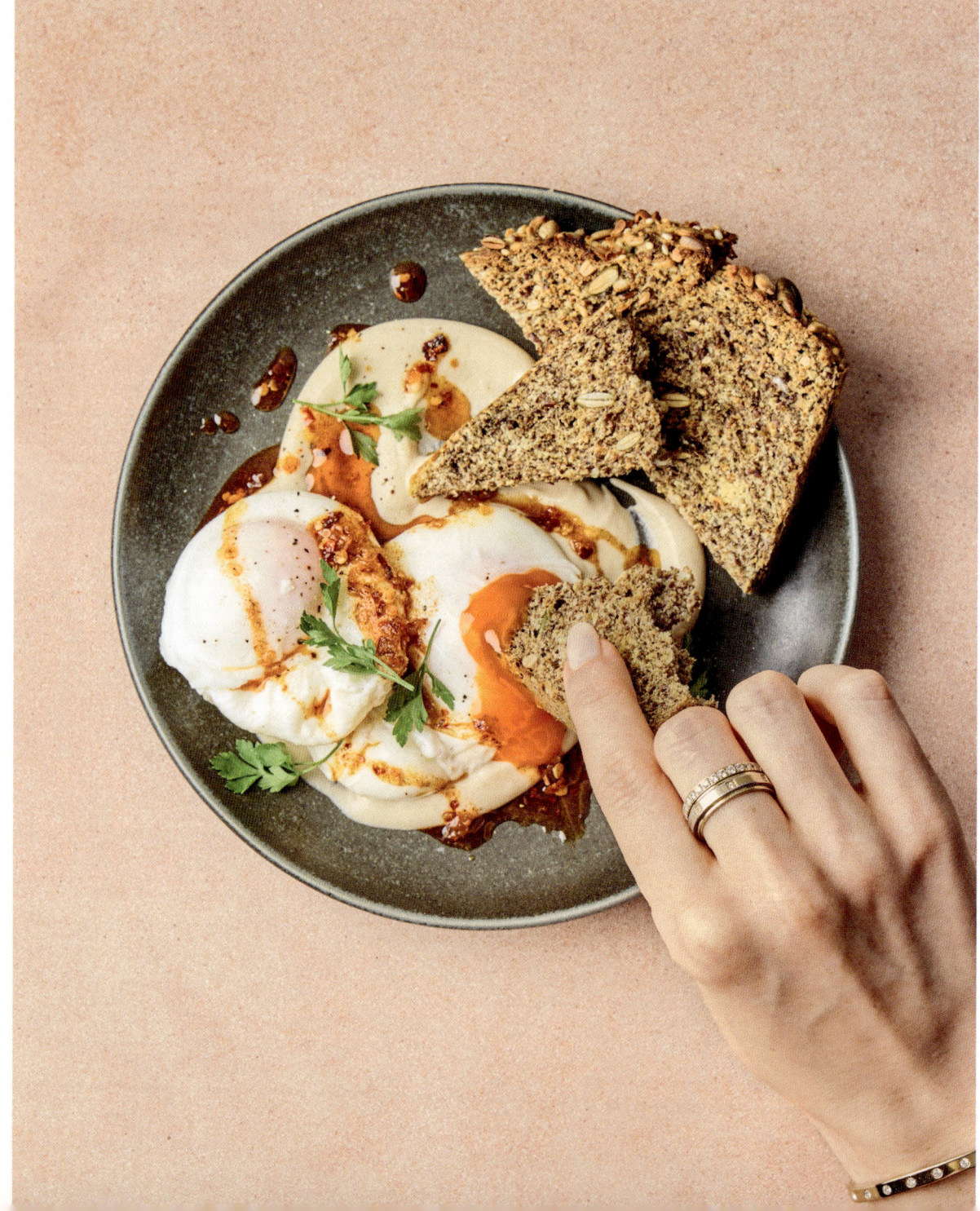

Whipped Tahini

with Poached Eggs & Chili Oil Drizzle

SERVES 2 ○ VEGETARIAN, HIGH PROTEIN

INGREDIENTS

4 tbsp tahini
¼ cup/60ml cold water
juice of ½ a lemon
1 small clove of garlic, finely grated
½ tsp sea salt
1 tbsp apple cider vinegar or white wine vinegar (for poaching)
4 large eggs

For the chili oil
2 tbsp olive oil or avocado oil
½ tsp smoked paprika
½ tsp chile flakes
¼ tsp sea salt

To garnish
chopped flat-leaf parsley (optional)

To serve
Grain-Free Seeded Bread (optional) (page 258)

Whisk together the tahini, cold water, lemon juice, garlic, and sea salt in a small bowl until thick, smooth, and slightly fluffy. Add a little more water, if needed, to reach a creamy consistency. Set aside while you poach your eggs.

Bring a medium saucepan of water to a gentle simmer. Add the vinegar. Crack each egg into a small cup. Swirl the water with a spoon and gently slide in the eggs. Poach for 3–4 minutes, until the whites are set but the yolks remain runny. Remove with a slotted spoon and drain on kitchen towels.

While the eggs are poaching, you can make the chili oil. In a small pan, heat the oil over medium heat. Stir in the smoked paprika, chile flakes, and sea salt. Heat for 30 seconds until fragrant but not burning.

When you are ready to plate up, spread the whipped tahini on serving plates. Top with the poached eggs, followed by a generous drizzle of the warmed chili oil, and garnish with parsley (if desired). Serve immediately, with slices of my Grain-Free Seeded Bread (if using).

TOP TIPS

Make ahead: the whipped tahini can be prepared in advance and stored in the fridge for up to 3 days.

Customize: add extra lemon juice for a tangier tahini, or swap the chile flakes for harissa for a different spice twist.

PROTEIN BOOSTERS

Increasing the eggs per serving from 2 to 3 will add 7g of protein.

1 tbsp of hemp seeds sprinkled on each serving will add 3g of protein.

1¾ oz/50g of smoked salmon per serving will add 11g of protein.

3 strips of nitrate-free bacon per serving will add 17g of protein.

2⅓ oz/65g of smoked mackerel per serving will add 13g of protein.

2⅔ oz/75g of organic tempeh per serving will add 16.5g of protein.

2⅔ oz/75g of smoked tofu per serving will add 12g of protein.

NUTRITIONAL INFORMATION *(Per Serving)*

Calories 444Kcals ○ Net carbohydrates 1.3g ○ Fiber 2g ○ Fat 40.5g ○ Protein 20.3g

Chia & Acai Split Bowl

SERVES 2 ○ VEGAN, HIGH FIBER, HIGH IN ANTIOXIDANTS, GRAIN-FREE

INGREDIENTS

⅓ cup/50g chia seeds
1 cup plus 1 tbsp/250ml unsweetened almond milk
½ tsp vanilla extract
1 tsp honey or maple syrup (optional)
⅓ cup/75g frozen mixed berries
1 tbsp acai powder
2 tbsp smooth peanut butter
¾ cup plus 1 tbsp/200ml unsweetened almond milk
1 tsp ground cinnamon

To garnish
fresh berries
coconut flakes
mint leaves

To prepare the chia seed pudding, mix the chia seeds with the almond milk, vanilla, and honey (if using). Stir, then leave to stand for at least 30 minutes, but ideally overnight.

When ready to make the acai element, place the rest of the ingredients in your blender and whizz until combined and smooth. Depending on your desired consistency, you may need to add more liquid.

To serve, spoon the chia seed mixture into one side of your bowl and pour the acai fruit mixture into the other side. Before serving, decorate with berries, coconut flakes, and mint leaves.

TOP TIP
If adjusting the consistency, add a little more almond milk as needed.

SERVING OPTIONS
If you prefer a sweeter acai mix, you can blend in a Medjool date or a teaspoon of honey.

This is a naturally high-fruit dish, so pairing it with added protein will help balance blood-sugar levels.

PROTEIN BOOSTERS
1 scoop (20g) of collagen or protein powder will add 10g of protein per serving.

Sprinkling 1 tbsp of hemp seeds on each serving will add 3g of protein.

NUTRITIONAL INFORMATION *(Per Serving)*

Calories 343Kcals ○ Net carbohydrates 20.7g ○ Fiber 15.1g ○ Fat 23.8g ○ Protein 11.4g

Bali in a bowl? This chia and acai split bowl isn't just perfectly Instagrammable, it's also a nutrient-dense, dairy-free twist on traditional yogurt pots. The bowl is designed to fuel you up for the day with healthy fats, fiber, and antioxidants, too. The chia pudding gives it a creamy, omega-rich base for anti-inflammatory goodness, while the acai blend is packed full of vitamins, minerals, and polyphenols for energy, brain power, and blood-sugar balance.

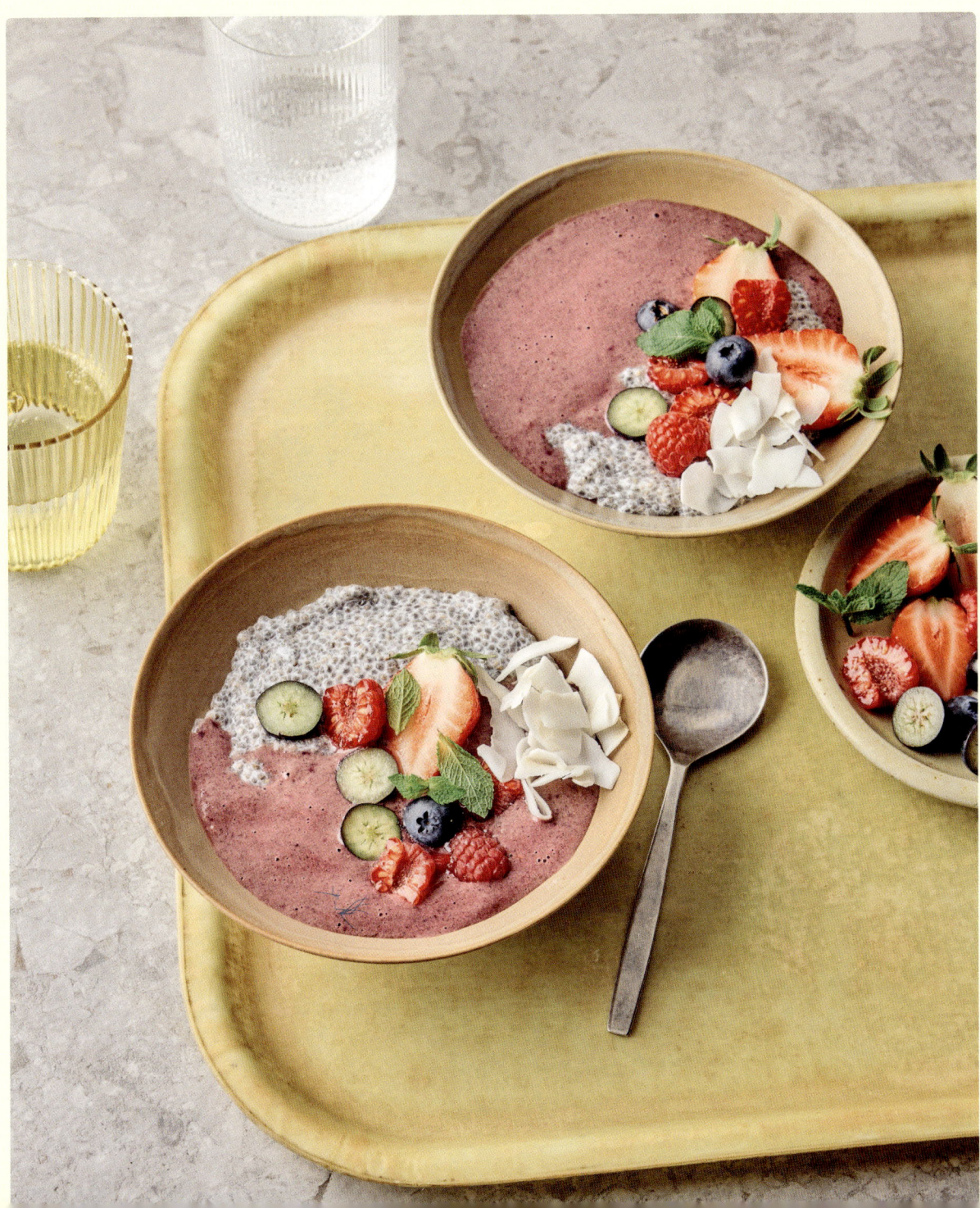

Who says you can't have cake for breakfast? Carrot cake is my all-time favorite, so when it came to "spicing" up my overnight oats, a carrot cake version was non-negotiable. It's creamy, nutritious, and bursting with healthy carbs and sweeteners from the oats and dates, while the pecans give it a tasty crunch! It's an effortless breakfast when prepped the night before, and allowing the oats to soak overnight will help with digestion, too. Simply mix, chill, and wake up to the perfect breakfast or pre-workout snack.

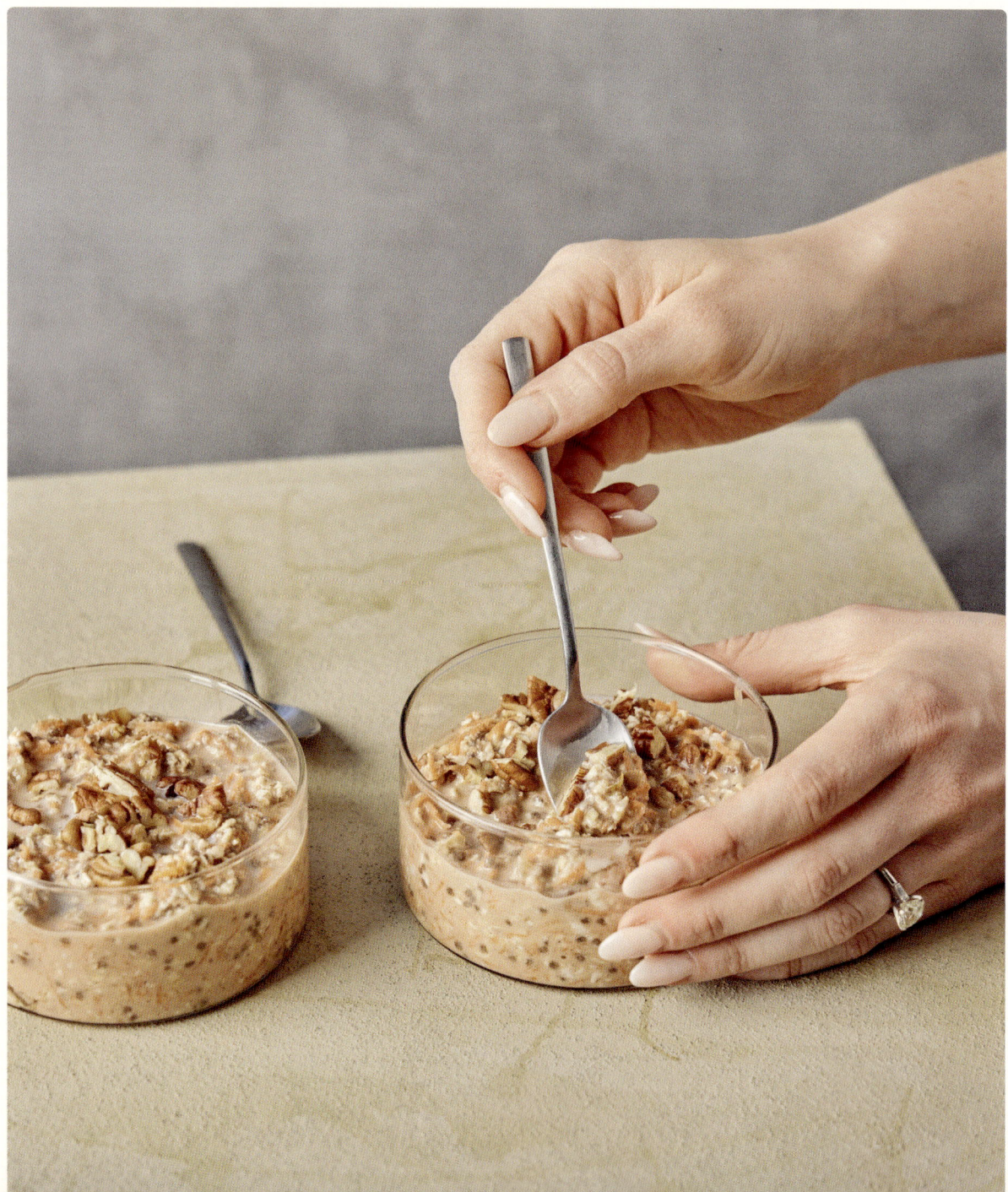

Spiced Carrot Cake Overnight Oats

SERVES 2   ○   VEGAN, GRAIN-FREE

INGREDIENTS

- ½ cup/75g gluten-free oats
- 1 small carrot, finely grated
- 1 tbsp chia seeds
- 1 tsp ground cinnamon
- ¼ tsp ground nutmeg
- ¼ tsp ground coriander
- ½ tsp vanilla paste
- 2 Medjool dates, finely chopped
- 1 cup plus 1 tbsp/250ml unsweetened almond milk
- 1 tbsp honey, or to taste
- 3–4 pecans, crushed

Combine the oats, carrot, chia seeds, spices, vanilla, and dates in a bowl.

Add the milk and honey and combine well.

Pour into two jars/glass dishes and cover. Leave overnight in the refrigerator.

When ready to eat, give it a good stir and add more milk if desired.

Serve with the crushed pecans on top.

TOP TIPS

The oats will keep in the fridge, in a sealed jar, for up to 3 days.

If you like a creamier breakfast, swap half the milk for coconut cream.

PROTEIN BOOSTERS *(Per Serving)*

1 scoop (20g) of collagen or protein powder will add 20g of protein (10g per serving).

1 tbsp of hemp seeds, sprinkled on top of each pot, will add 3g of protein.

NUTRITIONAL INFORMATION *(Per Serving)*

Calories 352Kcals   ○   Net carbohydrates 59g   ○   Fiber 9.7g   ○   Fat 11.6g   ○   Protein 7.6g

Green Shakshuka

SERVES 2   ○   VEGETARIAN, HIGH PROTEIN, HIGH FIBER

INGREDIENTS

- 1 tbsp olive oil or coconut oil
- 2 green onions, chopped, including green stems
- 1 clove of garlic, crushed
- 10 cups/300g greens (such as chard, spring greens, cabbage, baby-leaf spinach)
- 1 cup/150g frozen peas
- 1 tsp za'atar
- sea salt and freshly ground black pepper, to taste
- 4 eggs
- 2 tbsp tahini
- juice of ½ a lemon
- a drizzle of chili oil

Put the oil into a sauté pan. Add the green onions and garlic and cook for 1–2 minutes.

Add the greens and continue to cook on a moderate heat until they start to wilt slightly.

Add the peas and za'atar, season generously with salt and black pepper, and combine well.

Crack in the eggs, then cover the pan and continue to cook for 8–10 minutes, until the egg whites are set but the yolk remains soft.

Mix the tahini with the lemon juice and 1 tablespoon of water.

Place the eggs and vegetables on your serving plates and drizzle over the tahini paste, followed by a small drizzle of chili oil. Delicious with a slice of Grain-Free Seeded Bread (page 258).

PROTEIN BOOSTERS

Increasing the eggs per serving from 2 to 3 will add 7g of protein.

1 tbsp of hemp seeds sprinkled on each serving will add 3g of protein.

1¾ oz/50g of smoked salmon per serving will add 11g of protein.

3 strips of nitrate-free bacon per serving will add 17g of protein.

2⅓ oz/65g of smoked mackerel per serving will add 13g of protein.

2⅔ oz/75g of organic tempeh per serving will add 16.5g of protein.

2⅔ oz/75g of smoked tofu per serving will add 12g of protein.

NUTRITIONAL INFORMATION *(Per Serving)*

Calories 444Kcals   ○   Net carbohydrates 12.2g   ○   Fiber 9g   ○   Fat 33.9g   ○   Protein 23g

This "green goddess" twist on the traditional shakshuka makes a nutrient-packed breakfast (although I have it for lunch and dinner, too!). Full of greens, protein-rich eggs, and a dreamy tahini drizzle, this dish is as nourishing as it is delicious . . . so no more excuses for skipping your greens!

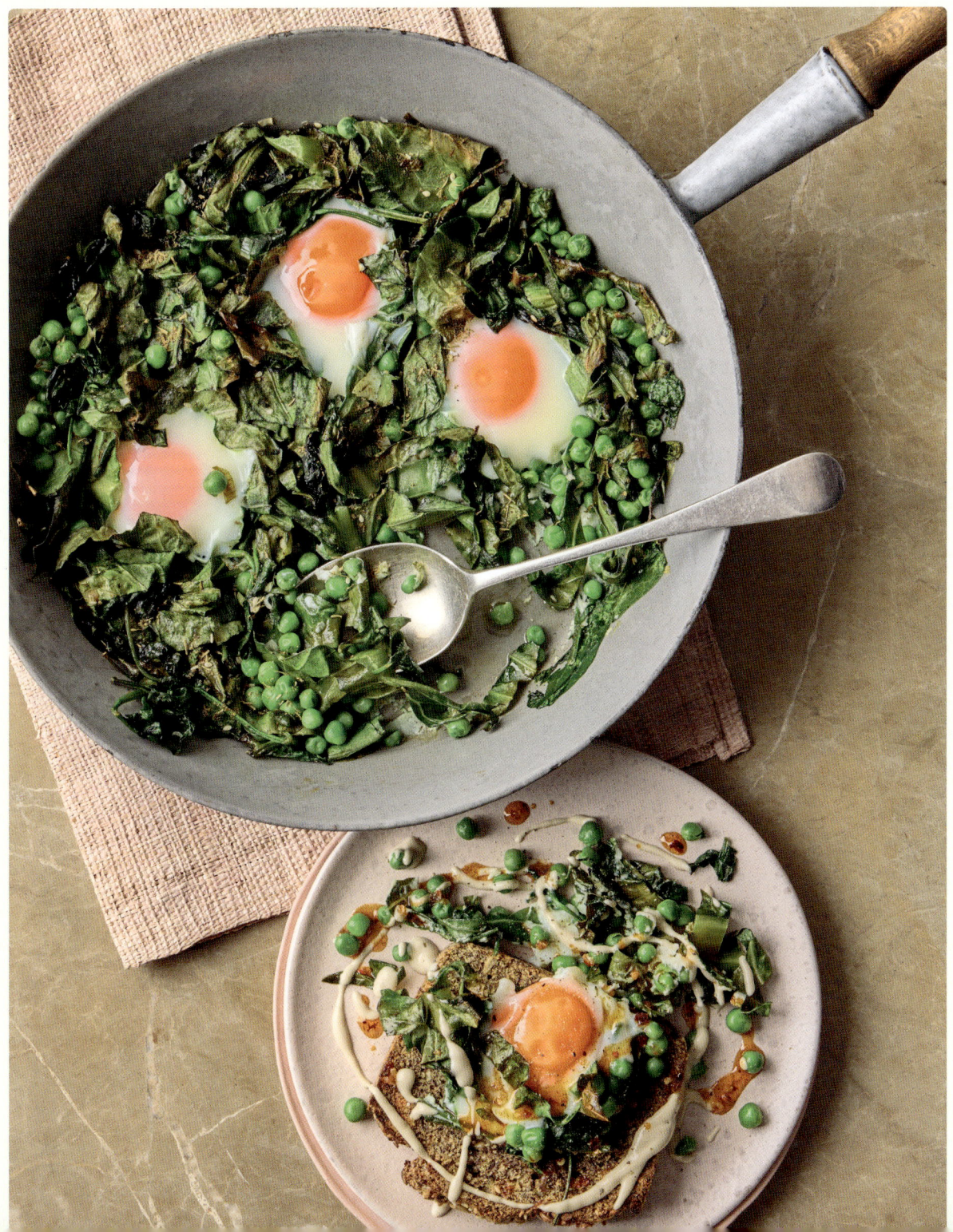

I shouldn't have favorites—BUT—this granola is definitely my most used and requested recipe! It's a delicious mix of crunchy nuts, seeds, coconut, and cozy spices with a hint of natural maple sweetness. The sprinkle of sea salt brings out all the flavors and makes it a dreamy sweet and savory snack or topping. Add it to your Natural Live Coconut Yogurt (page 299), smoothie bowls, or even eat it as a dessert! It keeps well in an airtight container for weeks, making it perfect for batch prepping.

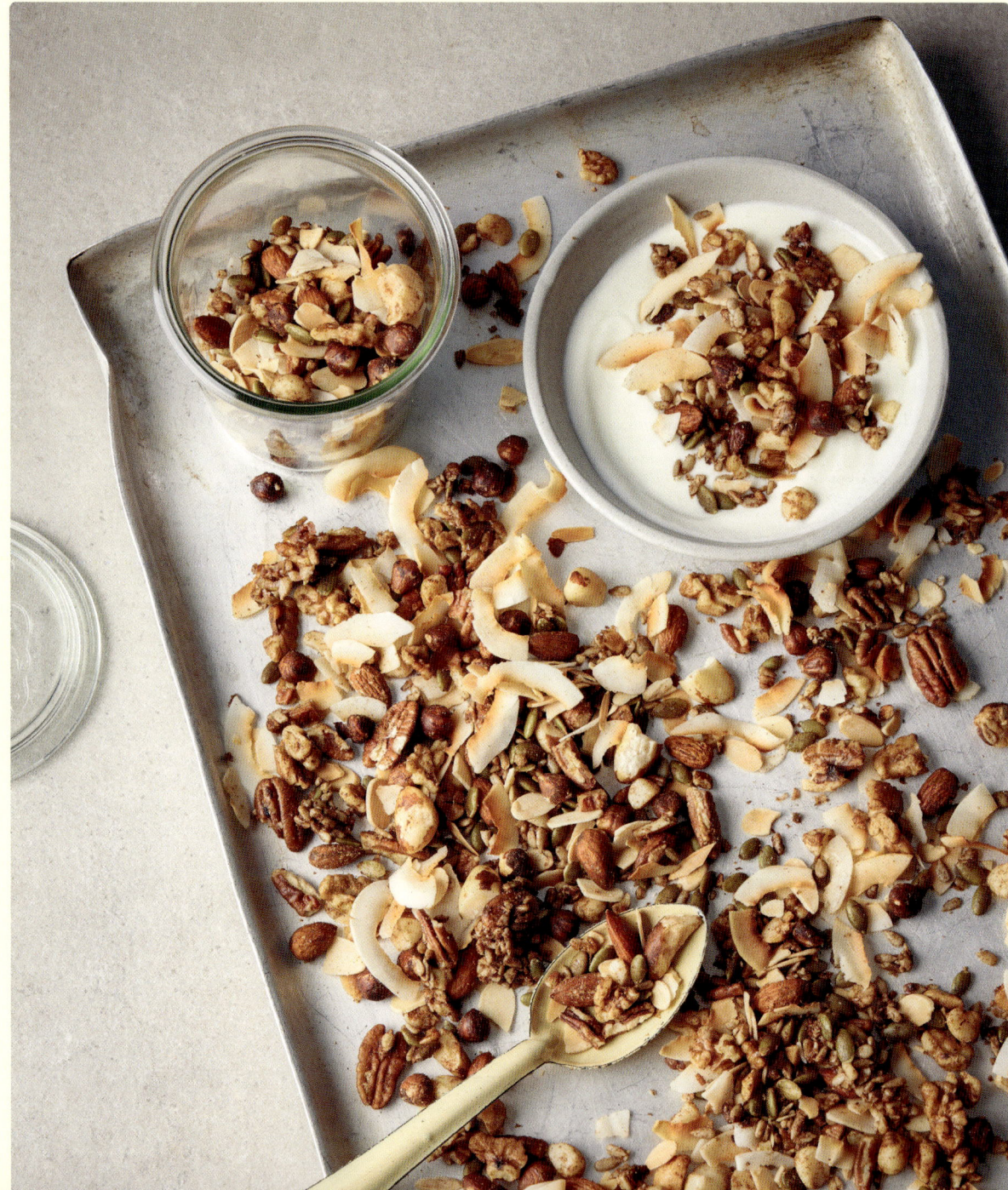

Salted Maple & Cinnamon Granola

MAKES 18 SERVINGS (BASED ON A 40G SERVING)   ○   VEGAN, GRAIN-FREE

INGREDIENTS

- 1 cup/100g walnuts
- ¼ cup plus 2 tbsp/50g Brazil nuts
- ¼ cup plus 2 tbsp/50g macadamia nuts
- ¼ cup plus 2 tbsp/50g almonds
- ½ cup/75g hazelnuts
- ¾ cup/100g pecans
- ⅔ cup/75g sliced almonds
- 1½ cups/75g unsweetened coconut flakes
- ½ cup/75g sunflower seeds
- ⅔ cup/75g pumpkin seeds
- 3 tbsp/40g coconut oil
- 2 tbsp maple or date syrup
- 1½ tsp ground cinnamon
- ½ tsp ground nutmeg
- ½ tsp ground ginger
- 1 tsp vanilla extract
- ½–1 tsp fine sea salt (or to taste)

Preheat the oven to 300°F (fan).

Place the whole nuts in a bag and bash with a rolling pin, or chop with a knife, until they are in bite-size pieces.

In a large bowl, combine the sliced almonds, coconut flakes, sunflower seeds, and pumpkin seeds with the crushed nuts.

Melt the coconut oil in a jug and combine it with the maple syrup, cinnamon, nutmeg, ginger, vanilla extract, and sea salt.

Pour this over the nut and seed mixture and combine well until it is evenly coated.

Spread the nut mixture on a large baking sheet (you may need two sheets), ensuring it is evenly distributed. Place in the oven and bake for 5 minutes.

Remove from the oven, stir well to combine, and return to the oven for another 5 minutes, making sure it does not burn.

Remove from the oven and allow to cool completely. Once cooled, place in an airtight container. If stored in a dry place, it should keep for 7–14 days.

PROTEIN BOOSTERS

Serve with protein yogurt, which can add up to 15g of protein per 200g serving.

Alternatively, add protein powder or collagen to your milk or yogurt.

Add 2 tbsp of cacao or cocoa powder to the coconut oil for a chocolate-spice flavor.

VARIATIONS

Add freeze-dried apple pieces for an apple and cinnamon granola.

Swap the cinnamon and nutmeg for ½ tsp each of cardamom, allspice, and black pepper for a chai spice flavor.

NUTRITIONAL INFORMATION *(Per Serving)*

Calories 281Kcals   ○   Net carbohydrates 4.4g   ○   Fiber 3.4g   ○   Fat 26.6g   ○   Protein 6.2g

Lemon & Blueberry Pots

SERVES 2 ○ VEGAN, GRAIN-FREE

INGREDIENTS

¾ cup/180g silken tofu
⅔ cup/150ml unsweetened coconut or almond milk
zest of 1 lemon
½ cup/75g blueberries, fresh or frozen
2 tbsp chia seeds
1 tbsp honey or maple syrup, or to taste
1 tsp vanilla extract
a pinch of sea salt

To garnish
fresh blueberries

Put all the ingredients into your blender and whizz until they are smooth and evenly combined.

Place in serving glasses and refrigerate for at least 15 minutes before serving.

Top with fresh blueberries and serve.

TOP TIPS

For a thicker pot, refrigerate for an hour or overnight.

To make a smoothie, add more coconut milk until you reach your desired consistency.

FLAVOR VARIATIONS

Swap the blueberries for raspberries.

For chocolate lovers, swap the lemon and blueberries for 1 tablespoon of cocoa or cacao powder. You may need to add a little more liquid to get the desired consistency.

PROTEIN BOOSTERS

1 scoop (20g) of collagen or protein powder will add 20g of protein (10g per serving).

1 tbsp of hemp seeds, sprinkled on each pot, will add 3g of protein per serving.

NUTRITIONAL INFORMATION *(Per Serving)*

Calories 201Kcals ○ Net carbohydrates 19.9g ○ Fiber 7.7g ○ Fat 9.3g ○ Protein 10.3g

Full of plant-based protein from silken tofu and chia seeds, these lemon and blueberry pots are creamy, super-satisfying, and nutrient-dense. The blueberries not only add a pop of color and natural sweetness, but are full of antioxidants, too, while the lemon zest keeps everything bright and refreshing. They take minutes to make and are full of healthy fats and fiber, making them the perfect blood-sugar-friendly start to your day.

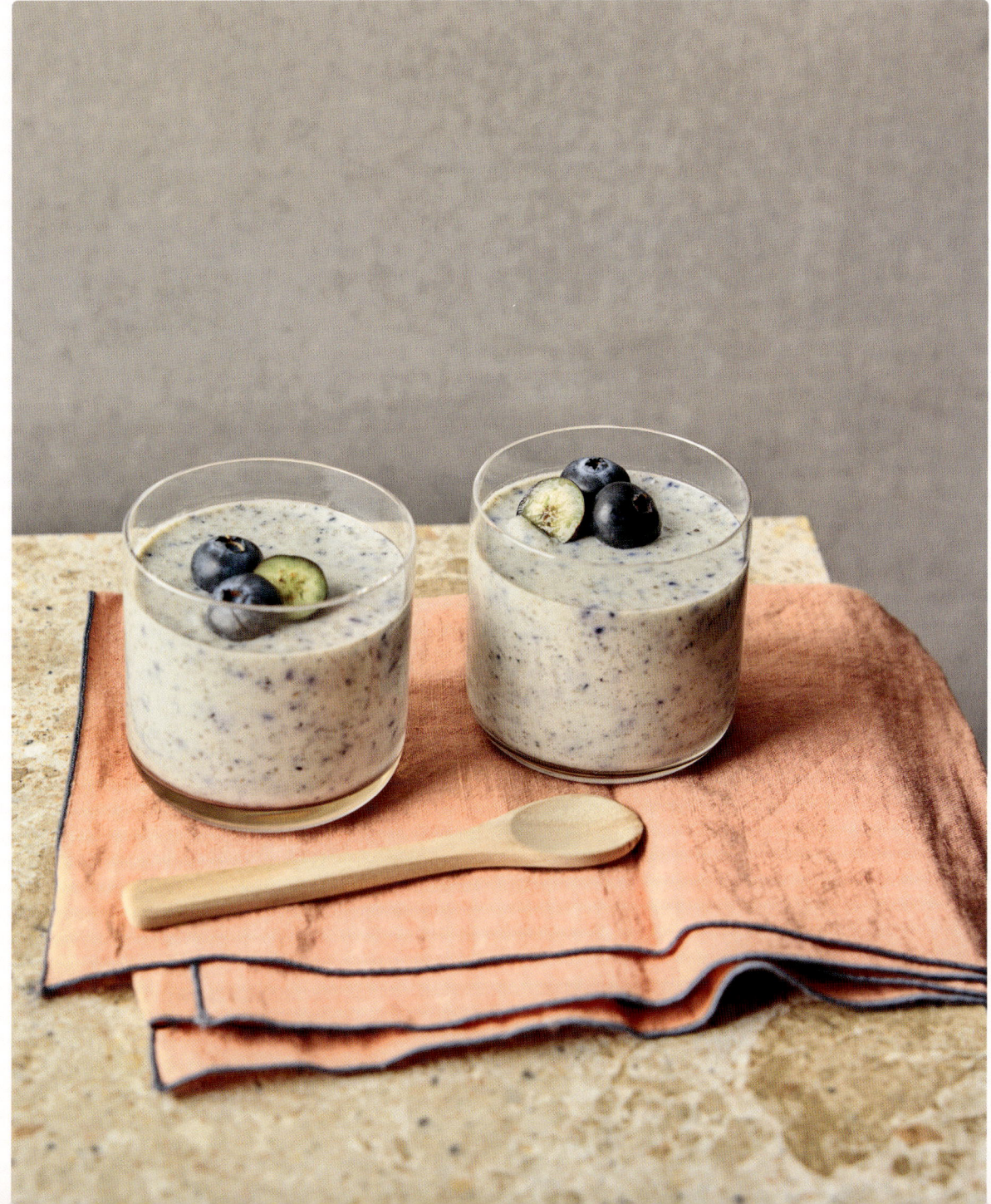

Crêpe-style pancakes that are gluten-free and full of protein? Yes, please! Served with my delicious Healthy Chocolate Spread (page 295), and filled with sliced banana... you've got yourself a naturally sweetened breakfast. I love adding a drizzle of Natural Live Coconut Yogurt (page 299) or a sprinkle of crushed nuts for a boost of flavor and healthy fats.

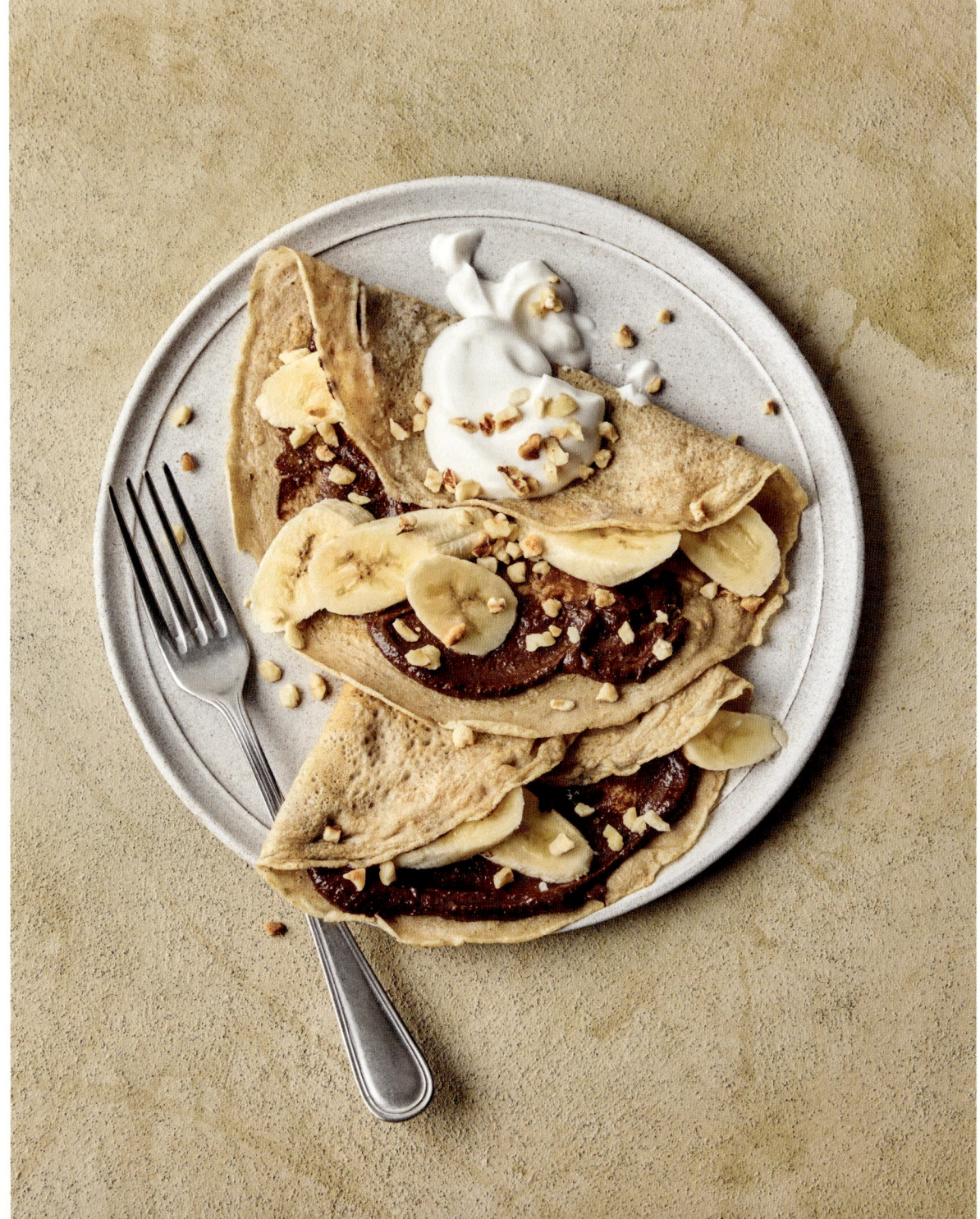

Banana & Chocolate Pancakes

SERVES 2 (4 MEDIUM PANCAKES) ○ NATURAL SWEETNESS, VEGETARIAN

INGREDIENTS

- 2 medium eggs
- ½ cup/100ml unsweetened almond milk
- 1 tsp vanilla extract
- a pinch of sea salt
- ¼ cup/40g buckwheat flour
- 1 tsp coconut oil
- 4 tsp Healthy Chocolate Spread (page 295)
- 1 ripe banana, thinly sliced

To serve
Natural Live Coconut Yogurt (page 299) and crushed nuts (optional)

In a mixing bowl, whisk the eggs, almond milk, vanilla, and sea salt.

Sift in the buckwheat flour and whisk until smooth and lump-free.

Heat a nonstick frying pan over medium heat and melt the coconut oil.

Pour in a quarter of the batter, swirling to coat the base. Cook for 1–2 minutes, until set, then flip and cook the other side. Repeat with the rest of the mixture, to make 4 pancakes.

Spread each pancake with 1 tsp of chocolate spread while still warm.

Add the banana slices and roll or fold into quarters.

Serve warm, topped with coconut yogurt and crushed nuts if you like.

TOP TIP

The pancakes freeze well, stacked between sheets of parchment paper. Reheat in a dry pan for 1–2 minutes each side.

NUTRITIONAL INFORMATION *(Per Serving)*

Calories 328Kcals ○ Net carbohydrates 27.3g ○ Fiber 3.3g ○ Fat 17.4g ○ Protein 14.4g

Lun

ch

This salad is everything a meal should be ... full of flavor, satisfying, and easy to make! Who doesn't love juicy grilled chicken with a rainbow of plant-based goodness, crisp textures, and a herby chimichurri? The roasted chickpeas and pumpkin seeds add an extra crunch and protein boost. It's a firm favorite of mine, and easily preppable, too.

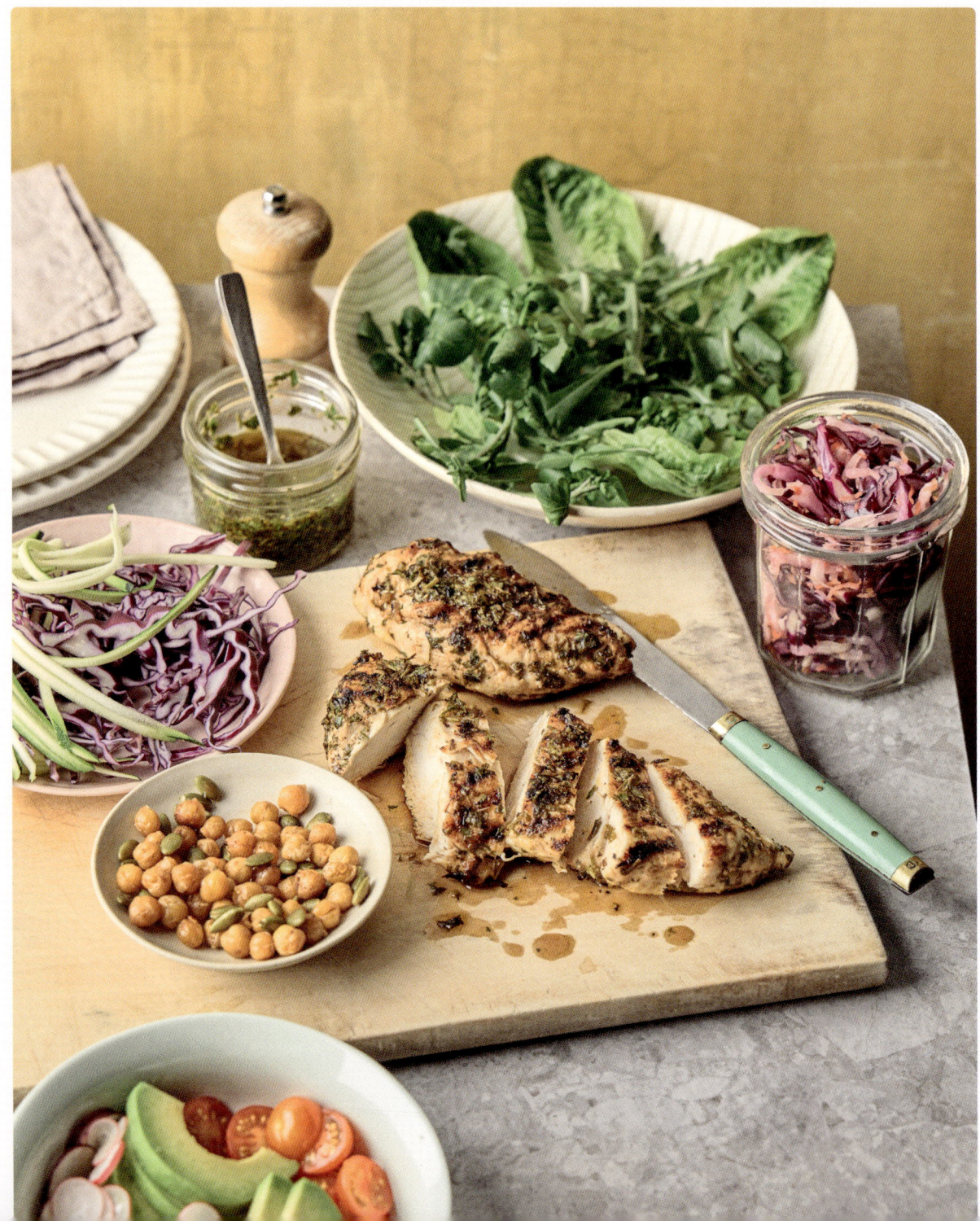

Grilled Chimichurri Chicken Salad

SERVES 2 ○ HIGH PROTEIN

INGREDIENTS

For the chimichurri sauce
¼ cup/60ml extra virgin olive oil
juice of ½ a lemon
2 tbsp red wine vinegar
1 small jalapeño, finely chopped (optional)
3 cloves of garlic, minced
1 cup/30g flat-leaf parsley, finely chopped
⅓ cup/10g fresh cilantro, finely chopped
½ tsp dried oregano
½ tsp smoked paprika
sea salt and freshly ground black pepper, to taste

10½ oz/300g skinless, boneless chicken breasts or thighs
sea salt and freshly ground black pepper, to taste

For the salad
4 cups/80g mixed salad greens (arugula, watercress, little gem)
½ cup/50g red cabbage, finely shredded
1½ cups/75g zucchini, spiralized or ribboned
¾ cup/100g cherry tomatoes, halved
1 small avocado, sliced
½ cup/30g radishes, thinly sliced
¼ cup/50g Roasted Chickpeas (page 255)
2 tbsps/15g toasted pumpkin seeds

To serve
1–2 tbsp Fermented Rainbow Kraut (page 291)

Prepare the chimichurri by combining the olive oil, lemon juice, red wine vinegar, jalapeño (if using), garlic, parsley, cilantro, oregano, smoked paprika, salt, and black pepper in a bowl. Stir well and set aside for at least 10 minutes to let the flavors infuse.

Season the chicken with salt and black pepper. Brush with the chimichurri and leave to marinate for at least 15 minutes, if time allows.

Heat a griddle pan over a medium-high heat and cook the chicken for 6–10 minutes on each side, or until cooked through and golden. Let rest, then slice.

Divide the salad greens, cabbage, zucchini, tomatoes, avocado, and radishes between 2 bowls. Add the Roasted Chickpeas and pumpkin seeds.

Place the grilled chicken slices on top, drizzle generously with the chimichurri, add a side of our Fermented Rainbow Kraut, and serve immediately.

TOP TIP

Make up a batch of chimichurri sauce. This can be used for our Chimichurri Steak with Grilled Vegetables (page 220) or as a dressing for your everyday salads.

GRAIN BOOSTERS

If you want to boost the grains or significantly increase the carbohydrates, you can add a grain of your choice to the salad, for example rice, quinoa, or buckwheat.

1 cup/150g of cooked basmati rice, 39.8g carbs (4g protein).

¾ cup/125g of cooked quinoa, 23.5g carbs (4.9g protein).

¾ cup/120g of cooked buckwheat, 16.9g carbs, (3.3g protein).

NUTRITIONAL INFORMATION *(Per Serving)*

Calories 604Kcals ○ Net carbohydrates 22.5g ○ Fiber 7.2g ○ Fat 34.7g ○ Protein 46.5g

Beet Falafel Bowl
with Lemon Tahini Drizzle

SERVES 4   ○   VEGAN, HIGH FIBER, HIGH PROTEIN

INGREDIENTS

2 fresh beets, peeled and chopped into chunks
2 tbsp olive oil
1 tbsp balsamic vinegar
sea salt and freshly ground black pepper, to taste
Two 14oz/400g cans of chickpeas, rinsed and drained
3 cloves of garlic, peeled
1 small red onion, quartered
2 tbsp tahini
1 tsp ground cumin
1 tsp ground coriander
1 tsp chili powder
a squeeze of lemon juice
1–2 tbsp chickpea flour (if needed to bind)

For the tahini dressing
3 tbsp tahini
juice of ½ lemon
1 tsp honey (optional)
2–3 tbsp water, as needed
a pinch of sea salt

For the salad
5 to 6 cups/100g mixed salad greens
½ cucumber, ribboned
1 red pepper, sliced
1 small avocado, sliced
¾ cup/100g cherry tomatoes, halved
2 tbsp hummus
2 tbsp pumpkin seeds
¼ cup/50g Roasted Chickpeas (optional) (page 255)

Preheat the oven to 375°F (fan) and line a baking sheet with parchment paper.

Place the beet chunks on another baking sheet and drizzle with 1 tbsp of the olive oil and the balsamic vinegar. Season well with salt and pepper.

Roast for 25 minutes, turning halfway, until tender. Remove from the oven and allow to cool slightly.

Put the roasted beets, chickpeas, garlic, onion, tahini, cumin, coriander, chili powder, lemon juice, salt, and pepper into a food processor and pulse until they form a thick, coarse paste. If it is too wet, stir in a little chickpea flour.

Form into 12 falafels and place them on the lined baking sheet. Brush lightly with olive oil and bake for 20 minutes, turning halfway, until they are crisp on the outside. Alternatively, you can pan-fry these until golden.

Mix the dressing ingredients together until smooth, adding water a little at a time to reach a drizzling consistency.

When ready to assemble, start with the salad greens, cucumber ribbons, and red pepper slices, then add the avocado, cherry tomatoes, and hummus. Top with the falafels, sprinkle with the seeds and, if using, Roasted Chickpeas and finish with a drizzle of tahini dressing.

TOP TIPS

Great for meal prep: store the falafels in the fridge for 3–4 days, or freeze them for up to 2 months.

Try wrapping the falafels and salad in a gluten-free wrap or in large romaine leaves for an easy lunch-to-go.

Add fermented veg such as sauerkraut or kimchi for extra gut-loving support.

NUTRITIONAL INFORMATION *(Per Serving)*

Calories 447Kcals   ○   Net carbohydrates 24.3g   ○   Fiber 6.9g   ○   Fat 25.5g   ○   Protein 30.5g

These oven-roasted beet falafels are not only stunning to look at, but they're also packed with flavor and with hormone-balancing nutrients such as manganese, fiber, and phytonutrients. Served with a zingy lemon tahini drizzle, vegetables, creamy hummus, and crunchy salad, this makes a well-balanced, filling lunch that's ideal for meal prep or alfresco dining.

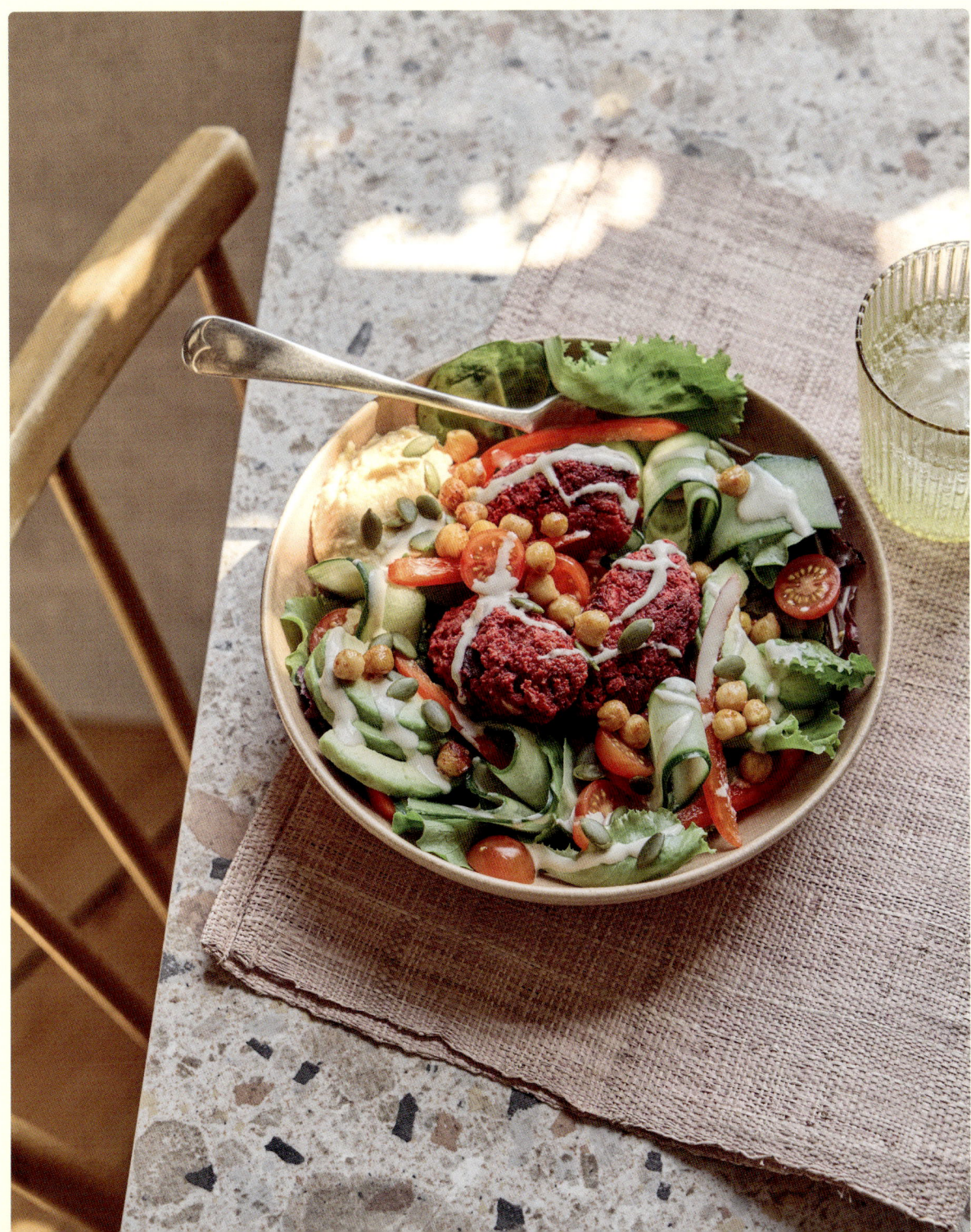

This fuss-free, quick and easy lunch is full of healthy fats, protein, and vibrant flavor. Creamy avocado halves are filled with a zesty tuna and green onion mix, dressed with a light lemony mayo. It's quick to make, nutrient-rich, and perfect for warm summer days.

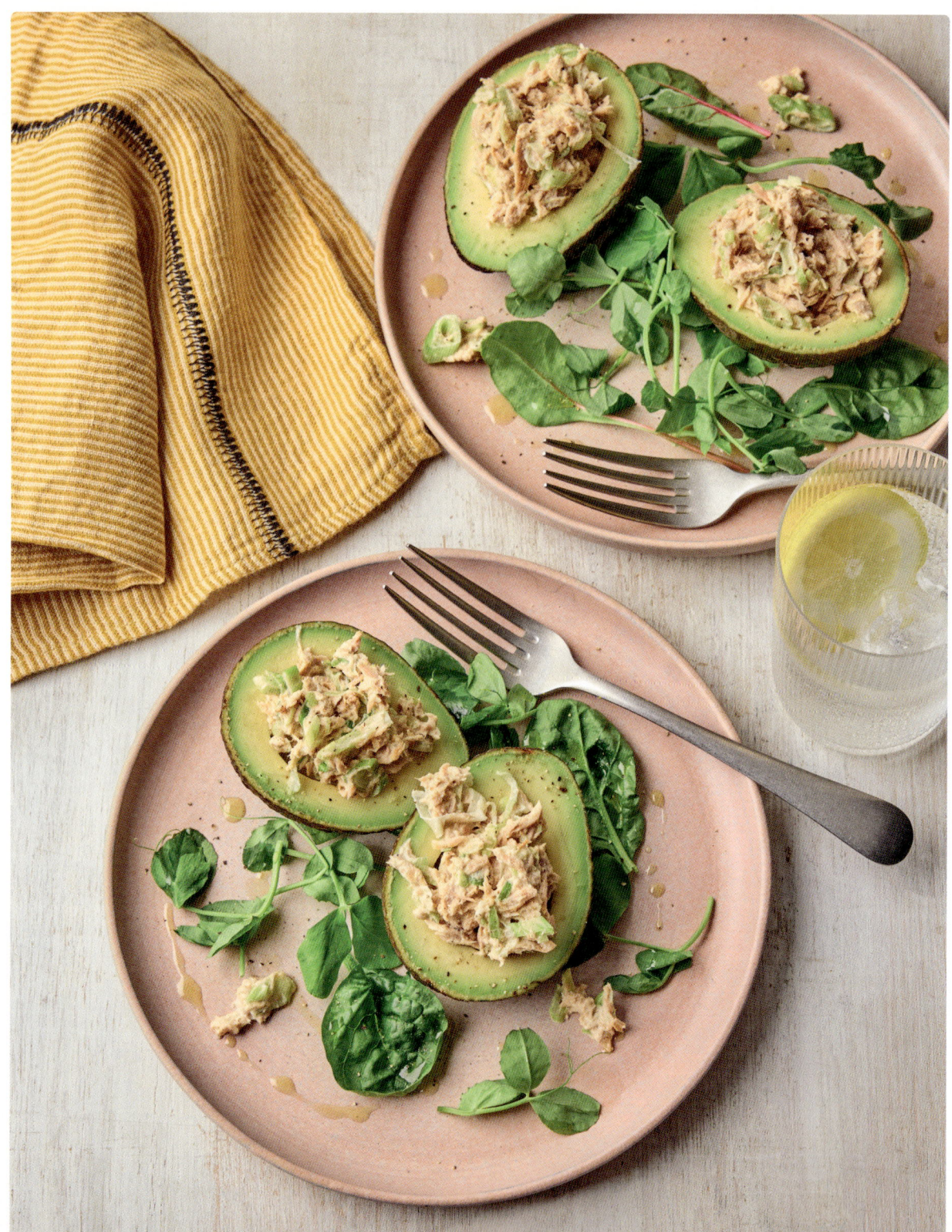

Stuffed Avocado
with Tuna & Lemon Mayo

SERVES 2 ○ HIGH OMEGA, HIGH PROTEIN, GRAIN-FREE

INGREDIENTS

2 medium avocados
One 3.8oz/110g can of tuna in spring water, drained
3 green onions, finely chopped, including greens
1 tbsp lemon juice
2 tbsp mayonnaise
sea salt and freshly ground black pepper, to taste
a handful of salad greens

Cut the avocados in half and remove the pits. Carefully scoop out a small spoonful from the center to create more room for the filling.

In a bowl, mix the tuna with the green onions, lemon juice, mayonnaise, salt, and black pepper.

Spoon the mixture into the avocado halves.

Serve immediately on a bed of salad greens.

TOP TIPS

Add a little Dijon mustard or chopped capers for extra tang.

Add 2–3 tbsp of sweet corn.

For extra texture, sprinkle with pumpkin seeds.

PROTEIN BOOSTER

For an extra protein boost, serve with a hard-boiled egg (an extra 7g of protein per egg).

NUTRITIONAL INFORMATION *(Per Serving)*

Calories 419Kcals ○ Net carbohydrates 4g ○ Fiber 5.2g ○ Fat 36.3g ○ Protein 18.8g

Roasted Vegetable Salad
with Lentils, Chickpeas & Tahini Dressing

SERVES 4 ○ VEGAN, HIGH FIBER, GLUTEN-FREE, PROTEIN BOOSTERS

INGREDIENTS

For the roasted veg
1 red onion, cut into wedges
2 medium carrots, peeled and chopped
1 zucchini, chopped
1 red pepper, sliced
1 yellow pepper, sliced
1⅓ cups/200g butternut squash, peeled and cubed
2 tbsp olive oil
½ tsp ground cumin
½ tsp smoked paprika
sea salt and freshly ground black pepper, to taste

For the tahini dressing
2 tbsp tahini
1 tbsp lemon juice
1 tsp honey
1 small clove of garlic, minced
3–4 tbsp water (if needed)

For the salad base
½ cup/100g cooked lentils (Puy or green)
One 14oz/400g can of chickpeas, drained and rinsed
2½ to 3 cups/75g arugula or spinach
1 tbsp chopped flat-leaf parsley
2 tbsp hemp seeds
2 tbsp pumpkin seeds

Preheat the oven to 375°F (fan).

Place the vegetables in a bowl. Add the olive oil, cumin, smoked paprika, salt, and black pepper and combine well until the vegetables are evenly coated in the oil.

Spread the vegetables in your roasting pan in a single layer and roast for 30 minutes, turning halfway through, until golden and tender.

While the veg are roasting, mix the tahini dressing ingredients in a small bowl or jar, adding enough water to reach a creamy but pourable consistency.

In a large bowl, combine the lentils, chickpeas, arugula or spinach, parsley, and seeds. Add the roasted vegetables once they are cooked.

Drizzle with the tahini dressing just before serving and toss gently to combine. Serve warm or at room temperature.

TOP TIPS

Roast extra veg while the oven's on and use in other meals throughout the week.

This salad also works well with roasted cauliflower, eggplant, or sweet potato.

PROTEIN BOOSTERS

Grilled chicken breast (3½oz/100g): 31g protein.

Grilled salmon (3½oz/100g): 25g protein.

2 hard-boiled eggs: 14g protein.

Roasted tofu (3½oz/100g): 23g protein.

Tempeh (3½oz/100g): 21g protein.

NUTRITIONAL INFORMATION *(Per Serving)*

Calories 378Kcals ○ Net carbohydrates 32.4g ○ Fiber 12.7g ○ Fat 21.2g ○ Protein 15.9g

This is a delicious plant-based salad packed with nutrients and is perfect for meal prepping. The fiber-rich hit from the chickpeas will get your gut going, and the creamy tahini dressing is to die for! Enjoy it warm or cold, and add an extra protein boost from the list opposite. Grilled chicken breast is always my favorite!

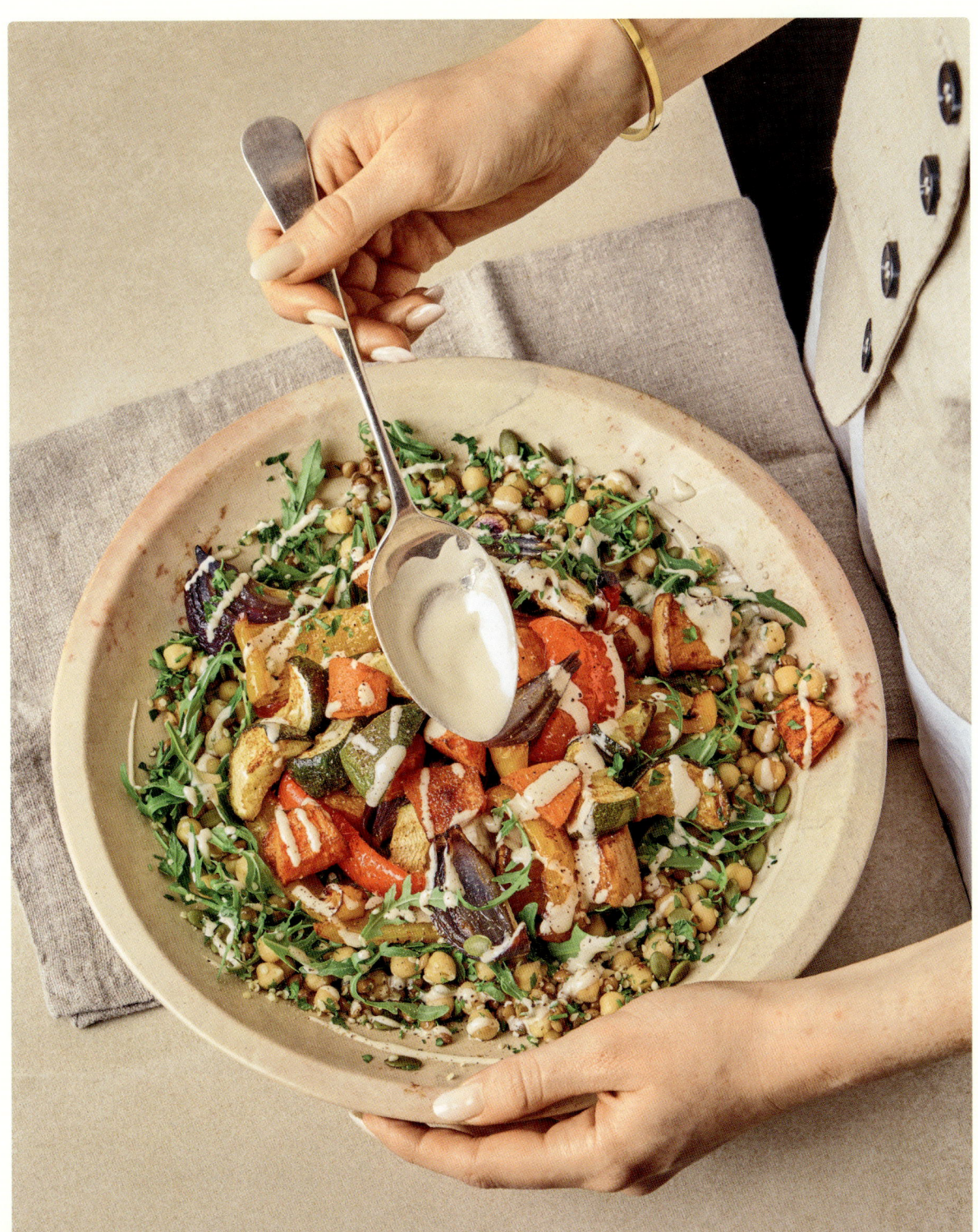

These fancy high-protein Scotch eggs elevate a classic recipe with an even better mushroom and walnut paste, which isn't just tastier than the original, but also adds depth, fiber, and a touch of umami. Coated in crumbled seeded bread, they're crisp and have a satisfying crunch while staying gluten-free—the dream! Served with a tangy mustard mayo, these are perfect for a tasty, nutrient-dense lunch or snack. PS. These are my partner's favorite!

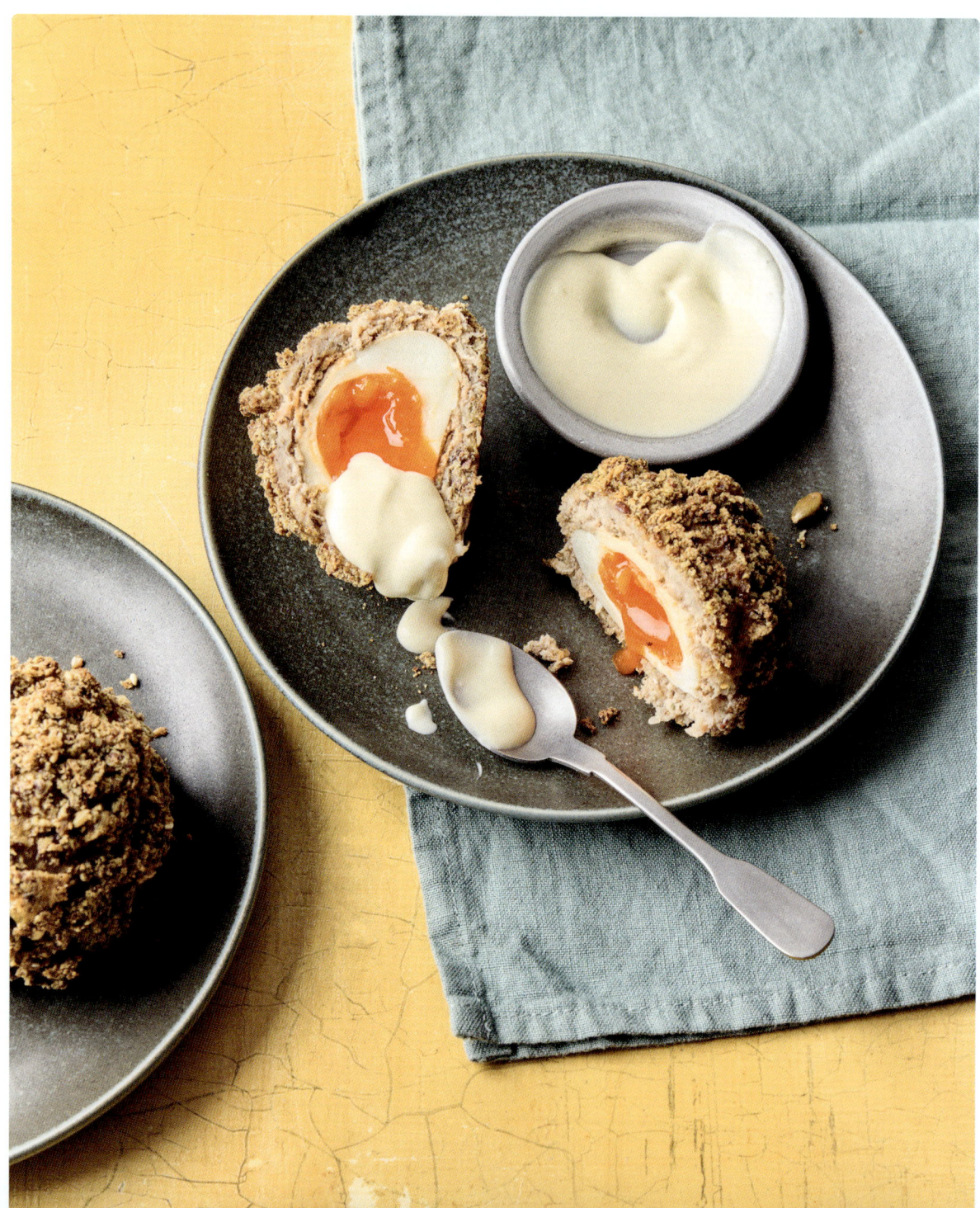

High-Protein Scotch Eggs

MAKES 4   ○   HIGH-PROTEIN, GRAIN-FREE

INGREDIENTS

5 eggs
1 tbsp olive oil
1 cup/100g chestnut mushrooms, finely chopped
⅓ cup/40g walnuts, toasted and finely chopped
1 clove of garlic, minced
1 tsp dried thyme
1 tsp tamari
1 tsp freshly ground black pepper
400g high-quality gluten-free sausage meat
1 tsp dried sage or rosemary
½ tsp garlic powder
a pinch of cayenne pepper (optional for an extra kick)
sea salt, to taste
1 beaten egg
2½ cups/100g crumbled Grain-free Seeded Bread (page 258) (alternative coatings: see Top Tips, below)

For serving
3 tbsp mayonnaise
1 tsp Dijon mustard
a squeeze of lemon juice

Preheat the oven to 400°F (fan).

Boil the kettle. Put 4 of the eggs in a saucepan and cover with boiling water. Simmer over medium heat for 6 minutes. Remove from the heat, drain, and run under cold water. Leave to cool before peeling.

To make the mushroom and walnut paste, heat the olive oil in a pan over a medium heat. Sauté mushrooms, walnuts, garlic, thyme, tamari, and ½ tsp of black pepper for 5 minutes until softened. Blend into a rough paste and let cool.

In a bowl, mix the sausage meat with sage or rosemary, garlic powder, cayenne (if using), salt, and another ½ tsp of black pepper. Divide into 4 equal portions.

Flatten each portion of sausage meat and spread with a thin layer of mushroom paste, then wrap it around a peeled egg, ensuring the egg is fully enclosed.

Beat the remaining egg, dip each sausage-wrapped egg into it, then roll in the crumbled seeded bread (or chosen coating).

Bake for 20–25 minutes, turning halfway through. They will take slightly less time if cooking in an air fryer.

Once cool, store in an airtight container in the fridge for up to 5 days. Reheat in an air fryer or oven for crispiness.

For serving, mix the mayonnaise with the Dijon mustard and a squeeze of lemon juice for a tangy dipping sauce.

TOP TIPS

Alternative coatings: try a mix of ground almonds and sesame seeds, crushed gluten-free crackers, or crushed good-quality pork rinds.

Frying option: heat about 2 inches of olive oil in a saucepan or use a deep-fat fryer at medium-high heat. Fry the Scotch eggs, turning frequently, until golden brown and crisp.

NUTRITIONAL INFORMATION *(Per Scotch Egg)*

Calories 679Kcals   ○   Net carbohydrates 11.4g   ○   Fiber 6.1g   ○   Fat 52g   ○   Protein 36.9g

Marinated Salmon Bowl

SERVES 4   ○   HIGH OMEGA, HIGH PROTEIN, GRAIN-FREE

INGREDIENTS

1 tbsp tamari
1 tsp sesame oil
1 tsp lime juice
1 tsp honey
1 clove of garlic, finely grated
½ tsp fresh ginger, grated
a pinch of chile flakes (optional)
sea salt and freshly ground black pepper, to taste
2 salmon fillets (approx. 5oz/150g each), diced

For the creamy miso dressing
1 tbsp white miso paste
2 tbsp tahini
1 tsp honey
1 tbsp apple cider vinegar
1 tsp fresh ginger, peeled and grated
1–2 tbsp water to loosen

For the salad
1 zucchini, spiralized or ribboned
1 small carrot, grated or ribboned
½ a cucumber, shaved into ribbons
1½ cup/100g red cabbage, very finely shredded
½ cup/60g edamame
1–2 tbsp beet sauerkraut or Fermented Rainbow Kraut (page 291)
1 avocado, sliced
½ cup/100g Roasted Chickpeas (page 255)
10 cherry tomatoes, halved
a small handful of mint and cilantro, finely chopped

Preheat the oven to 350°F (fan).

Mix the tamari, sesame oil, lime juice, honey, garlic, ginger, and chile flakes (if using) in a jug, and season to taste with salt and black pepper.

Place the diced salmon fillets on a lined baking sheet, touching, as this helps retain their moisture. Brush the salmon with the marinade until well coated.

Place in the oven and bake for 12–15 minutes, or until the salmon is starting to flake. Let it cool slightly, or if you like you can chill it and serve it cold.

Prepare the dressing by mixing all the ingredients together in a jug. Add water to help create a drizzle consistency.

Place the salad ingredients in 4 bowls. Top with the diced salmon, and finish with a drizzle of the creamy miso dressing.

GRAIN BOOSTERS

If you want to boost the grains or significantly increase the carbohydrates, you can add a grain of your choice to the salad, such as rice, quinoa, or buckwheat.

1 cup/150g of cooked basmati rice, 39.8g carbs (4g protein).

¾ cup/125g of cooked quinoa, 23.5g carbs (4.9g protein).

¾ cup/120g of cooked buckwheat, 16.9g carbs (3.3g protein).

NUTRITIONAL INFORMATION *(Per Serving)*

Calories 447Kcals   ○   Net carbohydrates 24.3g   ○   Fiber 6.9g   ○   Fat 25.5g   ○   Protein 30.5g

An Omega-3 supercharged lunch, full of flavor from delicious baked salmon, a rainbow of plant diversity, fermented veg, and a creamy miso dressing. It's rich in protein and fiber, tastes incredible, and makes the perfect nourishing lunch or dinner. Your taste buds and gut will love you for this one!

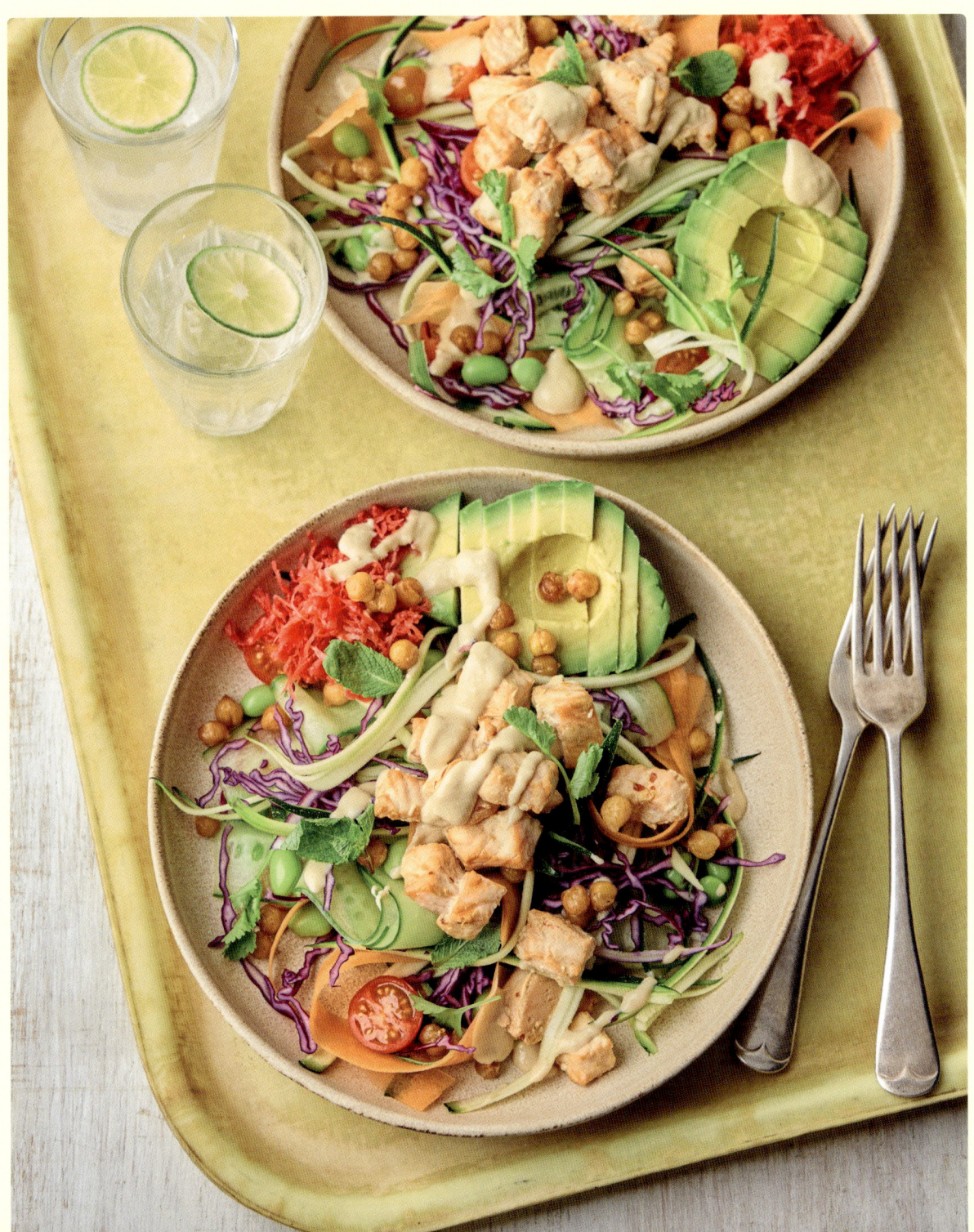

Don't be fooled by the word "soup"—this is a hearty, chunky, and incredibly satisfying dish inspired by Tuscan flavors. The slow-simmered tomatoes are deliciously rich, and paired with hearty beans and earthy kale they make this the perfect balance of comforting and nourishing. Whether it's a chilly winter evening or a light summer supper . . . this recipe is perfect for every season!

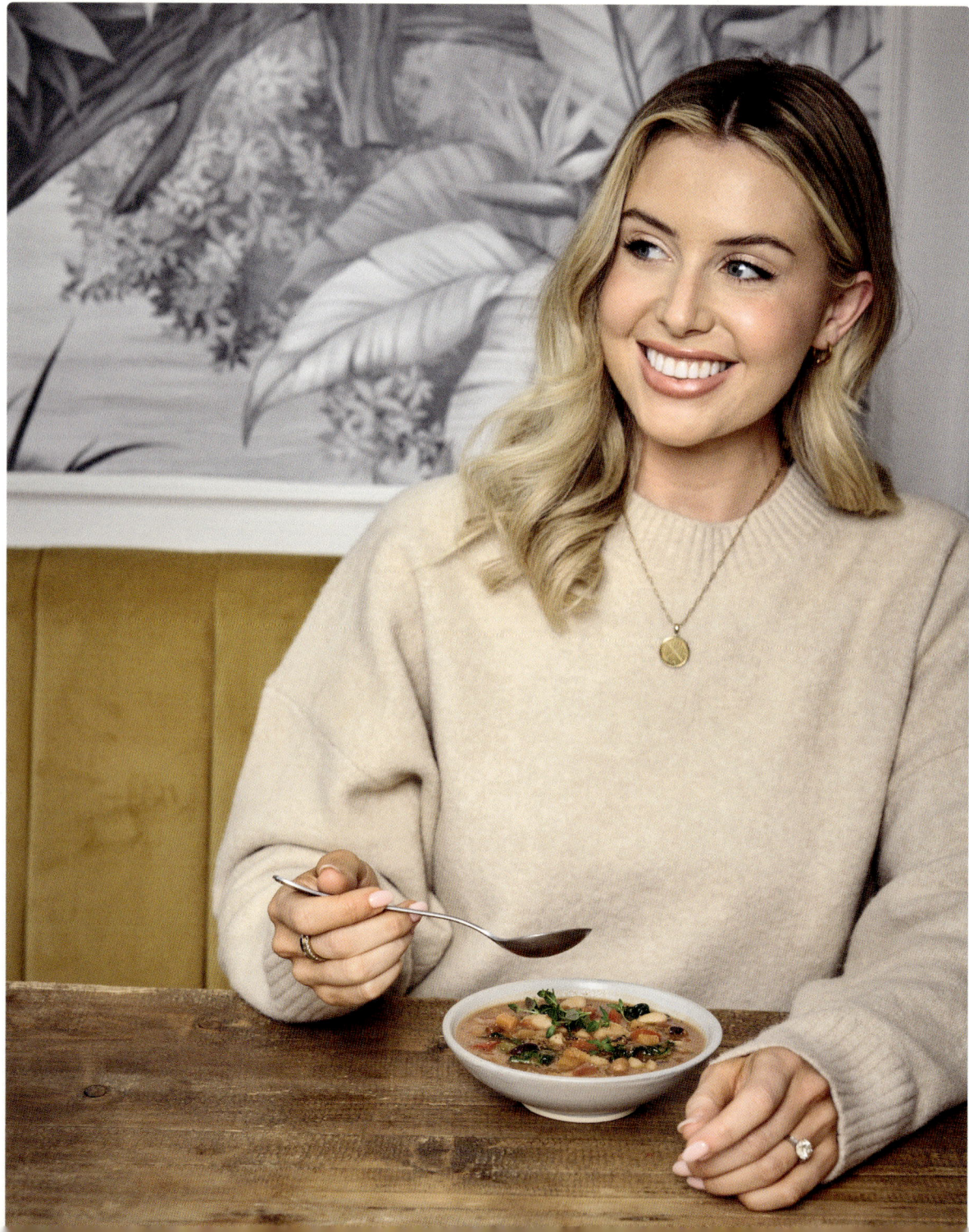

Tuscan Bean & Kale Soup

SERVES 4 ○ VEGAN, HIGH FIBER

INGREDIENTS

1 tbsp olive oil, plus more for drizzling
1 red onion, finely diced
2 cloves of garlic, crushed
1 carrot, diced
1 celery stalk, diced
½ a red pepper, diced
One 14oz/400g can of good-quality chopped tomatoes
1 tsp dried thyme
1 tsp dried oregano
2 cups plus 2 tbsp/500ml bone stock or vegetable stock
One 14oz/400g can of cannellini beans, drained and rinsed
One 14oz/400g can of mixed beans, drained and rinsed
3 to 4 cups/100g Tuscan kale (you can use curly kale), roughly chopped
sea salt and freshly ground black pepper, to taste
juice of ½ a lemon, to taste

To serve
fresh flat leaf parsley

Heat the olive oil in a large stock pot. Add the onion, garlic, carrot, celery, and red pepper and cook for a few minutes, until the vegetables start to soften slightly.

Add the tomatoes, thyme, oregano, stock, and beans and simmer gently for 15 minutes.

Five minutes before serving, stir in the kale and continue to cook until wilted but still vibrant in color. Season to taste with salt and black pepper and add the lemon juice.

Serve in bowls, drizzle with olive oil, and top with fresh parsley.

PROTEIN BOOSTER

Add 7oz/200g of shredded cooked chicken to the soup – this will increase the protein by 15g per serving.

NUTRITIONAL INFORMATION *(Per Serving)*

Calories 221Kcals ○ Net carbohydrates 25.5g ○ Fiber 13.2g ○ Fat 4.6g ○ Protein 15.6g

Elevated Poached Eggs
on Sweet Potato Toast

SERVES 2   ○   VEGAN, GRAIN-FREE, HIGH PROTEIN

INGREDIENTS

- 1 large sweet potato, skin on, sliced lengthwise into ½-inch slices
- 1 tbsp olive oil
- sea salt and freshly ground black pepper
- 4 eggs
- 1 tbsp apple cider vinegar
- a handful of arugula or microgreens
- ½ a small red onion, very finely sliced
- 1 avocado, mashed
- a pinch of dukkah
- ¼ cup/50g Roasted Chickpeas (page 255)
- 4 cherry tomatoes, quartered

Preheat the oven to 375°F (fan).

Brush the sweet potato slices lightly with olive oil and season well with salt and black pepper.

Place them on a lined baking sheet and roast for 20–25 minutes, flipping them halfway through, until soft in the middle and crisped at the edges.

To poach your eggs, bring a pan of water to a gentle simmer and add the apple cider vinegar. Crack each egg into a small bowl, then carefully slide them into the water. Poach for 3–4 minutes for a runny yolk, then remove with a slotted spoon and allow them to drain on kitchen towels.

Place the arugula on 2 plates, and top with the red onion. Spread the roasted sweet potato slices with avocado mash, then place on the arugula. Top with the poached eggs and season with dukkah. Finish with a scattering of Roasted Chickpeas and tomatoes.

TOP TIPS

Add a small heap of our Fermented Rainbow Kraut (page 291), for an energizing, probiotic hit.

You can roast extra sweet-potato slices in advance—they reheat beautifully in the toaster, air fryer, or oven.

PROTEIN BOOSTERS

Increasing the eggs per serving from 2 to 3 will add 7g of protein.

1 tbsp of hemp seeds sprinkled on each serving will add 3g of protein.

1¾oz/50g of smoked salmon per serving will add 11g of protein.

3 strips of nitrate-free bacon per serving will add 17g of protein.

2⅓oz/65g of smoked mackerel per serving will add 13g of protein.

2⅔oz/75g of organic tempeh per serving will add 16.5g of protein.

2⅔oz/75g of smoked tofu per serving will add 12g of protein.

NUTRITIONAL INFORMATION *(Per Serving)*

Calories 493Kcals   ○   Net carbohydrates 35g   ○   Fiber 8.4g   ○   Fat 30.4g   ○   Protein 21.6g

Sweet-potato toast is my all-time obsession, elevated with protein-packed poached eggs, a crunchy hit from the chickpeas, and a micronutrient gut-loving boost from the microgreens—this really is the ultimate healthy recipe! It's also lazy girl approved . . . you can cook your sweet potato "toast" in advance and pop it in the toaster when needed—just like bread!

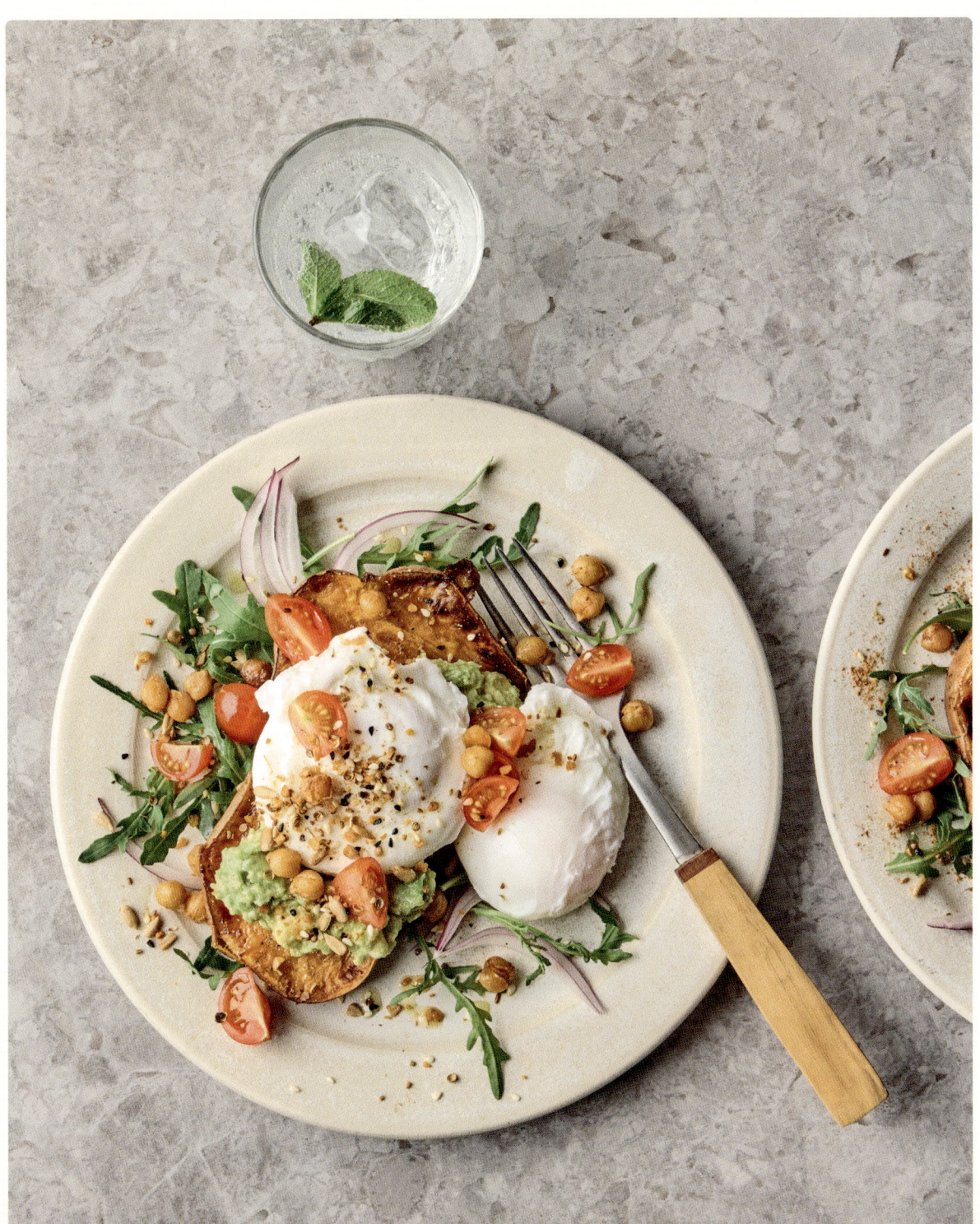

An anti-inflammatory twist on the classic BLT, this version swaps the bread for crispy, crunchy lettuce leaves that hold all the savory goodness together! It's perfect for lunch, and a super refreshing "wrap" that's light and easily customizable, too. You'll be kicking yourself for not trying it before.
For some extra protein inspiration, check out the variations opposite.

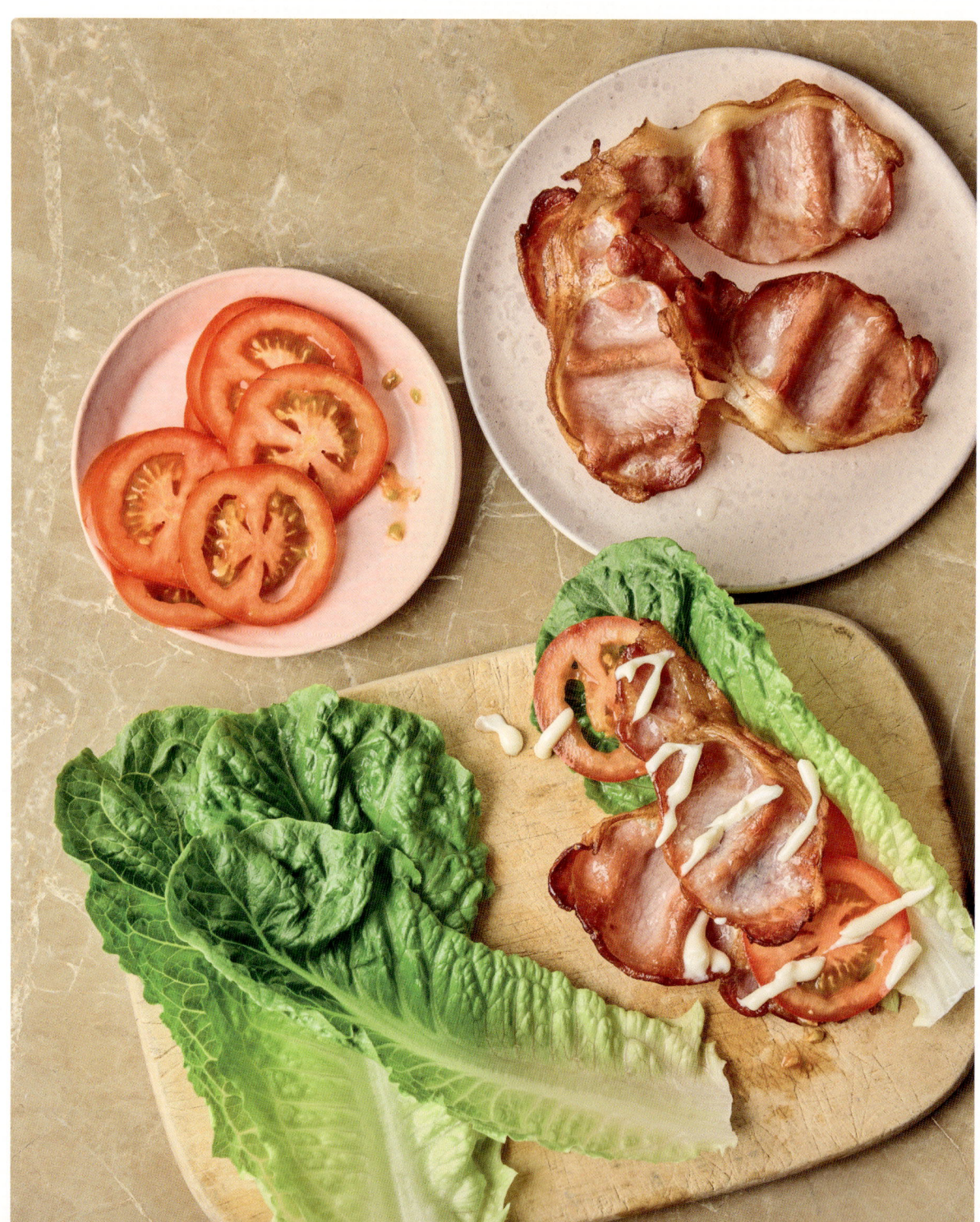

BLT Lettuce Wraps

SERVES 2 ○ HIGH PROTEIN, GRAIN-FREE

INGREDIENTS

6 strips of nitrate-free bacon
4 large lettuce leaves (such as romaine or gem)
2 medium tomatoes, sliced
mayonnaise

Cook the bacon until crisp. Once done, drain on paper towels and set aside.

Rinse and dry the lettuce leaves carefully to maintain their crunch.

On each lettuce leaf, lay out 1½ strips of bacon per wrap and top with the tomato slices. Drizzle with the mayonnaise.

Fold or roll the lettuce to enclose the filling and serve immediately.

TOP TIP

You can keep cooked bacon strips in the fridge for 3–4 days, ready to add to a salad or use for future wraps.

PROTEIN BOOSTERS

Top the wrap with a sliced hard-boiled egg for an extra protein punch (7g per egg).

Add 3½oz/100g of sliced chicken breast for 2, which will add another 15g of protein per serving.

FLAVOR BOOST

Gut boosting: Swap the tomato for a forkful of our Fermented Rainbow Kraut (page 291) for extra tang, crunch, and gut-friendly live cultures.

Extra crunch: Sprinkle toasted pumpkin or sunflower seeds inside the wrap for additional texture and a nutty flavor.

Avocado: Add slices of avocado or make an avocado mash with lime juice, salt, and chile flakes.

NUTRITIONAL INFORMATION *(Per Serving)*

Calories 438Kcals ○ Net carbohydrates 4.8g ○ Fiber 1.5g ○ Fat 40g ○ Protein 15.4g

Spiced Lentil & Chorizo Soup

SERVES 4   ○   COMFORTING AND NUTRITIONALLY BALANCED

INGREDIENTS

- 1 tbsp olive oil
- 5.3oz/150g diced, gluten-free chorizo
- 1 small red onion, finely chopped
- 1 clove of garlic, crushed
- 1 large carrot, diced
- 1 tsp smoked paprika
- ¼ tsp ground cumin
- ½ tsp ground coriander
- ¾ cup/175g red lentils
- One 14oz/400g can of chopped tomatoes
- 3 cups/800ml bone stock or vegetable stock
- freshly ground black pepper, to taste

To serve
chili oil
coconut cream
chopped flat-leaf parsley

Put the olive oil into a large pan. Add the chorizo and onion and cook on moderate heat for 5 minutes to release the oils and soften the onion.

Add the rest of the ingredients and combine well. Season with black pepper.

Bring to a gentle simmer and turn the heat down to low. Cook gently for 15–20 minutes, until the lentils have softened.

Cool slightly, then blend with a stick blender until lovely and smooth.

To serve, bring back up to heat. Spoon into bowls, with a drizzle of chili oil and a swirl of coconut cream, garnished with chopped parsley.

SERVING OPTIONS

Serve with Grain-Free Seeded Bread (page 258) or, if you can tolerate grain, with your favorite gluten-free bread.

NUTRITIONAL INFORMATION *(Per Serving)*

Calories 406Kcals   ○   Net carbohydrates 30.7g   ○   Fiber 10.5g   ○   Fat 19.7g   ○   Protein 28.6g

This rich, smoky, and super-satisfying soup is the perfect comfort meal when you need something warm, nourishing, and full of flavor. It's packed with protein from the lentils and spiced chorizo, making sure you're satisfied all day. Perfect for meal prep or a cozy night in... because let's be honest, nothing beats a warm hearty bowl of soup for the soul!

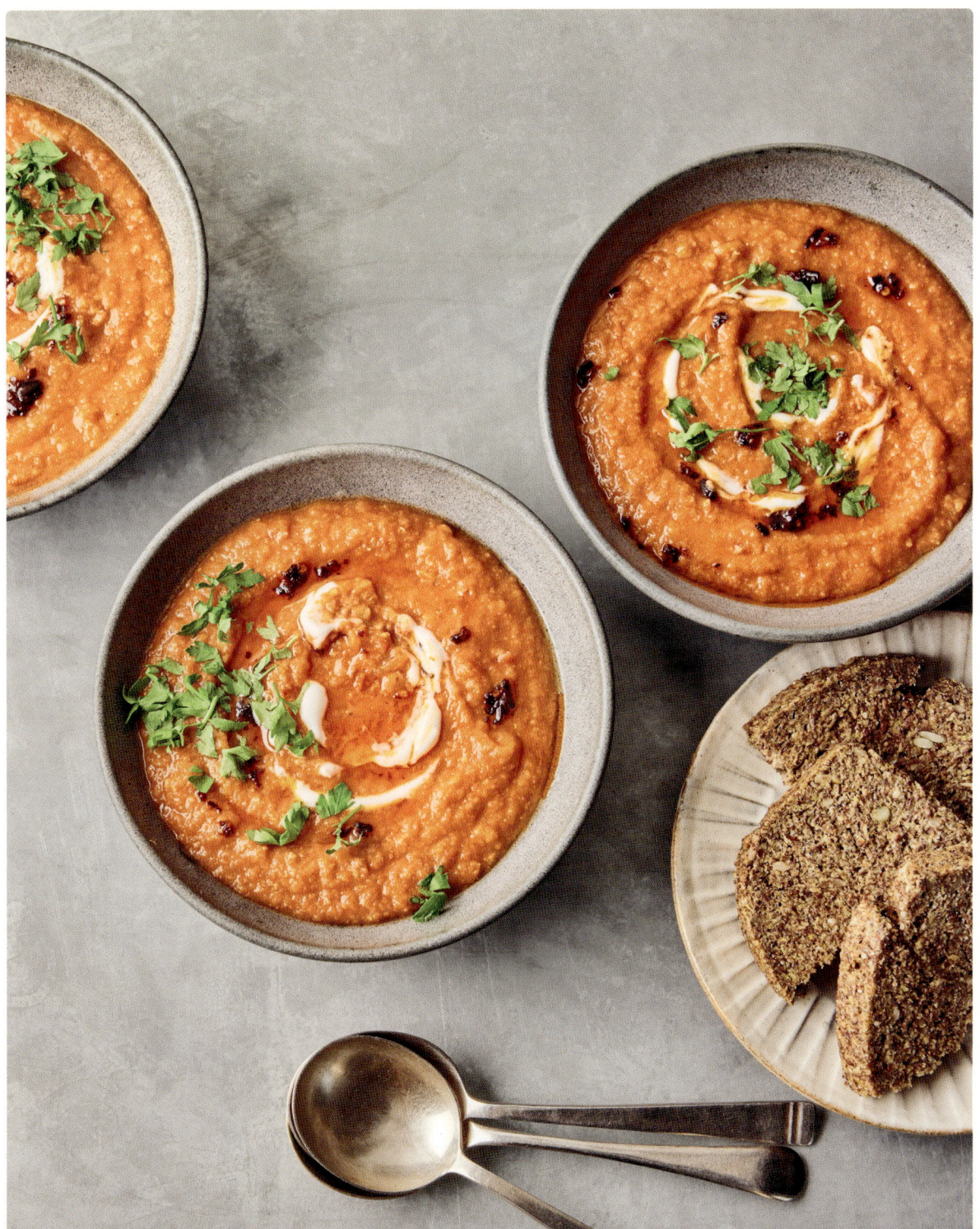

A fast, fuss-free lunch that's **BIG** on flavor! Juicy steaks are seared and served with a punchy, herby salsa verde and a colorful crunchy slaw—perfect for a nutrient-dense meal that's full of iron, and all made in less than 15 minutes.

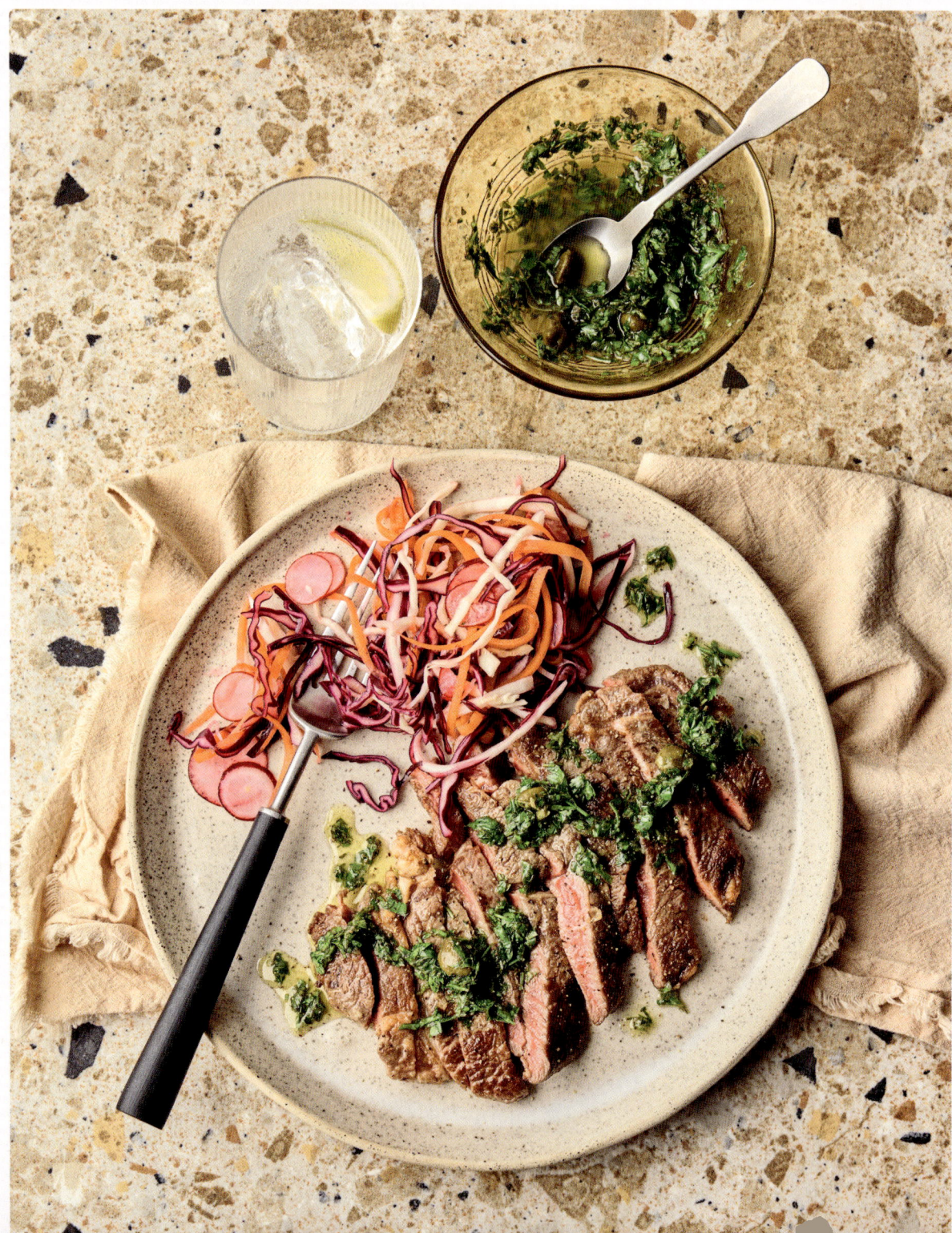

Minute Steak
with Herby Salsa Verde & Crunchy Slaw

SERVES 2 ○ HIGH PROTEIN, GRAIN-FREE

INGREDIENTS

For the salsa verde
¼ cup/10g flat-leaf parsley, finely chopped
10 capers, drained
1 clove of garlic, finely grated
1 tbsp lemon juice
1 tbsp olive oil
sea salt and freshly ground black pepper

For the crunchy slaw
1½ cups/100g mixed red and green cabbage, finely shredded
1 carrot, finely shredded
3 radishes, thinly sliced
sea salt and freshly ground black pepper
juice of ½ lemon
1–2 tbsp mayonnaise (optional)

1 tbsp olive oil
Two 4.4oz/125g minute steaks (or one large steak)
sea salt and freshly ground black pepper

Prepare the salsa verde by mixing the parsley, capers, garlic, lemon juice, and olive oil in a small bowl. Season to taste with salt and black pepper and set aside.

Prepare the slaw by combining the cabbage, carrot, and radishes in a bowl. Season lightly with salt and black pepper and toss with the lemon juice. If you prefer a creamy slaw, you can add 1–2 tbsp of mayonnaise.

Put the olive oil into a sauté pan and heat over a medium-high heat. Season the steak with salt and black pepper and cook for 1–2 minutes on each side (depending on thickness), then let rest for 2–3 minutes.

Slice the steaks thinly, divide between plates, and top with the salsa verde. Serve with the crunchy slaw on the side.

NUTRITIONAL INFORMATION *(Per Serving)*

Calories 299Kcals ○ Net carbohydrates 5.9g ○ Fiber 4.1g ○ Fat 17.6g ○ Protein 35.9g

Sun-Dried Tomato Frittata Muffins

with Quinoa Salad

SERVES 2*   ○   GLUTEN-FREE, HIGH PROTEIN, DAIRY-FREE OPTION

INGREDIENTS

- 3 eggs, beaten
- ½ cup/100ml unsweetened almond milk
- 2 tsp fresh chives, chopped
- ½ tsp dried oregano
- 2 tbsp nutritional yeast
- sea salt and freshly ground black pepper, to taste
- ⅓ cup/40g sun-dried tomatoes (in oil, drained and chopped)
- 2⅔oz/75g uncured ham, diced
- 2 green onions, finely chopped

For the quinoa salad
- 1 cup/150g cooked quinoa
- ⅓ cup/50g cucumber, finely diced
- One 14oz/400g can of chickpeas, drained
- 1 tbsp olive oil
- 1 tbsp lemon juice
- 1 tbsp finely chopped flat-leaf parsley
- sea salt and freshly ground black pepper, to taste

*(makes 4 muffins + 2 salad portions)

Preheat the oven to 375°F (fan) and grease a muffin pan, or use muffin liners.

Whisk together the eggs, almond milk, chives, oregano, nutritional yeast, salt, and black pepper in a jug.

Divide the sun-dried tomatoes, ham, and green onions between the muffin wells.

Pour the egg mixture over the fillings until each is around two-thirds full.

Bake for 18–20 minutes or until puffed and golden. Allow to cool slightly before removing from the pan.

To make the quinoa salad, toss all the ingredients together and season to taste with salt and black pepper. Serve chilled or at room temperature, alongside the muffins.

TOP TIPS

These muffins freeze brilliantly. Cool completely, then freeze in portions. Reheat in the oven at 300°F (fan) or in the microwave.

Try swapping sun-dried tomatoes for chopped olives, roasted peppers, or a spoonful of dairy-free pesto.

Change the flavors to suit. This works brilliantly with salmon and dill, or you can make this completely vegetarian by adding more vegetables.

NUTRITIONAL INFORMATION *(Per Serving)*

Calories 495Kcals   ○   Net carbohydrates 39.1g   ○   Fiber 13.9g   ○   Fat 23.4g   ○   Protein 32.1g

These frittata muffins have had an anti-inflammatory makeover. Full of Mediterranean flavors and paired with a nutty quinoa salad, this is the perfect lunch, packed full of protein and easily batched ahead of time. The sun-dried tomatoes and fresh herbs give these muffins a beautiful pop of color and richness, and they keep very well in the freezer—bonus!

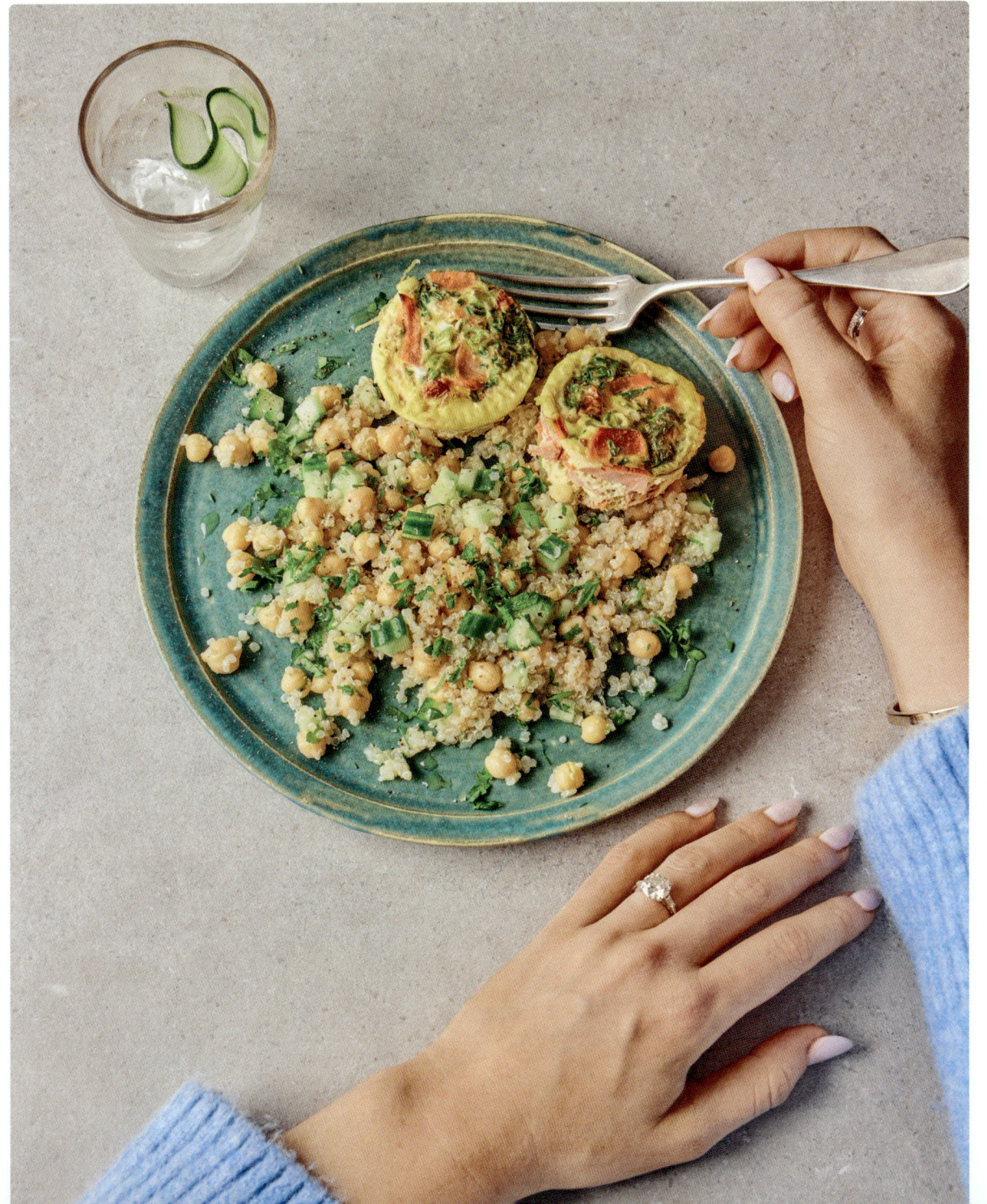

These speedy Thai Salmon Cakes are filled to the brim with flavor, protein, and healthy fats, ideal for lunch or dinner (I snack on them, too!). Served with a crunchy rainbow salad and a zingy dressing, you can prep these cakes well in advance and keep them in the fridge or freezer for a quick and easy meal throughout the week. It's a recipe I know you'll have on rinse and repeat.

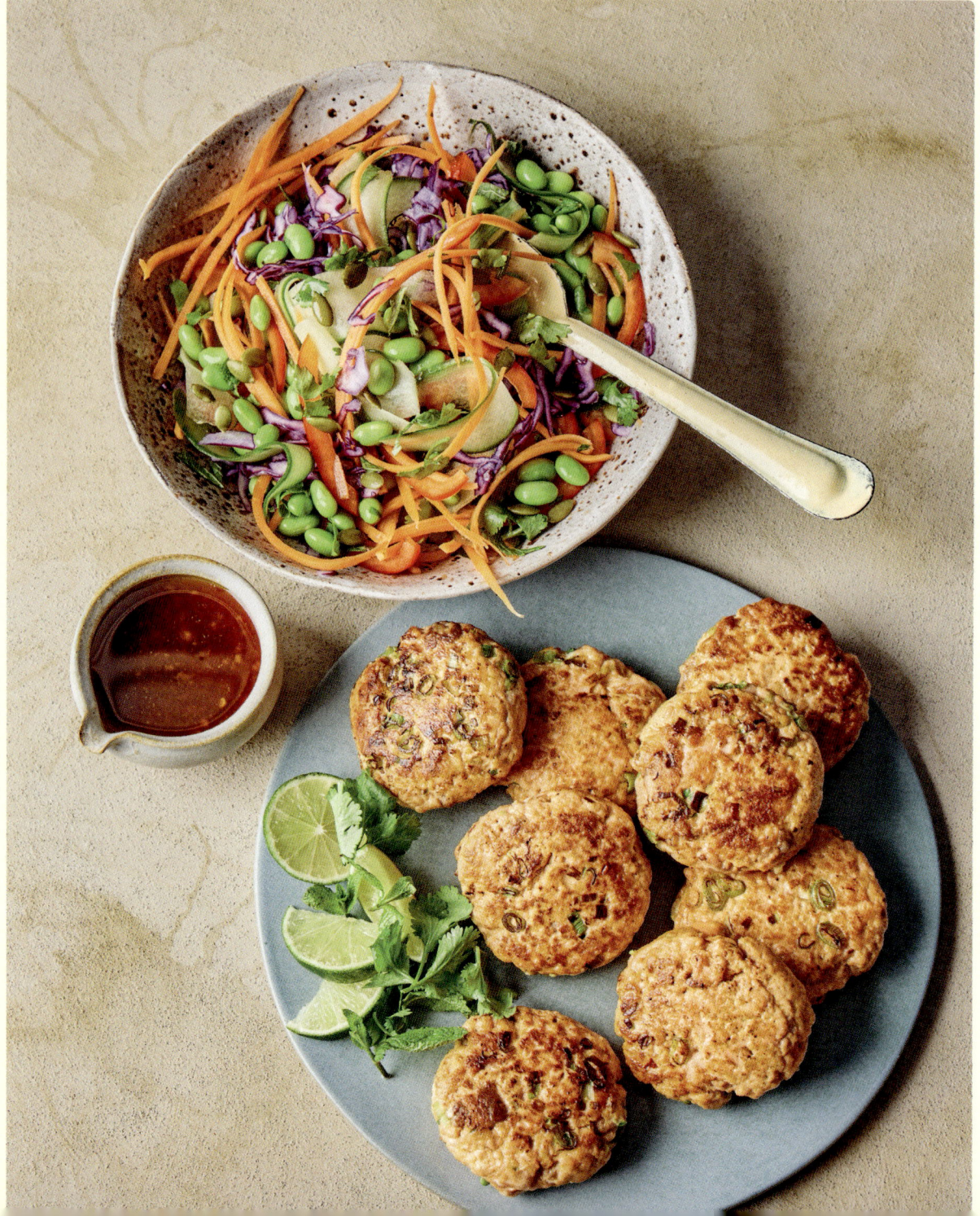

Thai Salmon Cakes

with Rainbow Crunch Salad

SERVES 4 ○ HIGH PROTEIN, HIGH OMEGA-3, FREEZER FRIENDLY

INGREDIENTS

17.6oz/500g fresh salmon fillets, skin removed
1 egg
½ a bunch of green onions, roughly chopped, including greens
2 tbsp Thai red curry paste
1 tsp lemongrass paste
zest of 1 lime
juice of ½ a lime
1 tbsp fish sauce
sea salt and freshly ground black pepper
1-2 tbsp coconut flour or chickpea flour (if needed)
olive oil

For the salad
1 carrot, cut into ribbons
½ a red pepper, finely sliced
¼ of a red cabbage, finely shredded
½ a cucumber, cut into ribbons
¾ cup/100g edamame
1 tbsp pumpkin seeds
a handful of fresh mint
a handful of fresh cilantro

For the dressing
1 tbsp sweet chili sauce
1 tsp tamari
juice of ½ a lime
1 tsp olive oil

Place the salmon, egg, green onions, Thai red curry paste, lemongrass paste, lime zest and juice, fish sauce, salt, and black pepper in a food processor and pulse in single bursts until the mix starts to come together. Don't over-blend—you want to retain some texture rather than create a purée. If the mix is too wet, add a little of your chosen flour.

Divide the mixture into 8 patties. Place on a sheet and chill for 10-15 minutes in the fridge to allow them time to firm up.

When ready to cook, heat a little olive oil in a sauté pan, add the fish cakes and cook on each side for 4-5 minutes, until golden.

While these are cooking, mix all of the salad ingredients in a large bowl. Mix the dressing ingredients in a small jug, then drizzle over the salad.

Place 2 salmon cakes on each plate with a generous portion of salad.

TOP TIPS

You can freeze the fish cakes raw on a sheet, then transfer to a bag or container. Defrost thoroughly before cooking.

You can swap the fresh salmon for canned (two 3.7oz/105g cans, drained). Reduce or omit the egg depending on the moisture, and add a tablespoon of flour if needed to bind.

GRAIN BOOSTERS

If you want to significantly increase the carbohydrates, you can add a grain of your choice to the salad.

1 cup/150g of cooked basmati rice—39.8g carbs (4g protein)

¾ cup/125g of cooked quinoa—23.5g carbs (4.9g protein)

¾ cup/120g of cooked buckwheat—16.9g carbs, (3.3g protein)

SERVING OPTIONS

Add a spoonful of kimchi or pickled veg on the side for an extra gut-friendly punch.

NUTRITIONAL INFORMATION *(Per Serving)*

Calories 523Kcals ○ Net carbohydrates 10.9g ○ Fiber 5.2g ○ Fat 35.5g ○ Protein 38.1g

Spanish Tortilla & Romesco Dip

SERVES 2   ○   HIGH PROTEIN, GRAIN-FREE

INGREDIENTS

- 1 tbsp olive oil
- 1 sweet potato, peeled and very thinly sliced
- 1 small red onion, finely sliced
- 1½ cups/50g baby-leaf spinach
- 4 eggs
- sea salt and freshly ground black pepper
- 1 tsp dried oregano
- arugula

For the romesco dip

- ½ cup/100g jarred roasted red peppers, drained
- 2 tbsp/15g almonds
- 1 clove of garlic
- 1 tbsp olive oil
- 1 tbsp lemon juice
- a pinch of smoked paprika
- sea salt and freshly ground black pepper, to taste

Heat the oil in a sauté pan. Sauté the sweet potato and red onion for 5–7 minutes, until softened.

Add the spinach and cook for 1–2 minutes, until wilted.

Whisk the eggs with a pinch of salt and black pepper and the oregano. Pour the eggs over the vegetables and stir very gently to combine.

Put a lid on your pan and leave the tortilla to cook slowly on a low heat for 15–20 minutes. When cooked, the base and edges should be golden and you should be able to flip it over easily without it falling apart. An easy way to do this is to place a plate over the pan, hold it securely and flip. Once flipped, slide it back into the pan for another few minutes until thoroughly cooked. If flipping feels tricky, you can finish it under the broiler for a couple of minutes instead.

While the tortilla is cooking, place all the dip ingredients in a blender and blend until smooth. Add a splash of water if necessary to get your desired consistency.

Remove the tortilla from the pan and cut into wedges. Serve hot or cold, with arugula and a generous dollop of romesco.

TOP TIPS

Add leftover cooked chicken or chickpeas for extra protein.

Swap the almonds for sunflower seeds to make the dip nut-free.

NUTRITIONAL INFORMATION *(Per Serving)*

Calories 419Kcals   ○   Net carbohydrates 24.1g   ○   Fiber 6.2g   ○   Fat 28.4g   ○   Protein 17.3g

This wholesome Spanish-inspired tortilla is packed with eggs, sweet potato, red onion, and spinach and is served with a vibrant romesco dip made from roasted red peppers, garlic, and almonds. It's simple to prepare and is ideal hot or cold for lunch, meal prep, or picnics.

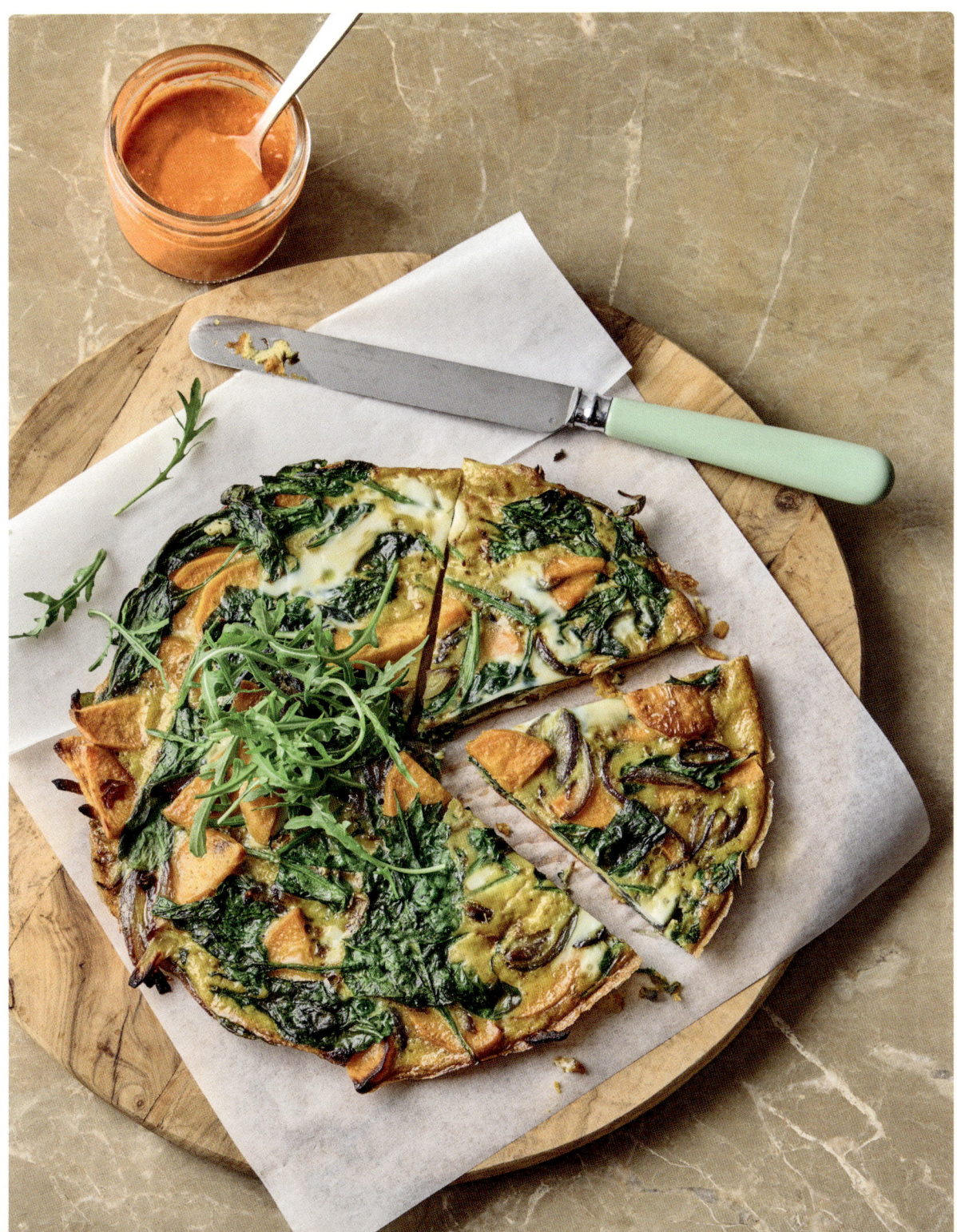

Main meal

S

Yes, food needs to be tasty, but it needs to have substance, too! This comforting spin on a family favorite delivers not only on taste, but also on nutrition—keeping you fuller for longer. You've got the classic hearty meaty sauce that's been jazzed up with extra nutrients from walnuts, fresh vegetables, and a hint of balsamic vinegar, tossed over zucchini spaghetti (don't knock it until you try it!), so you get all the goodness of a traditional spaghetti bol, without the heaviness of pasta!

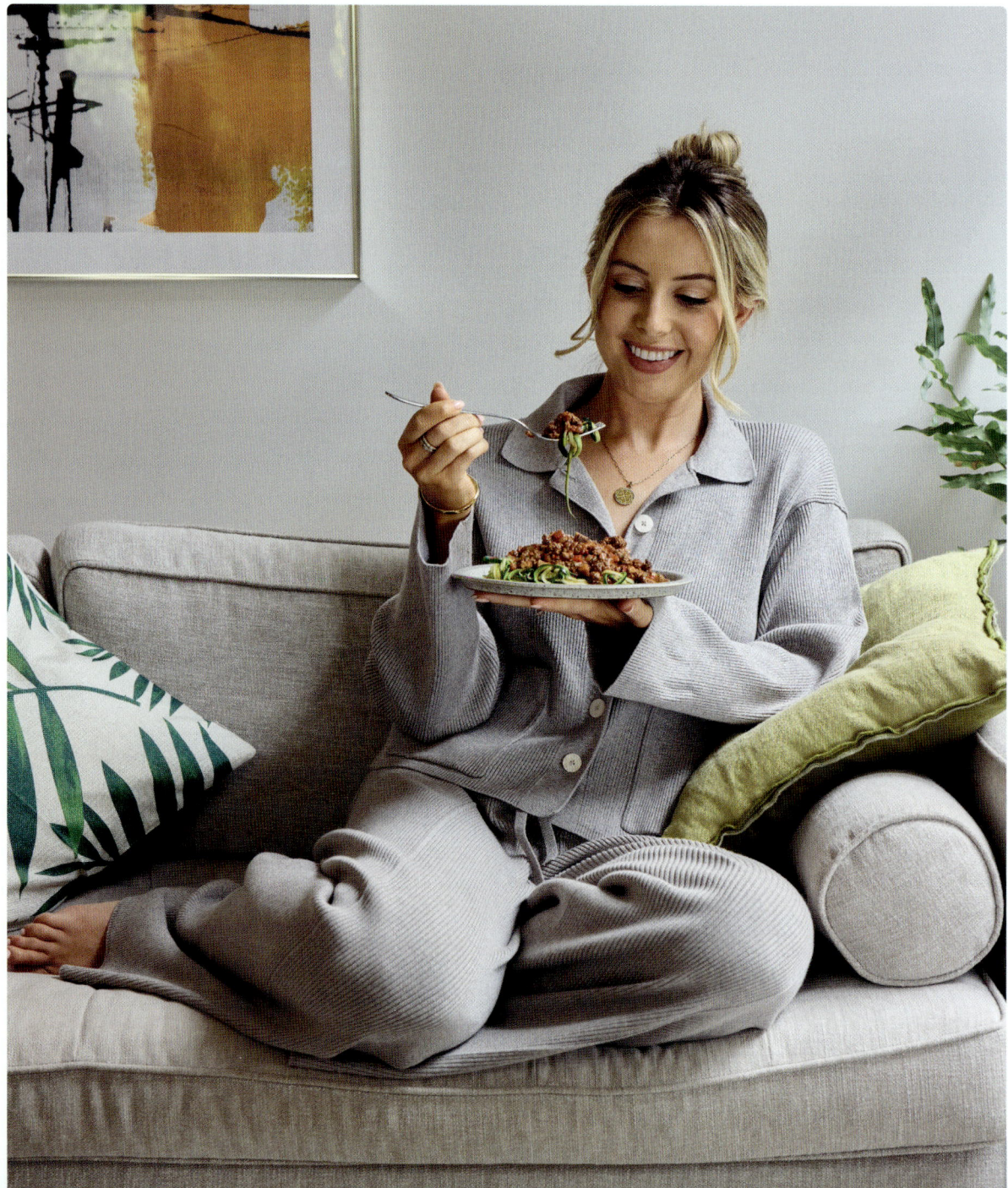

Rich & Nutritious Zucchini Bolognese

SERVES 4 ○ HIGH PROTEIN, GRAIN-FREE, NUTRIENT DENSE

INGREDIENTS

- 1 tsp coconut oil or olive oil
- 1 red onion, finely chopped
- 1 carrot, finely diced
- 1 celery stalk, finely diced
- 2–3 cloves of garlic, finely chopped
- 1 red pepper, finely chopped
- ⅔ cup/100g diced pancetta
- 2½ cups/400g ground beef
- ½ cup/50g walnuts, finely chopped
- ¾ cup/200ml beef bone stock (or red wine)
- One 14oz/400g can of chopped tomatoes
- 1 tbsp tomato paste
- ¾ cup/75g mushrooms, diced
- 1 heaped tsp dried oregano
- ½ tsp paprika
- ½ tsp dried thyme
- 1 tbsp balsamic vinegar
- ½ tsp ground cinnamon
- sea salt and freshly ground black pepper, to taste
- about 2 medium zucchini
- chile flakes (optional)

To garnish *(Optional)*
- dairy-free Parmesan
- a sprinkle of Savoury Soft Crumble (page 300)

Heat the coconut oil or olive oil in a sauté pan over medium heat. Add the onion, carrot, and celery and cook for 5 minutes, stirring occasionally. Add the garlic and red pepper and cook for another 2 minutes, until softened.

Stir in the pancetta and ground beef, cooking until browned. Add the walnuts, then the stock, and bring to a gentle simmer.

Stir in the chopped tomatoes, tomato paste, mushrooms, oregano, paprika, thyme, balsamic vinegar, cinnamon, salt, and black pepper. Lower the heat and simmer for 15–20 minutes, stirring occasionally.

While the Bolognese is cooking, spiralize the zucchini. You should have 4 cups/400g noodles. Put them in a colander, sprinkle with salt, and leave them for 10 minutes to help remove excess liquid.

When ready to serve, lightly toss the noodles with olive oil and black pepper, then heat a small sauté pan and cook them for 3–5 minutes. to soften. You can add some chile flakes if you like a bit of heat.

Place the zucchini on the plates and top with the Bolognese. If you like, scatter with dairy-free Parmesan or a spoonful of Savoury Soft Crumble over the top.

TOP TIPS

Add extra vitamins and minerals by mixing in some minced chicken liver with your ground beef.

The Bolognese sauce can be stored in the fridge for up to 3 days or frozen for up to 3 months.

The Bolognese base can be used to make a healthy lasagne. Swap pasta sheets for butternut squash sheets. To make a dairy-free white sauce, blend cooked cauliflower with unsweetened almond milk, garlic, nutritional yeast, and a touch of olive oil until smooth. Layer with the Bolognese and bake until golden and bubbling.

NUTRITIONAL INFORMATION *(Per Serving)*

Calories 386Kcals ○ Net carbohydrates 14.9 g ○ Fiber 5g ○ Fat 22.1g ○ Protein 32.5g

Salade Niçoise

SERVES 2 ○ HIGH OMEGA, HIGH PROTEIN, HIGH FIBER, GRAIN-FREE

INGREDIENTS

- 5 new potatoes
- ½ cup/50g asparagus tips
- 2 eggs
- ½ tbsp capers, rinsed and chopped
- ½ tsp Dijon mustard
- ½ tsp apple cider vinegar
- juice of ¼ of a lemon
- ¼ tsp honey (optional)
- 1–2 tbsp extra virgin olive oil
- sea salt and freshly ground black pepper
- 2 fresh tuna steaks (approx. 5.3oz/150g each)
- 2 to 3 cups/50g mixed salad greens
- 5 cherry tomatoes, halved
- ¼ of a red onion, very finely sliced
- ¼ cup/30g Kalamata olives, pitted and halved
- a small handful of fresh mint, finely chopped
- a small handful of flat-leaf parsley, finely chopped

Steam the new potatoes for 15–20 minutes, until tender. In the final 2–3 minutes, add the asparagus tips to the steamer. Once just tender, plunge the asparagus into a bowl of cold water to retain its bright color. Set the potatoes aside to cool slightly.

While the potatoes are cooking, boil the eggs for 8 minutes. When cooked, place the saucepan under the cold tap and continue to run the water until the eggs cool. This will help with peeling and will also prevent them from continuing to cook.

In a small bowl or jar, whisk together the capers, Dijon mustard, vinegar, lemon juice, honey (if using) and olive oil. Season with salt and black pepper to taste.

Brush the tuna with olive oil and season with black pepper. Heat a frying pan over a medium-high heat and sear the tuna for 1–2 minutes each side for medium-rare, or longer if you prefer the tuna cooked through. Let rest for 1 minute, then slice thickly.

Arrange the salad greens on a large platter. Scatter over the cooled potatoes, cherry tomatoes, red onion, olives, blanched asparagus, chopped herbs, and halved eggs. Top with the sliced tuna and drizzle over the dressing and sprinkle with parsley. Serve immediately.

TOP TIPS

Make ahead: The eggs, potatoes, dressing, and even the tuna can be prepped in advance—serve cold or at room temperature.

Vary it: Swap the tuna for grilled salmon or leftover roast chicken.

Vegan twist: Try marinated grilled tofu or tempeh, and skip the eggs.

New potatoes have the lowest amount of starch (sugars) of all the potato family. Sweet potatoes have the highest (hence the name), so new potatoes are a better option for those wishing to reduce inflammation and lower blood sugar.

NUTRITIONAL INFORMATION *(Per Serving)*

Calories 414Kcals ○ Net carbohydrates 12.3g ○ Fiber 3.1g ○ Fat 19.7g ○ Protein 47g

This isn't your everyday salad . . . this is the ULTIMATE feel-good feast! A fresh take on the classic Niçoise salad, this recipe is packed with protein, healthy fats, and fiber, while giving all of the Mediterranean vibes. The seared tuna steak packs a protein punch, while the salad gives you a pop of color that's not only great to look at, but feeds your gut, too. It's easy enough to throw together for a weekday lunch, but fancy enough for your next dinner party!

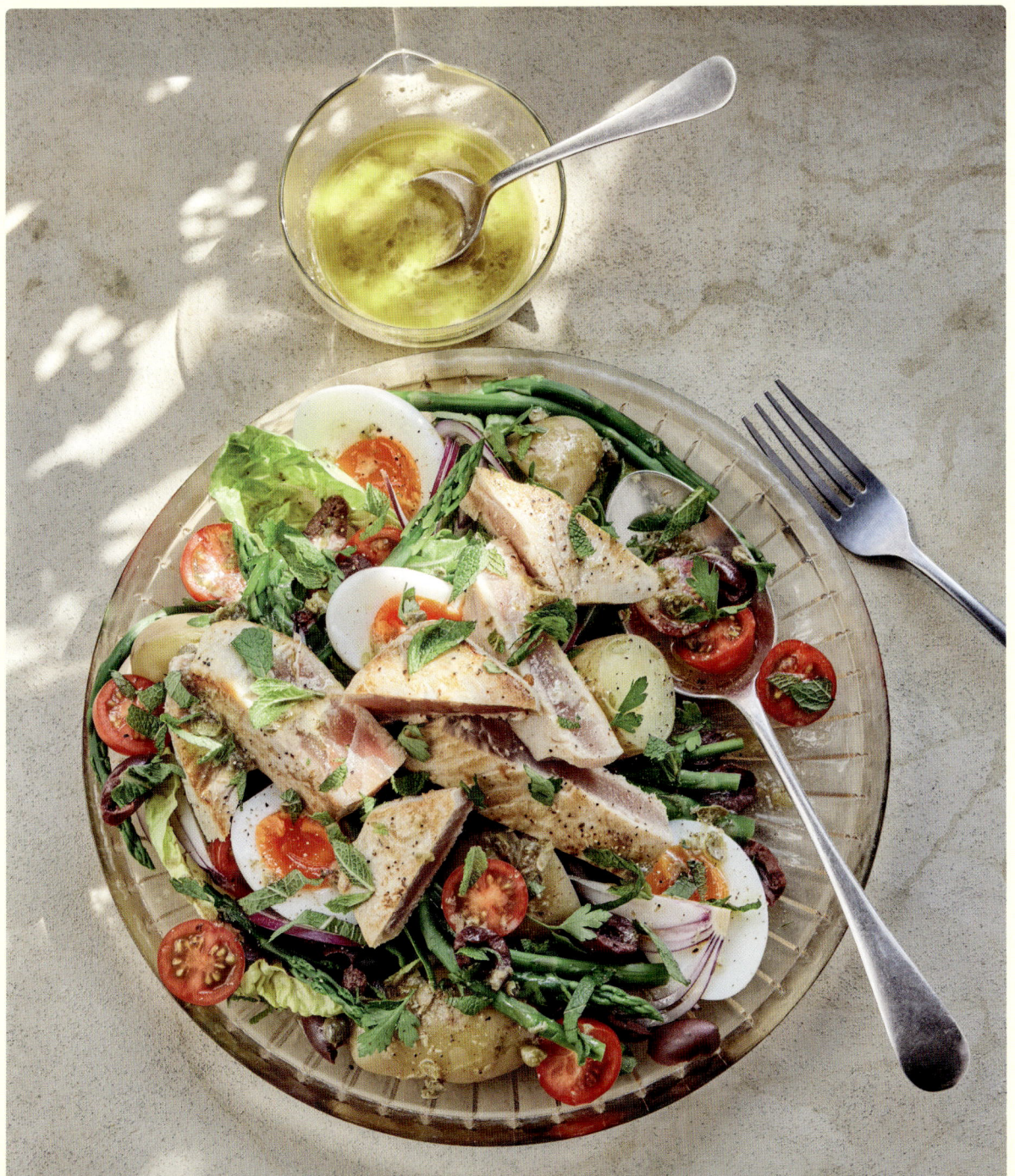

This curry is rich, cozy, and packed with flavor—and gives you a little taste of Malaysian-style cuisine. It's got melt-in-your-mouth beef, creamy coconut-spice sauce, and it honestly couldn't be easier. Everything goes into a blender and one pot! Serve it with fluffy coconut cauliflower rice, and this high-protein grain-free recipe will be a winner. FYI: like with most curries . . . it tastes even better the next day.

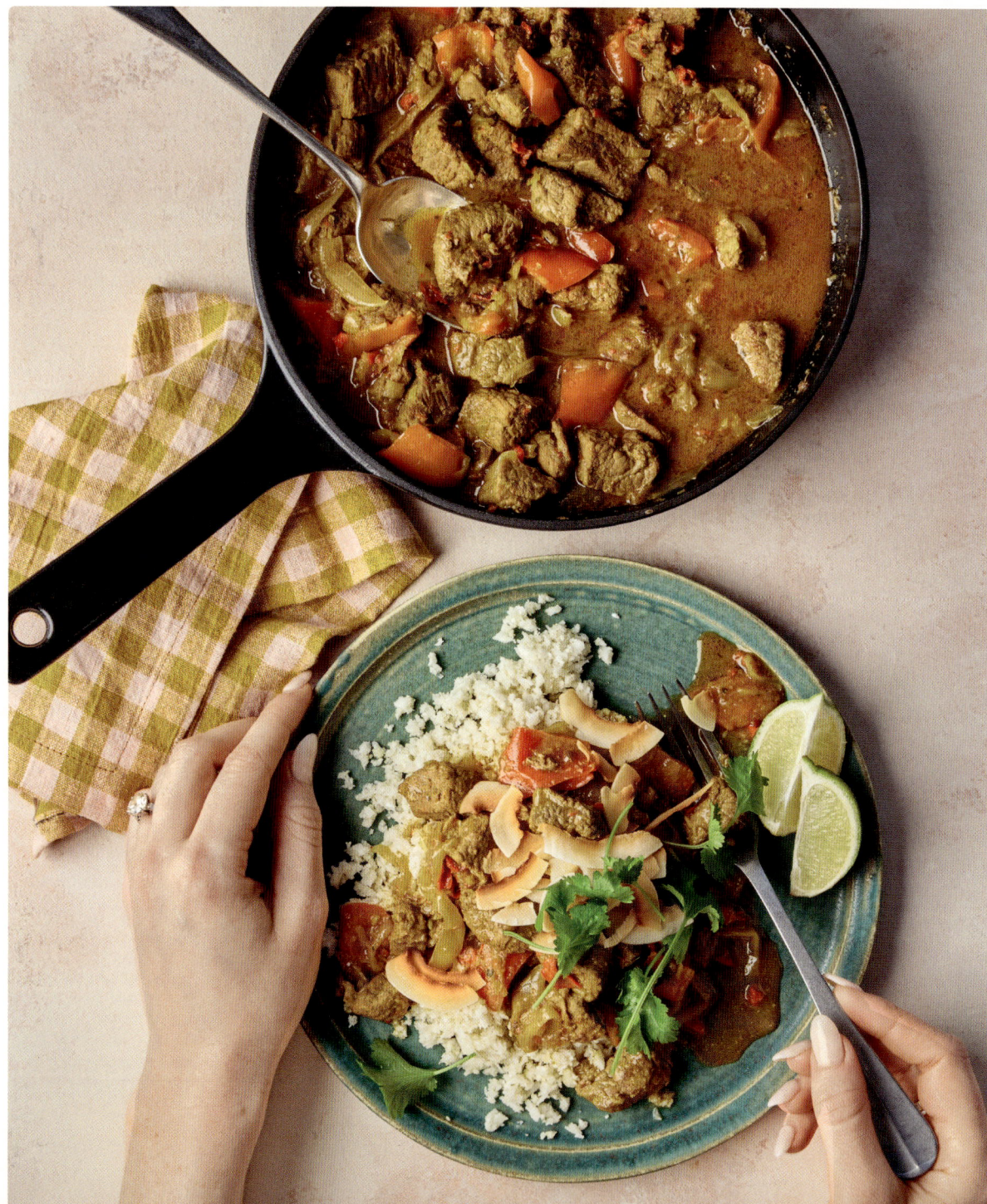

Fragrant Beef Rendang
with Coconut Cauliflower Rice

SERVES 4 ○ HIGH PROTEIN, GRAIN-FREE

INGREDIENTS

For the curry paste
1½in/4cm piece of fresh ginger, peeled
4 cloves of garlic, peeled
3 red chiles, deseeded
2 lemongrass stalks, tough outer layer removed
1½in/4cm fresh galangal
seeds from 4 cardamom pods
4 kaffir lime leaves
1 tsp fennel seeds
2 tsp coriander seeds
1 tsp cumin seeds
zest and juice of 1 lime
2 tsp ground cinnamon
½ tsp ground ginger
1 tsp ground turmeric
1 tbsp honey
One 13.5oz/400ml can of full-fat coconut milk

2 tsp coconut oil
750g stewing steak or beef shin, diced
1 large onion, thickly sliced
2 red peppers, cut into chunks
30g unsweetened coconut flakes, toasted
a handful of fresh cilantro, chopped

For the coconut cauliflower rice
1 small cauliflower, cut into florets
1 tsp coconut oil
1 tbsp desiccated coconut
a pinch of sea salt
a squeeze of lime juice

Put all the curry paste ingredients into a food processor or blender and blend until smooth. Set aside.

Heat the coconut oil in a large, heavy-based pan on medium heat, and brown the beef in batches for 3–4 minutes until well seared. Set aside.

Using the same pan, reduce the heat to medium and add the onion. Cook for a few minutes until soft, then add the red peppers and cook for another 2 minutes.

Stir in the curry paste and cook for a few minutes to release the fragrance and deepen the flavor.

Add the beef and stir everything until evenly coated. Bring to a simmer, then reduce to a low heat. Cover and simmer gently for 2–3 hours, stirring occasionally, until the beef is meltingly tender.

While the beef is slow cooking, place the coconut flakes in a dry frying pan and toast gently over a medium heat until golden. Shake often to avoid burning. Set aside to cool.

Prepare the coconut cauliflower rice. Blitz the cauliflower in a food processor until it resembles rice. Heat 1 tsp of coconut oil in a large frying pan. Add the cauliflower rice, desiccated coconut, and a pinch of salt. Sauté over a medium heat for 4–5 minutes, stirring frequently. Finish with a squeeze of lime.

When the beef is ready, serve with the coconut cauliflower rice and garnish with the toasted coconut and chopped fresh cilantro.

TOP TIPS
The paste can be frozen for up to 3 months.
No galangal? Use more ginger and an extra squeeze of lime.

GRAIN BOOSTERS
For those who can tolerate grains you can use:
Jasmine rice—slightly sticky and fragrant.
Basmati rice—lighter and fluffier, slightly lower GI than jasmine.

NUTRITIONAL INFORMATION *(Per Serving)*

Calories 594Kcals ○ Net carbohydrates 24.3g ○ Fiber 7.5g ○ Fat 33.8g ○ Protein 48.6g

Smoky Chorizo Beef

SERVES 4 ○ HIGH PROTEIN, GRAIN-FREE

INGREDIENTS

- 1 tbsp olive oil
- 3.5oz/100g chorizo, diced
- 1lb 2oz/500g stewing beef
- 1 onion, finely chopped
- 1 red pepper, roughly chopped
- 2 cloves of garlic, minced
- 1 red chile, deseeded and finely chopped
- ½ tsp dried oregano
- 1 tsp smoked paprika
- 1 tsp ground cumin
- 1 tsp ground coriander
- ½ tsp ground cinnamon
- 1 tbsp tomato paste
- One 14oz/400g can of good-quality chopped tomatoes
- 1 cup plus 1 tbsp/250ml beef bone broth (or beef stock)
- ⅔ cup/150ml red wine (optional but adds depth—if not used, add ⅔ cup/150ml more stock)
- 1 tbsp apple cider vinegar
- 1 tbsp coconut aminos
- 1 bay leaf
- sea salt and freshly ground black pepper, to taste
- 2 tbsp/20g 85% dark chocolate, finely chopped

Heat the olive oil in a large pan. Over medium heat, add the chorizo and cook for 2 minutes until it releases its oils. Add the beef and continue to cook until all sides are browned. Remove the meat from the pan, retaining the oil.

Add the onion and red pepper to the oil in the pan and soften for 2–3 minutes, then add the garlic, chile, herbs, and spices.

Stir for 1 minute to heat the spices and release the flavors, then add the remaining ingredients (apart from the dark chocolate), along with the beef and chorizo. Season to taste with salt and black pepper.

Bring to a gentle simmer, then turn the heat to low, and continue to cook for 2–2½ hours, until the beef is tender. (Other options: place it in the oven at 300°F for 2–3 hours, or in your slow cooker for 6 hours on low and 4 hours on high.)

Add the dark chocolate in the last 10 minutes before serving and stir well until fully melted.

TOP TIPS

Can be batch cooked and frozen for up to 3 months.

You can adjust the chile to taste. This is a mild heat, as I have removed the seeds, allowing the flavor of the other spices to come through.

SERVING OPTIONS

I recommend serving with cauliflower rice with fresh cilantro, lime zest, and avocado slices, but you could swap it for your choice of grain, sautéed greens, potato wedges, or gluten-free flatbreads.

Optional: dairy-free coconut yogurt for topping.

NUTRITIONAL INFORMATION *(Per Serving)*

Calories 413Kcals ○ Net carbohydrates 10.6g ○ Fiber 3.7g ○ Fat 21g ○ Protein 38.9g

Get ready for your kitchen to smell like pure heaven! This dish is rich, smoky, and full of flavor, with slow-cooked beef packed with deep earthy flavors, a hint of dark chocolate (trust me—it's insane), and chorizo for an extra punch. It's comfort food with a little bit of spice, and perfect for when you want a hearty meal without the heaviness.

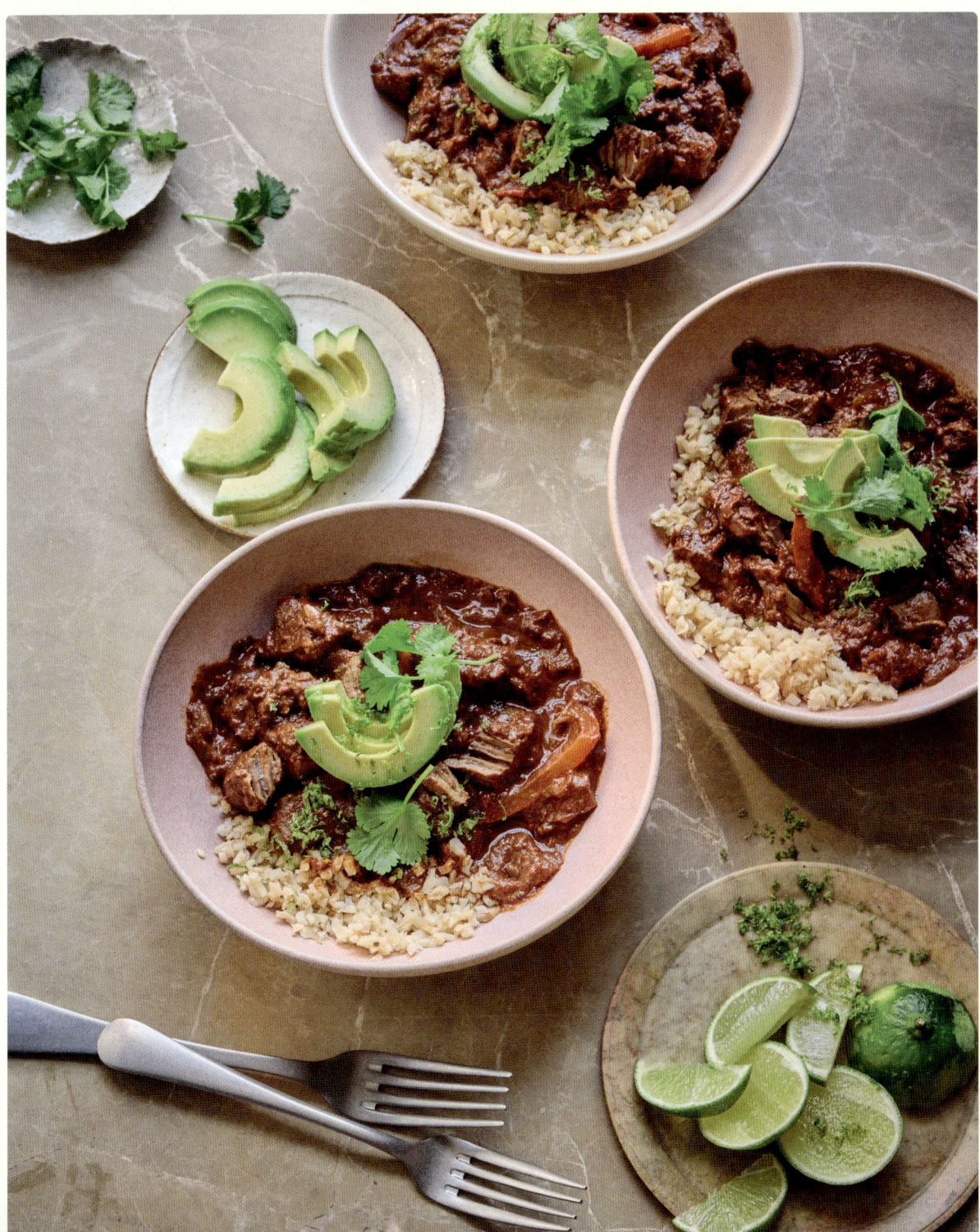

A quick and easy, nutrient-dense twist on the traditional egg fried rice. Using cauliflower instead of rice can help those who are grain-sensitive, without losing any of the protein punch or taste. Great on its own, or as a side to some juicy chicken.

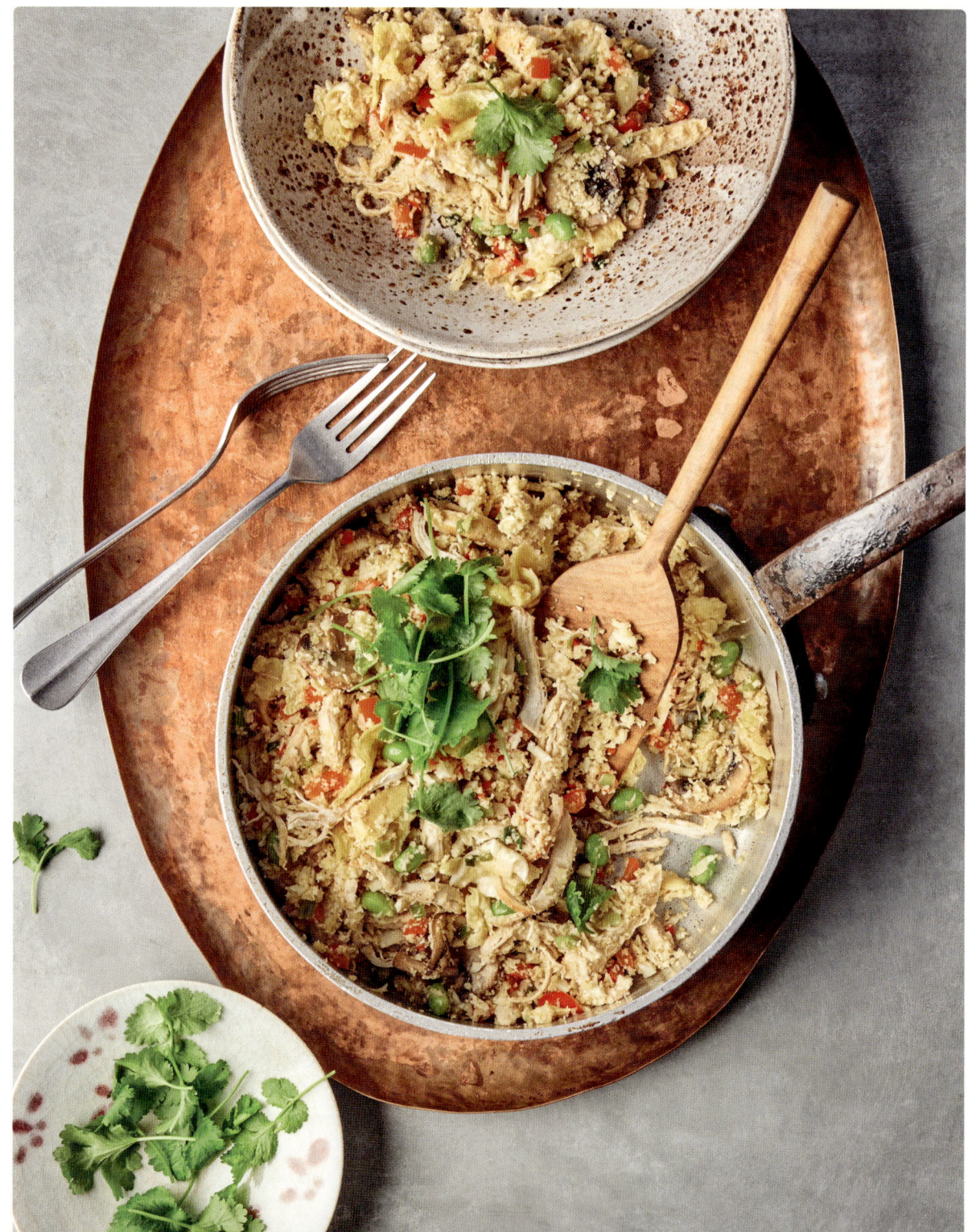

High-Protein Cauli-Egg Fried Rice

SERVES 2　○　HIGH PROTEIN, GRAIN-FREE

INGREDIENTS

- 1 tbsp coconut or olive oil
- 1 to 1⅛ inches fresh ginger, peeled and grated
- 1 red chile, deseeded and finely chopped
- 1 clove of garlic, crushed
- 3 green onions, finely sliced, including greens
- ½ a red pepper, finely chopped
- 3 medium eggs
- 3½ cups/300g cauliflower rice (you can use frozen, defrosted)
- ¾ cup/75g cremini mushrooms, sliced
- a handful of edamame beans
- 1 tbsp tamari
- 7oz/200g shredded cooked chicken (or try salmon, tuna, tempeh, marinated tofu)
- sea salt and freshly ground black pepper

To garnish
chopped red chiles
fresh cilantro

Heat the oil in a large wok or sauté pan.

Add the ginger, chile, garlic, green onions, and red pepper. Cook for a couple of minutes to soften, then remove from the pan.

Add a little more oil if needed. Add the eggs and scramble until only just softly set.

Add the cauliflower rice, onion mix, mushrooms, edamame beans, tamari, and your chosen protein and stir-fry for 3–4 minutes, until heated through.

Season to taste with salt and black pepper and sprinkle with extra chiles and fresh cilantro before serving.

GRAIN BOOSTERS

If you can tolerate grains, you can swap the cauliflower rice for a grain of your choice.

Basmati rice will increase carbs by 41g.

Buckwheat will increase carbs by 26g.

Quinoa will increase carbs by 28g.

NUTRITIONAL INFORMATION *(Per Serving)*

Calories 401Kcals　○　Net carbohydrates 7.9g　○　Fiber 7.5g　○　Fat 17.5g　○　Protein 49.8g

Grilled Spiced Salmon

with Coconut-Lime Drizzle

SERVES 4 ○ HIGH OMEGA, HIGH PROTEIN

INGREDIENTS

For the sweet potatoes
2 sweet potatoes, cut into wedges
1 tbsp melted coconut oil
2 tbsp lime juice
a pinch of ground cinnamon
sea salt and freshly ground black pepper

For the yogurt drizzle
⅔ cup/150ml thick coconut yogurt or coconut cream
2 tbsp lime juice
1 tsp lime pickle (optional)
1 small clove of garlic, grated
½ tsp honey
a pinch of sea salt

For the salmon
1 tbsp olive oil
1 tsp fresh ginger, peeled and grated
½ tsp ground cumin
½ tsp ground coriander
zest of 1 lime
freshly ground black pepper
4 salmon fillets (approx. 7oz/200g each)

To garnish
1 tbsp chopped fresh cilantro
6 cups/120g arugula or baby-leaf spinach
extra lime wedges

Preheat the oven to 375°F (fan).

Put the sweet potatoes into a bowl and add the coconut oil, lime juice, and cinnamon. Season to taste with salt and black pepper. Combine well to ensure the potatoes are evenly coated. Bake in the oven for 25–30 minutes, until golden, turning halfway through to ensure they are evenly cooked.

While the sweet potatoes are cooking, prepare the drizzle by mixing the yogurt with the lime juice, lime pickle (if using), garlic, honey, and salt to taste. Leave to chill in the fridge.

In a small bowl, mix the oil, ginger, cumin, coriander, lime zest, and black pepper to form a paste. Brush this over your salmon fillets. Heat your griddle or grill (or sauté pan) and cook for 3–4 minutes on each side, or until cooked to your liking.

Remove the sweet potatoes from the oven and garnish with the chopped cilantro. Serve the salmon with the roasted sweet potato wedges, a handful of arugula or baby-leaf spinach, extra lime wedges, and a generous drizzle of the coconut lime sauce.

TOP TIPS
The drizzle can be made up to 3 days ahead and stored in the fridge.
The salmon can be marinated and frozen raw in advance.
For a vegan version, swap the salmon for grilled tempeh or tofu, or cauliflower steaks.

GRAIN BOOSTER
You can serve this with rice instead of sweet potatoes.

SERVING OPTIONS
Swap the salmon for prawns or cod fillets if preferred.

NUTRITIONAL INFORMATION *(Per Serving)*

Calories 496Kcals ○ Net carbohydrates 18.3g ○ Fiber 4.2g ○ Fat 32.6g ○ Protein 33.1g

The definition of wholesome on a plate, this creamy, zingy, and tropical salmon dish has been on rinse and repeat in my house. The salmon is packed with anti-inflammatory omega-3 as well as protein, and the roasted sweet potato not only tastes delicious, but gives you a wonderful hit of healthy carbs and energy. The coconut lime drizzle? Well, let's just say you'll want to put it on everything. It's a proper show-off dinner that's secretly easy, naturally dairy- and gluten-free, and guaranteed to impress.

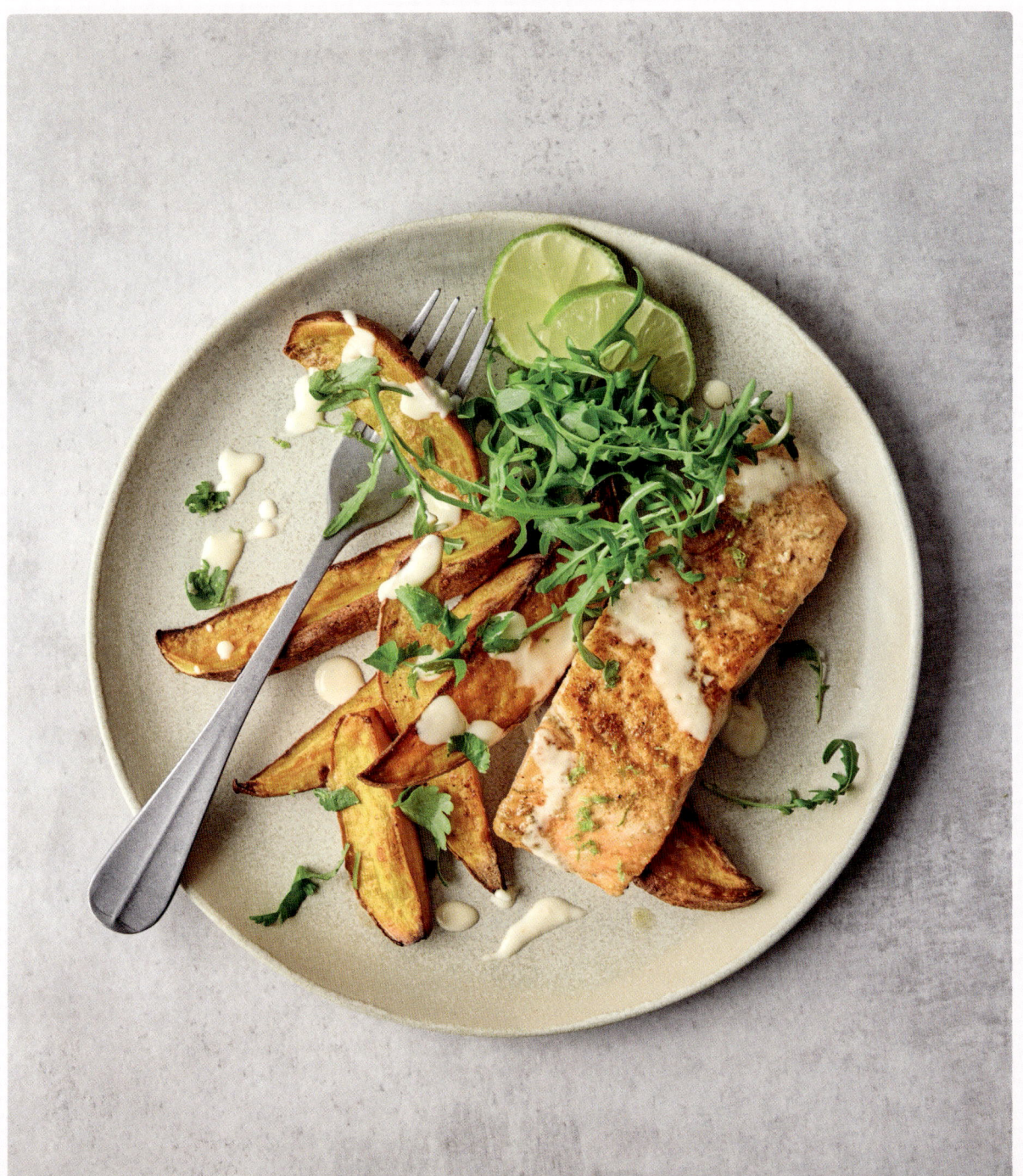

This is how a nut roast should REALLY taste. It's rich, warming, and packed with flavor, and will have even dedicated meat eaters coming back for seconds (or thirds!). Whether it's a special occasion or you want a satisfying plant-based dinner, it's the G.O.A.T of nut roasts—and as a bonus, it's freezer-friendly, too.

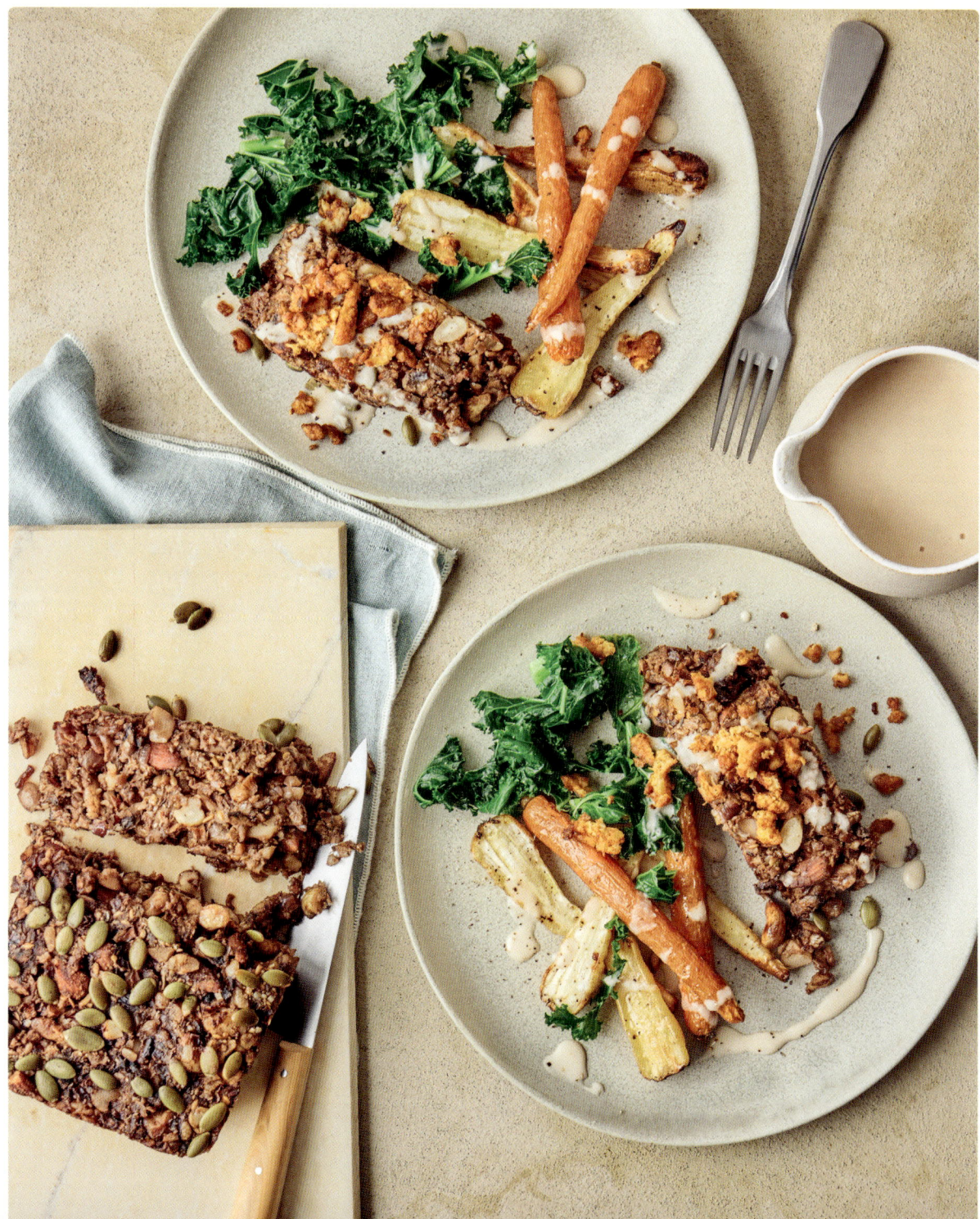

The Ultimate Nut Roast
with White Bean & Miso Dressing (optional Smoky Tempeh Crumble)

SERVES 6 ○ VEGAN, GRAIN-FREE

INGREDIENTS

- 2 tbsp flaxseeds
- 2 tbsp chia seeds
- 2 tbsp hemp seeds
- ⅓ cup/75ml of water
- 2 tsp coconut oil
- 1 red onion, finely chopped
- 2 cloves of garlic, crushed
- 2½ cups/250g mushrooms, chopped
- ⅔ cup/75g Brazil nuts, chopped
- ¾ cup/75g walnuts, chopped
- ¾ cup/75g almonds, chopped
- ½ cup/50g cashews, chopped
- 1 tsp dried oregano
- 1 tsp fresh thyme leaves (or ½ tsp dried)
- 2 tbsp nutritional yeast flakes (optional)
- 3 tsp yeast extract
- 1 tbsp balsamic vinegar
- 2 tbsp sun-dried tomatoes, finely chopped
- sea salt and freshly ground black pepper, to taste
- ¼ cup/25g ground almonds
- 2 tbsp/20g pumpkin seeds

For the dressing
- ½ cup/100g cannellini beans
- 1 tsp white miso
- ½ tsp garlic powder
- juice of ½ a lemon
- 1 tbsp olive oil
- 3 tbsp water (for adjusting to desired consistency)

To serve
Smoky Tempeh Crumble (see Protein Booster)

Preheat the oven to 375°F (fan). Line a loaf pan with parchment paper.

Place the flaxseeds, chia seeds, and hemp seeds in a small bowl and add ⅓ cup/75ml of water.

Heat the coconut oil in a pan, add the onion and garlic, and fry until soft and translucent. Stir in the mushrooms and cook until they release moisture and reduce in size.

Add the chopped nuts, oregano, thyme, nutritional yeast (if using), yeast extract, balsamic vinegar, and sun-dried tomatoes. Season to taste with salt and black pepper and cook for 5 minutes, stirring occasionally. Stir in the ground almonds and rehydrated seeds and mix well to combine.

Spoon into the lined pan, pressing down firmly. Top with the pumpkin seeds. Bake for 40 minutes, or until golden brown and firm to the touch.

Meanwhile, blend all the dressing ingredients until smooth, adding water as needed to reach the desired consistency.

Remove the nut roast from the oven and let it cool slightly before slicing—it holds together better this way! Serve drizzled with the dressing and optional smoky tempeh crumble.

TOP TIPS

To freeze before baking, wrap tightly in plastic wrap and foil and freeze for up to 3 months. Thaw overnight in the fridge before baking.

To freeze after baking, slice into portions, store in airtight containers, and freeze for up to 3 months. Reheat in the oven at 350°F (fan) for 10-15 minutes.

PROTEIN BOOSTERS

For an extra 6g of protein per serving, add this Smoky Tempeh Crumble. Heat 2 tsp of olive oil in a pan, then add 1 cup/200g of tempeh, seasoned with 1½ tsp of smoked paprika, 1 tsp of tamari, and 1 tsp of garlic powder. Cook over a medium heat for 5-7 minutes, until golden and crispy. Sprinkle over the nut roast before serving.

NUTRITIONAL INFORMATION *(Per Serving)*

Calories 446Kcals ○ Net carbohydrates 12.3g ○ Fiber 9.3g ○ Fat 36.4g ○ Protein 15.7g

Spiced Red Lentil Dahl
with Chickpea Flatbreads

SERVES 4   ○   VEGAN, HIGH FIBER

INGREDIENTS

For the flatbreads
2 cups/250g chickpea flour (gram flour)
½ tsp cumin seeds
½ tsp garlic powder
½ tsp sea salt, or to taste
1 tbsp olive oil (plus extra for cooking)
approx. 1½ cups/400ml warm water

For the dahl
1 tbsp coconut oil
1 large onion, finely chopped
2 cloves of garlic, crushed
1-inch piece of fresh ginger, peeled and grated
1 tsp ground cumin
1 tsp ground coriander
1 tsp garam masala
1 tsp ground turmeric
½ tsp chile flakes
¾ cup/200g red lentils, rinsed
One 13.5oz/400ml can of coconut milk
One 14oz/400g can of finely chopped tomatoes
2 cups plus 2 tbsp/500ml bone or vegetable stock
sea salt and freshly ground black pepper

To serve
Natural Live Coconut Yogurt (page 299)
flaked coconut
cilantro leaves

To make the flatbreads, place the flour, cumin seeds, garlic powder, and salt in a bowl.

Add the oil to the warm water and pour this into the dry ingredients. Stir well until combined. Set aside to rest to improve texture and digestibility, until ready to cook. The batter can be made several hours in advance.

Heat an oiled frying pan over medium heat. Cook each flatbread just like a pancake for 1–2 minutes, then flip over until both sides are golden. They can be made in advance and reheated when needed, or cooked fresh once the dahl is cooked.

To make the dahl, heat the oil in a saucepan over medium heat. Add the onion and sauté until soft and golden.

Add garlic, ginger, and spices. Stir for 1–2 minutes until fragrant.

Stir in the lentils, then pour in the coconut milk, tomatoes, and stock. Season to taste.

Bring to a gentle simmer.

Simmer on low heat, uncovered, for 20–25 minutes, stirring regularly to avoid sticking, until the lentils are soft and the dahl has thickened.

Serve warm, with coconut yogurt topping, flaked coconut, and fresh cilantro with the flatbreads alongside for dipping.

TOP TIPS

Add chopped fresh cilantro, flat-leaf parsley, or nigella seeds, to the flatbread batter for extra flavor.

Both the dahl and the flatbreads can be made ahead. Reheat the flatbreads in a dry pan or warm oven.

NUTRITIONAL INFORMATION *(Per Serving)*

Calories 653Kcals   ○   Net carbohydrates 72.5g   ○   Fiber 15.6g   ○   Fat 25.1g   ○   Protein 34.4g

Now **THIS** will be one of your favorites—I'm sure of it. This gently spiced red lentil dahl is the kind of recipe your friends will be begging for. It's super comforting, satisfying, and packed with plant protein and fiber. It's perfect either on its own, or served with my delicious chickpea flatbreads for scooping up that dahl goodness. Incredible for batch cooking, and even tastier the next day.

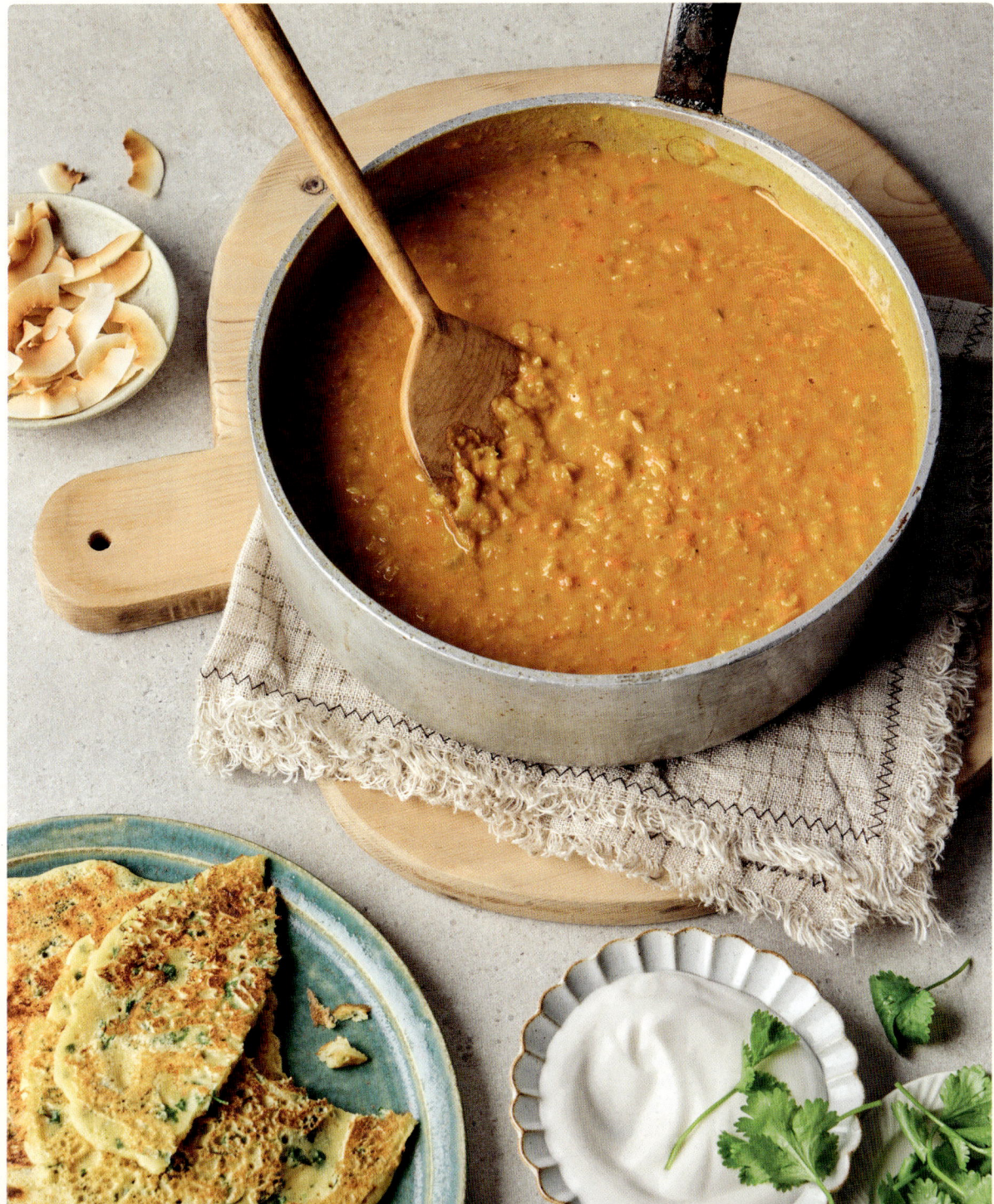

No more ordering Greek takeout—you've got everything you need right here! This Greek-style dish is perfect for any season, and the herby lamb chops can be paired with virtually anything. My preference is sweet roasted vine tomatoes, caramelized onions, and melt-in-your-mouth eggplant. It's packed with protein, rich in flavor, and so easy to prep!

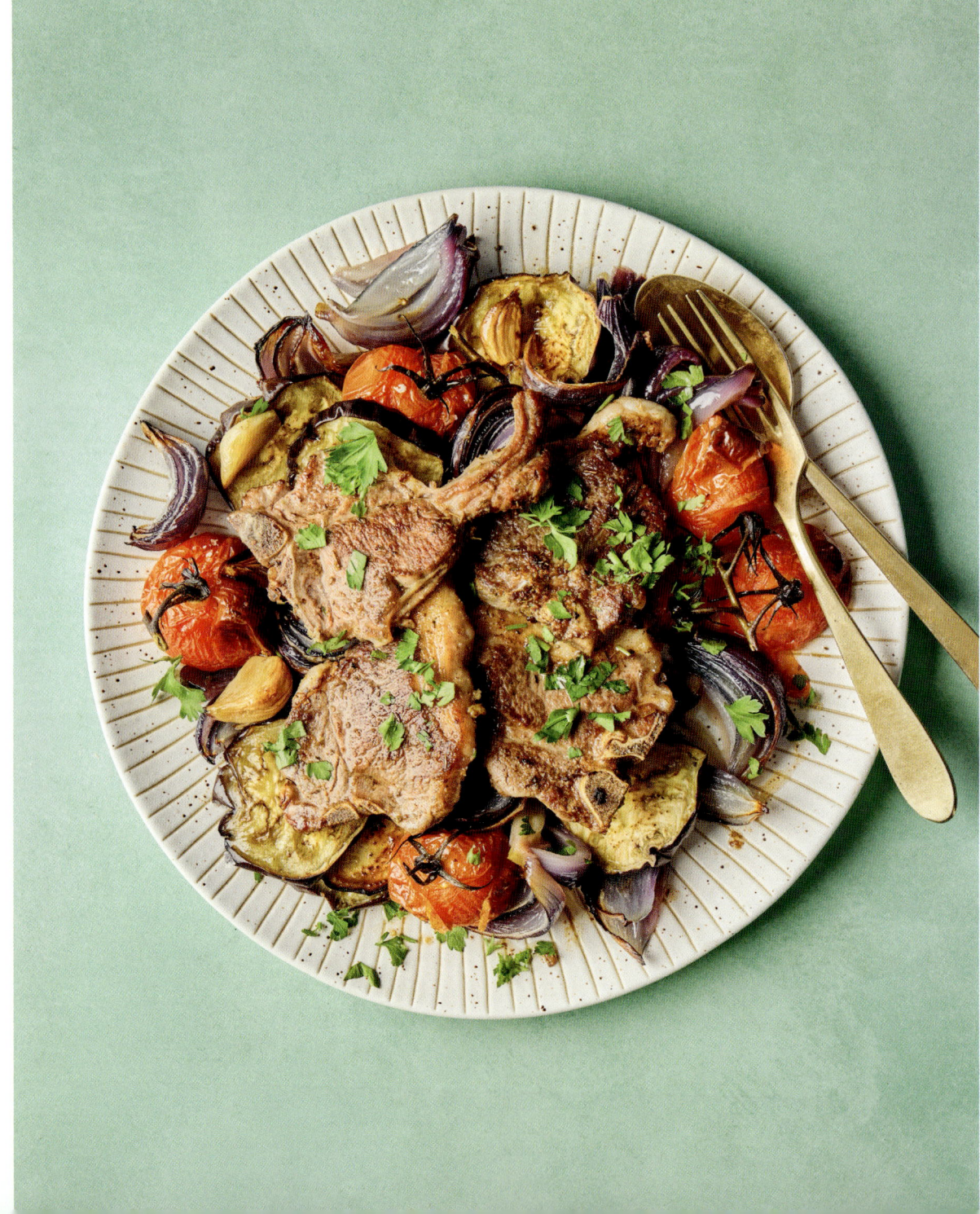

Greek-Style Lamb Chops

with Roasted Vegetables

SERVES 2   ◦   HIGH PROTEIN, GRAIN-FREE

INGREDIENTS

- 4 tbsp olive oil
- 2 cloves of garlic, crushed
- 1 tsp dried oregano
- 1 tsp dried thyme
- ½ tsp sea salt
- freshly ground black pepper, to taste
- 4 lamb chops (approx. 2⅔oz/75g each chop)
- 1 eggplant
- 2 red onions, cut into wedges
- 3-4 cloves of garlic, peeled
- 1½ cups/250g vine tomatoes, left whole

To garnish
chopped flat-leaf parsley

Put 2 tbsp of the olive oil into a small bowl with the garlic, herbs, salt, and black pepper to taste and combine well.

Rub the marinade all over the lamb chops and leave them to rest for at least 30 minutes. They can be left in the fridge overnight, but make sure they are covered.

Preheat the oven to 350°F (fan).

Chop the eggplant into thick slices and place in a roasting dish. Add the red onions, garlic, and vine tomatoes. Drizzle with the remaining 2 tbsp of olive oil and roast in the oven for 20-25 minutes.

Ten minutes before the vegetables finish roasting, heat a sauté pan over medium-high heat. Sear the lamb chops for 3-4 minutes per side, until golden or cooked to your liking.

Remove the vegetables from the oven and put them into your serving dish. Add the lamb chops and garnish with chopped parsley.

NUTRITIONAL INFORMATION *(Per Serving)*

Calories 545Kcals ◦ Net carbohydrates 10.3g ◦ Fiber 4.2g ◦ Fat 42.6g ◦ Protein 30g

Chimichurri Steak
with Grilled Vegetables

SERVES 2 ○ HIGH PROTEIN, GRAIN-FREE

INGREDIENTS

Two 7oz/200g sirloin or rib-eye steaks
1 tbsp olive oil
sea salt and freshly ground black pepper, to taste

For the chimichurri sauce
¼ cup/60ml extra virgin olive oil
juice of ½ a lemon
2 tbsp red wine vinegar
1 small jalapeño, finely chopped (optional for spice)
3 cloves of garlic, crushed
¾ cup/30g flat-leaf parsley, finely chopped
⅓ cup/10g fresh cilantro, finely chopped
½ tsp dried oregano
½ tsp smoked paprika
sea salt and freshly ground black pepper, to taste

For the grilled vegetables
1 zucchini, peeled into ribbons
1 red pepper, thickly sliced
1 small eggplant, thickly sliced
1 tbsp olive oil
½ tsp smoked paprika
½ tsp dried oregano
sea salt and freshly ground black pepper, to taste

To garnish
roasted pumpkin seeds

Remove the steaks from the fridge 30 minutes before cooking, to bring them to room temperature. Rub the steaks with olive oil, salt, and black pepper, and leave to rest.

Prepare the chimichurri by combining all the ingredients in a bowl. Stir well and set aside for at least 10 minutes to let the flavors infuse.

Preheat your grill and heat your sauté pan. We are aiming to cook the steak and the vegetables simultaneously, but if that is challenging for you, cook the vegetables first, and cover them with foil to keep warm while you cook the steak.

Toss the zucchini, red pepper, and eggplant slices with the olive oil, smoked paprika, oregano, salt, and black pepper. Grill over medium heat for 3–5 minutes per side, until slightly charred and tender.

While the vegetables are grilling, heat your sauté pan over high heat. Sear the steaks for 2–3 minutes per side for medium-rare, or longer if desired.

While the steaks rest, make sure the vegetables are cooked to your liking.

Serve immediately sprinkled with pumpkin seeds and enjoy!

TOP TIPS

This recipe serves 2 to deliver a higher-protein meal, ideal post-workout, but it could serve 4 if you want a lighter meal.

Chimichurri sauce tastes even better after a few hours in the fridge. It is also delicious with other dishes, so I always have a jar in my fridge.

SERVING OPTION

Slice the steak. Arrange the grilled vegetables on a plate and top with toasted pumpkin seeds. Place the sliced steak on top, and drizzle generously with the chimichurri sauce.

NUTRITIONAL INFORMATION *(Per Serving)*

Calories 832Kcals ○ Net carbohydrates 11.3g ○ Fiber 6.3g ○ Fat 61.3g ○ Protein 58.9g

This recipe is a game-changer. Nothing is nicer than a perfectly seared steak drizzled with a fresh, herby chimichurri sauce. Forget the chips. We're pairing it with grilled Mediterranean vegetables, which have much more flavor and nutrients, but you can serve it with a delicious salad for a lighter meal, too. It's perfect for BBQs, meal prep, or a quick midweek dinner.

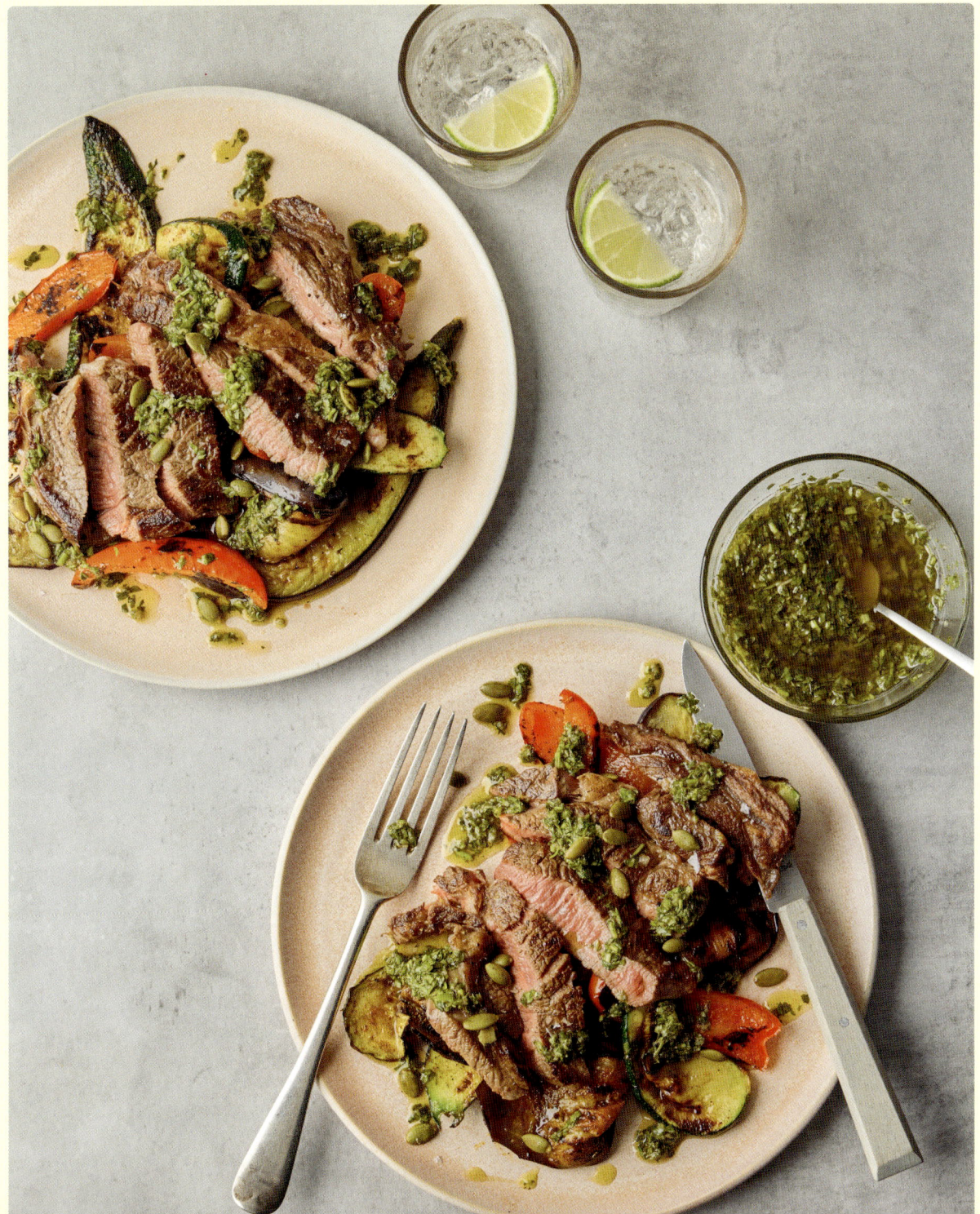

Cauliflower steaks were something I used to be skeptical about—until I made this recipe, which changed my mind! Thick, heavy slices of roasted cauliflower on a delicious harissa-spiced marinade, with a super tender core. Paired with a creamy chickpea mash and a dollop of tahini drizzle, this is the ultimate plant-based feast that ticks the texture and flavor boxes, and plant points, too! Gorgeous as a main, but I prefer this as a side, paired with a protein of choice.

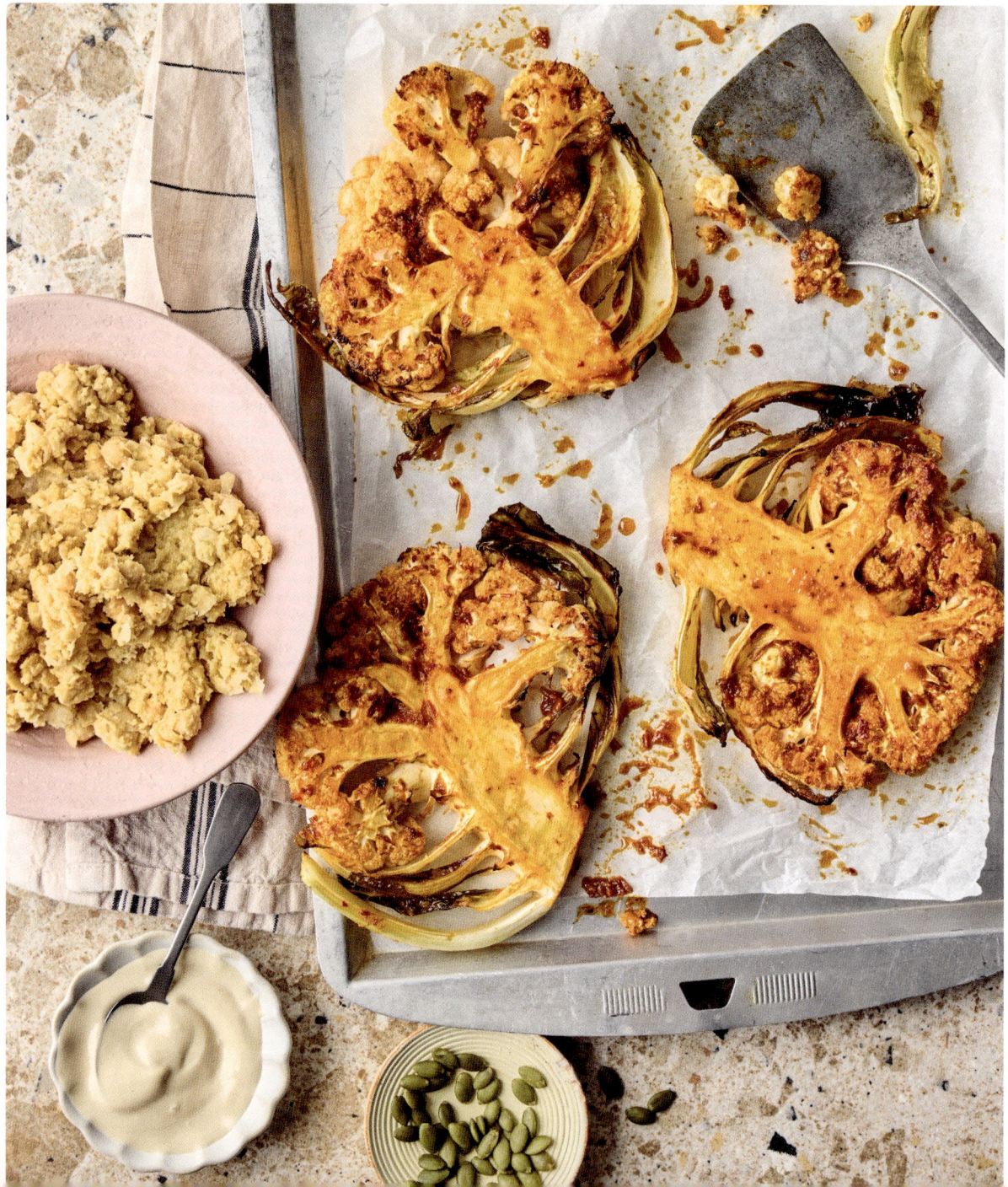

Harissa Cauliflower Steaks
with Chickpea Mash

SERVES 2 ○ VEGAN, HIGH FIBER

INGREDIENTS

2 tbsp olive oil
1 tbsp harissa paste
½ tsp ground coriander
½ tsp ground turmeric
½ tsp onion powder
sea salt and freshly ground black pepper, to taste
1 cauliflower, trimmed and cut into steaks
3 tbsp/30g pumpkin seeds

For the chickpea mash
3 tsp olive oil
2 cloves of garlic, crushed
1 tsp ground cumin
½ tsp ground cinnamon
two 14oz/400g cans of chickpeas, drained
juice of ½ a lemon
½ cup/100ml warm water
sea salt and freshly ground black pepper, to taste

For the tahini drizzle
2 tbsp tahini
juice of 1 lemon
3-4 tbsp water

Preheat your oven to 350°F (fan).

Mix the olive oil, harissa paste, coriander, turmeric, onion powder, salt, and black pepper to taste in a small bowl.

Brush both sides of the cauliflower steaks with the harissa mixture and place them on a lined baking sheet.

Roast for 20–25 minutes, turning halfway through to make sure they are evenly cooked.

Five minutes before the steaks are ready, prepare the chickpea mash and tahini drizzle. First, heat the olive oil in a small pan, add the garlic, cumin, and cinnamon, and heat gently for 1 minute.

Add the chickpeas, lemon juice, and water and warm through, then mash and season with salt and black pepper to taste.

To make the tahini drizzle, mix the tahini, lemon juice, and water to make a smooth and pourable drizzle consistency.

When the steaks are cooked, remove them from the oven. Place the mash on the plate, followed by the cauliflower. Finish with a drizzle of the tahini mixture and a sprinkle of pumpkin seeds.

SERVING OPTIONS

Sprinkle our Savory Soft Crumble (page 300) over the cauliflower before roasting, or use it as a garnish.

Sprinkle with pomegranate seeds, fresh mint, and toasted almonds or sesame seeds for extra flavor and crunch.

Serve with a good protein source or a selection of salads.

NUTRITIONAL INFORMATION *(Per Serving)*

Calories 675Kcals ○ Net carbohydrates 56.7g ○ Fiber 23.8g ○ Fat 37.7g ○ Protein 30.7g

Chicken Karahi
with Quinoa

SERVES 4   ○   HIGH PROTEIN

INGREDIENTS

- 1 tbsp coconut oil or olive oil
- 1 large red onion, finely chopped
- 3 cloves of garlic, crushed
- 1-inch piece of ginger, peeled and grated
- 2 jalapeños, deseeded and finely chopped
- 1lb 9oz/700g boneless, skinless chicken thighs, cut into chunks
- 1 tsp ground cumin
- 1 tsp ground coriander
- ½ tsp ground turmeric
- 1 tsp smoked paprika
- 1 tsp garam masala
- 1 tsp chile powder
- ½ tsp sea salt (or to taste)
- ½ tsp freshly ground black pepper
- one 14oz/400g can of chopped tomatoes
- 2 tbsp tomato paste
- ½ cup/100ml chicken bone broth
- juice of ½ a lemon
- a small handful of fresh cilantro, chopped
- 150g quinoa
- 1⅓ cups/300ml water or chicken bone broth

Heat the coconut or olive oil in a deep sauté pan over a medium-high heat. Add the onion and cook until softened. Stir in the garlic, ginger, and most of the chopped jalapeños, sautéing for 1–2 minutes until fragrant.

Add the chicken pieces and cook for a few minutes, stirring occasionally.

Stir in the cumin, coriander, turmeric, paprika, garam masala, and chile powder, and season with salt and black pepper. Cook for 1 minute, to toast the spices. Pour in the chopped tomatoes and tomato paste, stirring well. Simmer for 10 minutes, until the sauce thickens.

Add the chicken bone broth and simmer uncovered for another 10–15 minutes, until the sauce reduces and the chicken is tender, then stir in the lemon juice and half the cilantro leaves.

Rinse the quinoa in cold water. Put it into a saucepan and add 1⅓ cups/300ml of water or bone broth. Bring to the boil and simmer gently for 12–15 minutes, or until the liquid is absorbed, being careful not to let the quinoa stick or burn.

Fluff up the quinoa and serve, garnished with the rest of the cilantro and the remaining sliced jalapeños.

TOP TIPS
This dish tastes even better the next day, so make a double batch! Freezes for up to 3 months.

SERVING OPTIONS
Swap the quinoa for your choice of grain, cauliflower rice, sautéed greens, or gluten-free flatbreads.

Note: *150g quinoa will add 139kcals, 24g carbs, 2.3g fat, 4.9g protein.*

NUTRITIONAL INFORMATION *(Per Serving)*

Calories 416Kcals   ○   Net carbohydrates 36.2g   ○   Fiber 6g   ○   Fat 7.5g   ○   Protein 50.6g

This recipe is full of flavor and is the perfect option for a cozy evening in. Chicken Karahi is spicy, vibrant, and rich in all the nutritional heroes like garlic, ginger, and jalapeños, and the warming spices cooked down in a thick tomatoey sauce make this the perfect meal for curry lovers. It's easy to make and pairs well with quinoa, sautéed greens, or a gluten-free flatbread . . . anything that will soak up that sauce!

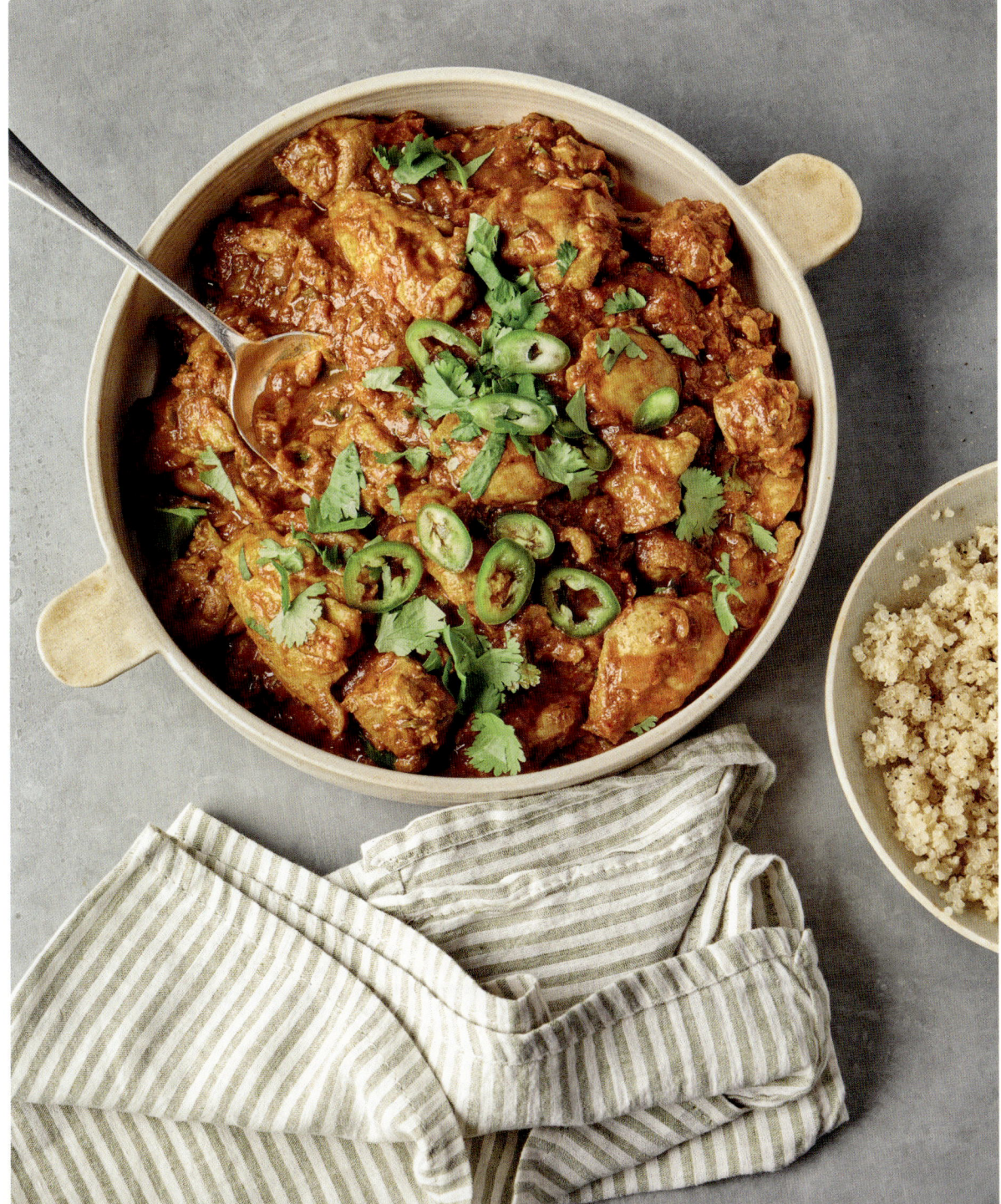

Nando's lovers, I've got you! Juicy chicken thighs seasoned with a peri peri mix, served with creamy avocado and a charred corn salsa. It's full of color, super zesty, and packed with protein and healthy fats. Perfect for a big family dinner.

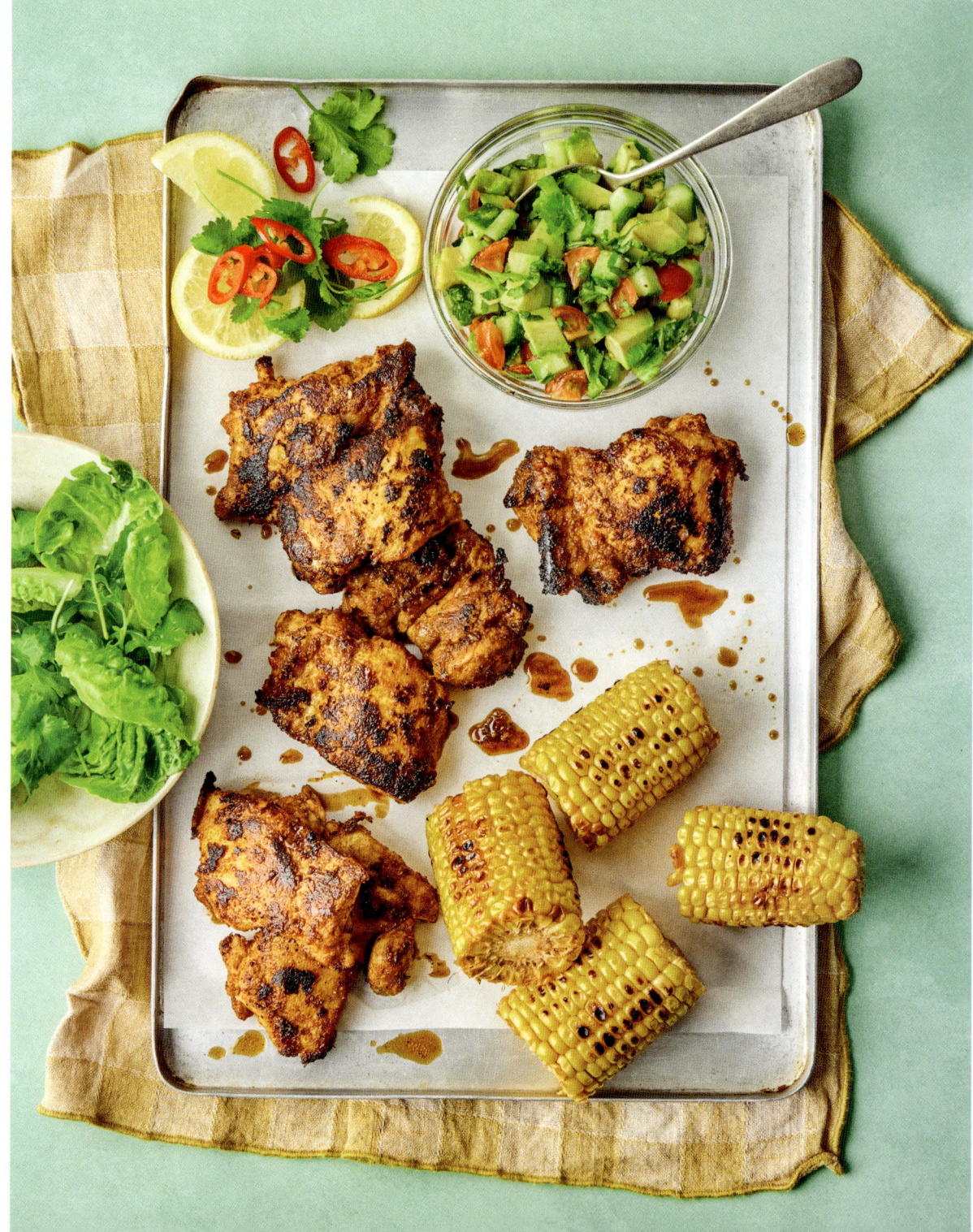

Peri Peri Chicken Thighs
with Charred Corn & Avocado Salsa

SERVES 4 ○ HIGH PROTEIN

INGREDIENTS

For the marinade
2 tsp ground coriander
2 tsp onion powder
1 tsp dried oregano
1½ tsp smoked paprika
½ tsp cayenne pepper
1–2 tbsp olive oil
2 cloves of garlic, crushed
juice of 1 lemon
1 tsp chopped flat-leaf parsley
1 red chile, deseeded and finely chopped
sea salt and freshly ground black pepper, to taste

1lb 5oz/600g skinless, boneless chicken thighs
4 sweet corn cobettes
1–2 tbsp olive oil

For the salsa
⅔ cup/100g avocado, diced
3 green onions, finely chopped, including greens
5 cherry tomatoes, diced
1½ inch cucumber, diced
1 tbsp lemon juice
1 tbsp finely chopped fresh cilantro
sea salt and freshly ground black pepper, to taste

Combine all the marinade ingredients in a bowl. Add the chicken thighs, coat well, and leave to marinate for at least 15 minutes (or overnight for more depth).

Place a large pan of boiling water on the stovetop. Add the sweet corn and boil for 6–7 minutes or until tender. Drain and set aside.

Heat a sauté pan over a medium-high heat. Add the chicken and cook for 12–15 minutes, turning regularly until the chicken is cooked through.

While the chicken is cooking, prepare the salsa. Mix the avocado, green onions, cherry tomatoes, cucumber, lemon juice, and cilantro, and season to taste with salt and black pepper.

When the chicken is almost ready, heat the olive oil in a griddle or sauté pan on a high heat. Add the sweet corn and turn until all sides are very slightly charred.

Serve the chicken with charred corn and a generous spoonful of avocado salsa, with cauliflower rice, quinoa, or a crisp green salad alongside.

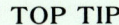
TOP TIP
For extra heat, add more chile or cayenne pepper.

NUTRITIONAL INFORMATION *(Per Serving)*

Calories 340Kcals ○ Net carbohydrates 10.1g ○ Fiber 5.8g ○ Fat 14.7g ○ Protein 40.2g

Zesty Buckwheat & Chickpea Salad

SERVES 4   ○   VEGAN

INGREDIENTS

- ¾ cup/150g buckwheat, rinsed
- ½ a cucumber, diced
- 4 green onions, diced, including greens
- 1 red chile, deseeded and very finely diced
- a small handful of mint, finely chopped (you can use 1 tsp dried)
- a small handful of flat-leaf parsley, finely chopped
- ½ tsp dried thyme
- One 14oz/400g can of chickpeas, drained
- ⅔ cup/100g sweet corn (canned or frozen)
- 6 sun-dried tomatoes, chopped
- zest and juice of 1 lemon
- 2 tbsp olive oil
- sea salt and freshly ground black pepper, to taste

Place the buckwheat in a saucepan. Cover with water and simmer gently for 15–20 minutes, until tender but still with texture and bite. Drain and rinse under cold water.

Place the drained buckwheat in a large bowl. Add the rest of the ingredients and combine well. Season to taste.

Cover and place in the fridge until ready to eat.

TOP TIP
The salad will keep in the fridge for up to 4 days.

SERVING OPTIONS
This salad can be eaten on its own, served with a protein source of your choice, or as part of a salad.

For extra crunch, sprinkle with some toasted nuts and seeds when serving.

NUTRITIONAL INFORMATION *(Per Serving)*

Calories 314Kcals   ○   Net carbohydrates 47g   ○   Fiber 8.5g   ○   Fat 10.8g   ○   Protein 9.5g

Salads aren't just for summer, and this one is a perfect example of a hearty, flavorful protein-packed meal. It's naturally gluten-free, thanks to using buckwheat, and gives a nutty bite that pairs well with the crispy cucumber and juicy sweet corn. Mint, parsley, and thyme bring a burst of freshness, while the touch of chile gives it that little kick of heat. Perfect as a light lunch or a side dish, it can be easily made ahead of time for those days where you're rushing around!

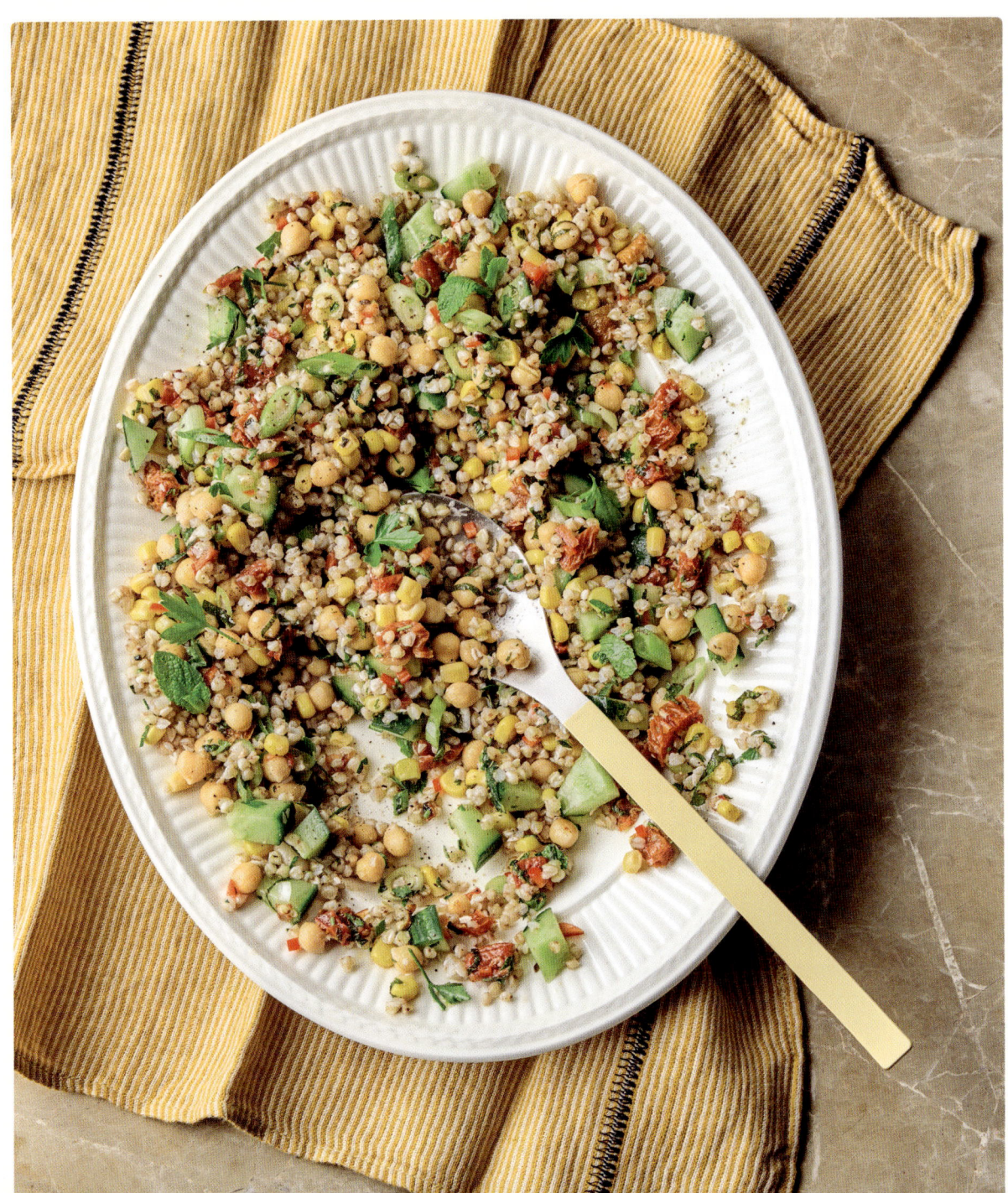

We've all fallen in love with the "Dubai" pistachio chocolate trend—but what about bringing a touch of pistachio magic to your main meals? This crunchy pistachio, cumin, and lemon crust adds the most gorgeous color, texture, and flavor to protein-packed cod fillets. It's beautifully balanced with a sweet red pepper sauce, and as a bonus it's quick and easy but elegant, all at the same time!

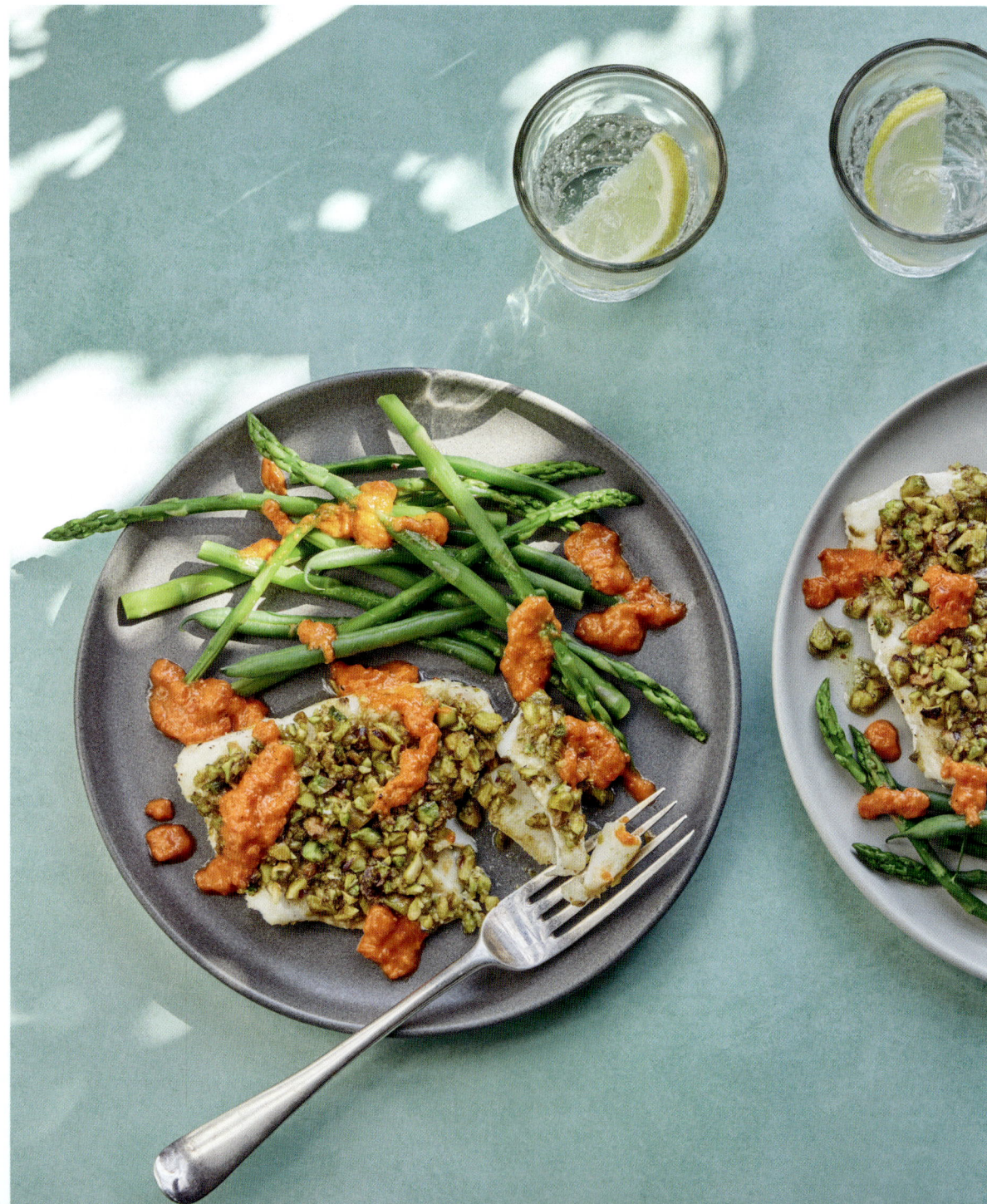

Pistachio-Crusted Cod
with Roasted Pepper Sauce

SERVES 2 ○ HIGH PROTEIN, GRAIN-FREE

INGREDIENTS

¼ cup/30g pistachios, chopped
1 tsp ground cumin
1 clove of garlic, grated
zest of ½ a lemon
freshly ground black pepper, to taste
2 cod fillets
1 tbsp olive oil

For the roasted pepper sauce

½ cup/100g jarred roasted red peppers, drained
1 tbsp lemon juice
1 tbsp olive oil
sea salt and freshly ground black pepper, to taste

Preheat the oven to 400°F (fan) and line a baking sheet with parchment paper.

In a small bowl, combine the pistachios, cumin, garlic, and lemon zest, and season with black pepper.

Place the cod fillets on the lined baking sheet. Rub them with olive oil and press the pistachio mixture on top of each fillet.

Bake for 12–15 minutes, or until the fish flakes easily and the crust is golden.

While the fish is cooking, blend the roasted peppers with the lemon juice, olive oil, salt, and black pepper. Once blended, warm gently before serving if preferred.

Serve the cod with a spoonful of sauce and a side of salad or greens.

TOP TIP
Swap the cod for any other fish of your choice.

GRAIN BOOSTER
If you're including grains and are not concerned about blood-sugar balance, this pairs beautifully with basmati or wild rice.

NUTRITIONAL INFORMATION *(Per Serving)*

Calories 324Kcals ○ Net carbohydrates 5.1g ○ Fiber 1.7g ○ Fat 23.1g ○ Protein 24g

Dess

ert

These beautifully poached pears are gently simmered with maple syrup, orange zest, and warm spices, making the perfect dessert—light, comforting, and effortlessly elegant. Serve them warm or chilled, drizzled with the spiced syrup from the pan and with a big dollop of Velvety Vanilla Custard (page 304) for a creamy finish.

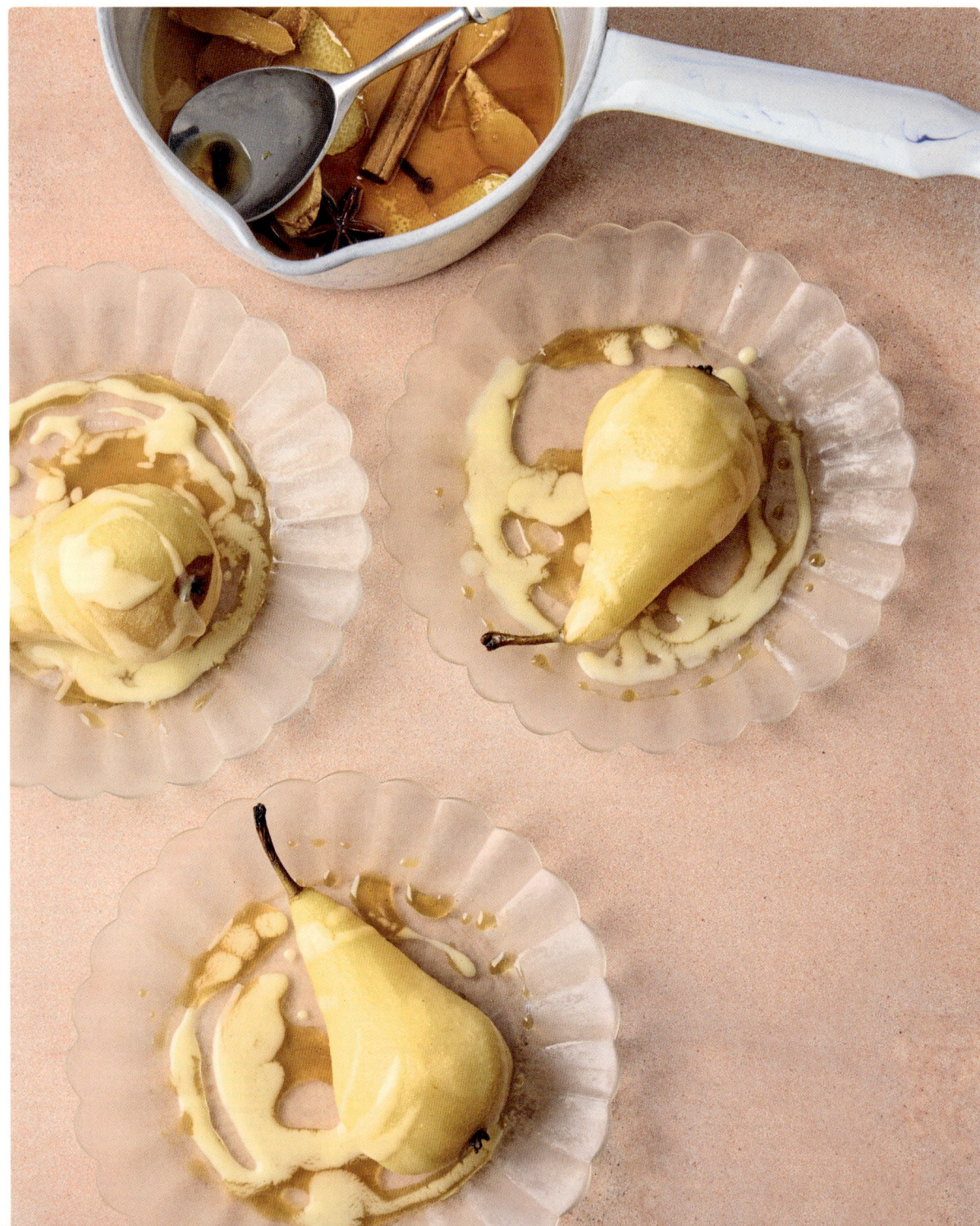

Maple Spiced Poached Pears
with Citrus Zest

SERVES 4   ○   VEGAN, GRAIN-FREE

INGREDIENTS

- 2 cups plus 2 tbsp/500ml water
- ½ cups/100ml maple syrup
- zest and juice of 1 orange
- zest of 1 lemon
- 1 cinnamon stick
- 3 cloves
- 1 star anise
- 1-inch piece of ginger, peeled and sliced
- 1 tsp vanilla paste
- 4 firm Conference or Bosc pears, peeled

In a saucepan large enough to hold the pears upright or side by side, combine the water, maple syrup, orange zest and juice, lemon zest, cinnamon, cloves, star anise, ginger, and vanilla.

Bring to a simmer, then add the peeled pears. Cover and simmer gently for 20–25 minutes, turning occasionally to ensure even poaching.

The pears are done when tender but still holding their shape.

Remove the pears and set aside. Increase the heat and reduce the poaching liquid for 10–15 minutes until slightly syrupy.

Serve the pears warm or chilled, drizzled with the reduced syrup.

TOP TIPS

Serve with our Velvety Vanilla Custard (page 304) or a dollop of Natural Live Coconut Yogurt (page 299).

Garnish with toasted chopped nuts or pomegranate seeds.

This recipe can be made 1–2 days in advance and stored in the syrup in the fridge.

NUTRITIONAL INFORMATION *(Per Serving)*

Calories 145Kcals   ○   Net carbohydrates 35.4g   ○   Fiber 5.1g   ○   Fat 1.3g   ○   Protein 1g

Sticky Toffee Pudding
with Caramel Sauce

SERVES 4–6   ○   GRAIN-FREE, NATURALLY SWEET

INGREDIENTS

- 2 medium eggs
- ⅓ cup plus 1 tbsp/80g coconut sugar
- 3 tbsp/40g coconut oil, melted, plus extra for greasing the dish
- ⅓ cup/80g Natural Live Coconut Yogurt (page 299) or plant-based yogurt
- 1 tsp date syrup
- 1 tsp vanilla extract
- 1¼ cups/150g ground almonds
- 1 tsp baking powder
- ⅔ cup/100g Medjool dates, pitted and finely chopped

To serve
Caramel Sauce (page 294)

Preheat the oven to 340°F (fan). Grease a medium ovenproof dish or individual ramekins with coconut oil.

In a bowl, beat the eggs, coconut sugar, melted coconut oil, yogurt, date syrup, and vanilla until combined.

Add the ground almonds and baking powder to the wet mixture. Add the chopped dates and make sure they are evenly distributed in the batter.

Spoon the mixture into the ovenproof dish or ramekins. Bake for 20–25 minutes (15–20 if using ramekins), until golden and just set.

While the pudding is cooking, prepare or heat up the caramel sauce.

Serve the pudding warm, with a generous serving of the caramel sauce.

TOP TIPS

The pudding will freeze well. Defrost, and reheat at 300°F for 8–10 minutes before serving.

To make ahead, prep the pudding and sauce in advance, then reheat the sauce on low heat gently before serving.

Serve with a dollop of my Natural Live Coconut Yogurt (page 299) or my Velvety Vanilla Custard (page 304) for extra indulgence.

NUTRITIONAL INFORMATION *(Per Serving)*

Calories 442Kcals   ○   Net carbohydrates 40g   ○   Fiber 3.5g   ○   Fat 28.4g   ○   Protein 9.1g

This is the ultimate comfort dessert—rich, squidgy, and sweet in all the right ways, but made without grains, dairy, or refined sugar. Packed with soft Medjool dates and topped with a dreamy coconut caramel sauce, it's a feel-good healthy treat that doesn't compromise on flavor. Serve warm with a dollop of coconut yogurt or dairy-free ice cream . . . and ENJOY!

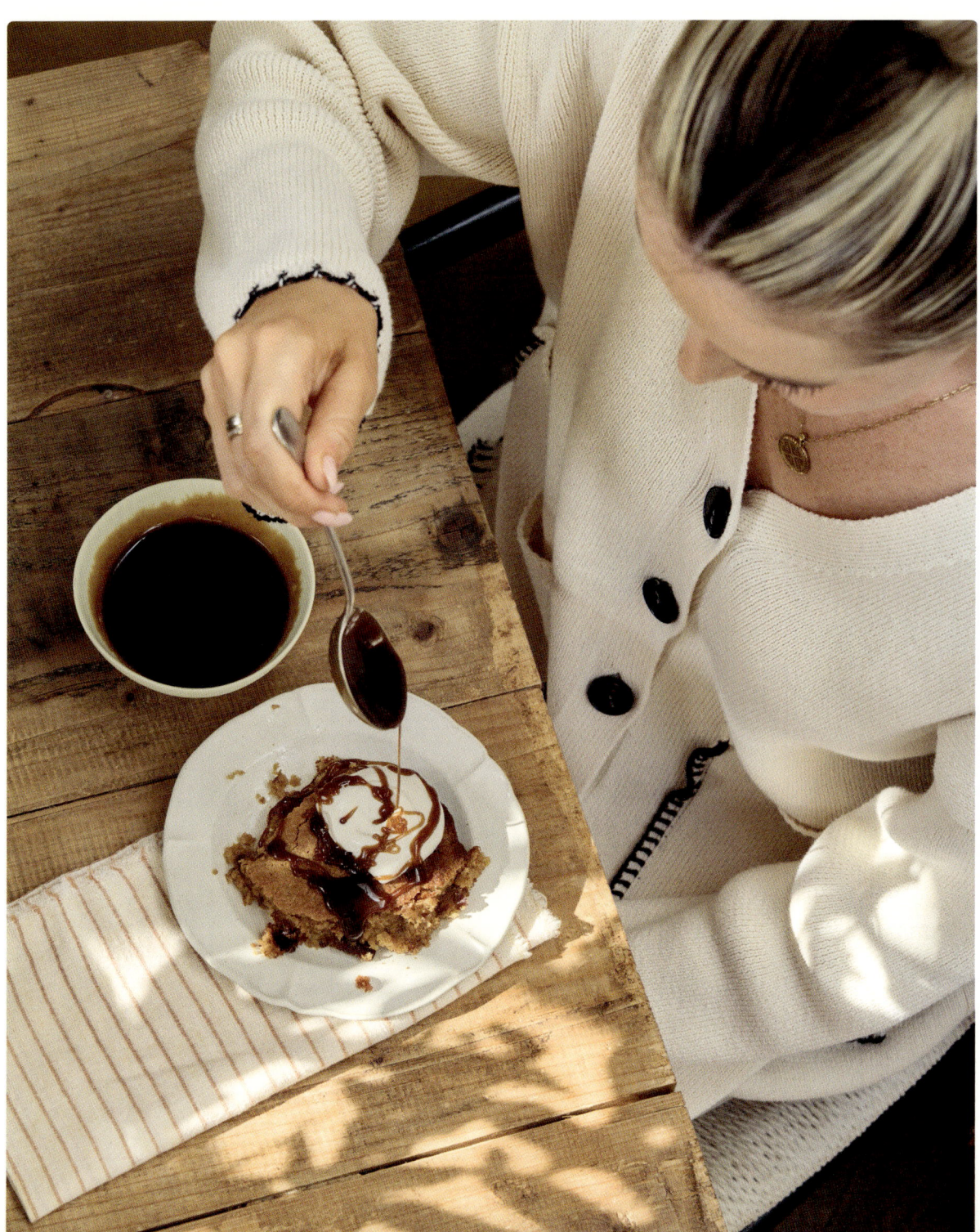

This rich and creamy mousse, a silky blend of avocado, cocoa, and a touch of coconut cream, is perfect for when you fancy a guilt-free, indulgent treat. It's nutritious, packed with fiber and healthy fats, takes minutes to make and is easy to customize, so you'll never get bored.

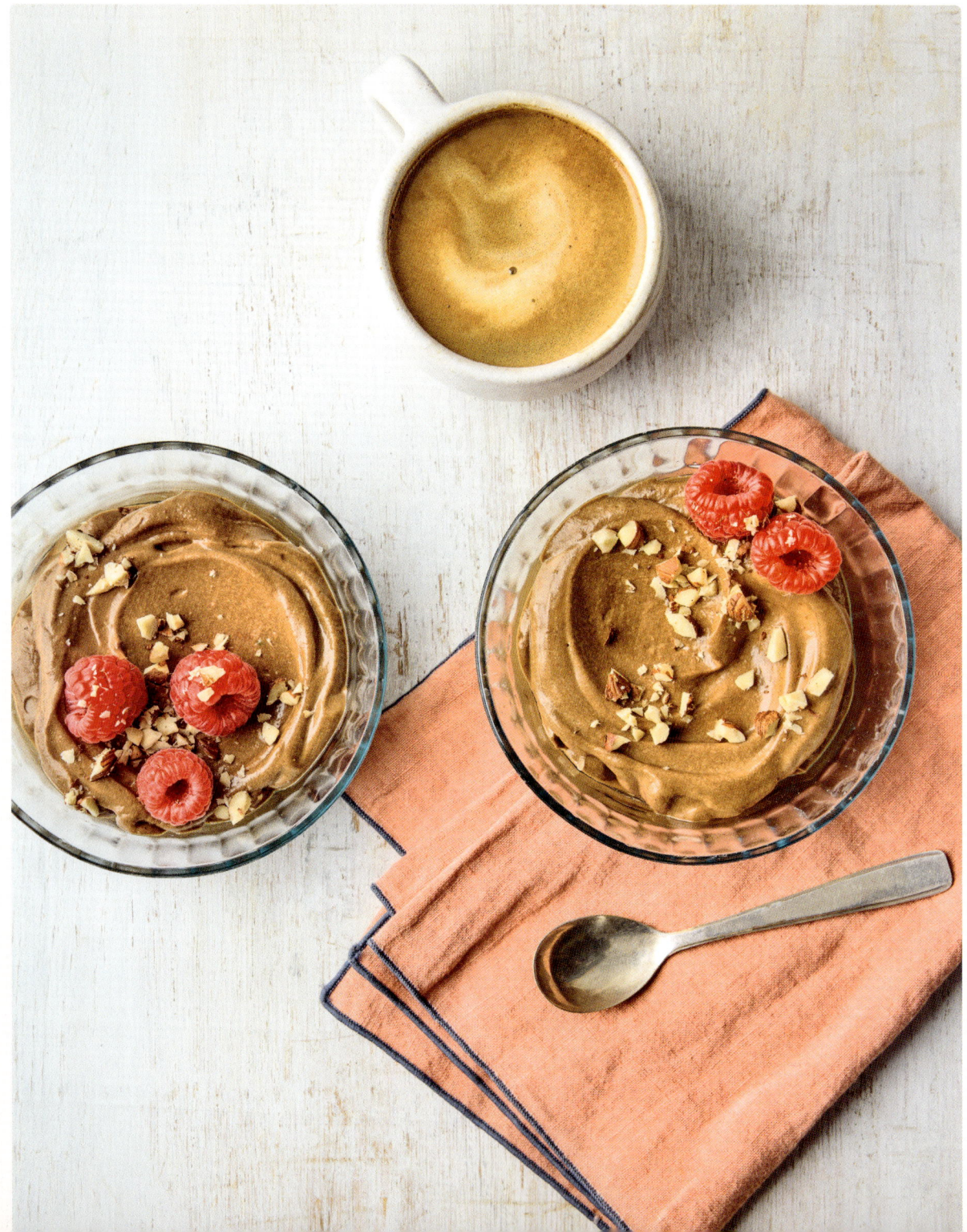

Rich & Creamy Chocolate Mousse

SERVES 2   ○   GRAIN-FREE, NO-COOK, DAIRY-FREE, GLUTEN-FREE

INGREDIENTS

- 1 ripe avocado
- 2 tbsp cocoa powder
- ½ cup/100ml unsweetened almond milk
- 1 tbsp maple syrup, or to taste
- 2 tbsp coconut cream
- 1 tsp vanilla extract
- a pinch of sea salt
- 4 hazelnuts, finely chopped

To garnish
fresh raspberries

Place all the ingredients (apart from the hazelnuts) in a blender or food processor.

Blend until completely smooth, scraping down the sides if needed. Adjust the almond milk to get your desired consistency.

Taste and adjust the sweetness to your preference. Do not skip the sea salt, as it enhances the flavor.

Spoon into ramekins or small glasses and sprinkle over a few chopped hazelnuts. Chill for at least 30 minutes.

Garnish with fresh raspberries and serve.

TOP TIPS

Keeps in the fridge for 2-3 days.

For a firmer texture, chill for longer or freeze for 10-15 minutes before serving.

PROTEIN BOOSTERS

Add 1 tablespoon of chocolate collagen or good-quality protein powder to enhance the protein.

Stir in a tablespoon of smooth peanut butter.

SERVING OPTIONS

Swap the vanilla extract for mint or orange, for a flavor variation.

Serve with my Chocolate, Hazelnut & Orange Biscotti (page 281) for dipping.

NUTRITIONAL INFORMATION *(Per Serving)*

Calories 261Kcals   ○   Net carbohydrates 9.1g   ○   Fiber 6.9g   ○   Fat 21.4g   ○   Protein 5.2g

Rhubarb, Strawberry & Elderflower Crumble

with Velvety Vanilla Custard

SERVES 6 ○ HIGH FIBER

INGREDIENTS

- 250g rhubarb, cut into ¾- to 1-inch lengths
- 1½ cups/200g strawberries, hulled and halved
- 2 tbsp elderflower cordial
- ¼ cup/50g coconut sugar
- 1¼ cups/100g oats
- 1 cup/100g ground almonds
- ½ cup/50g pecans or walnuts, roughly chopped
- 2 tbsp/20g flaxseeds
- 2 tbsp/20g chia seeds
- 1 tbsp hemp seeds
- 3 tbsp/40g mixed seeds (e.g., pumpkin, sunflower, sesame)
- 1 tbsp coconut oil
- 2 tbsp honey or maple syrup
- a sprinkle of flaked almonds (optional)

To serve
Velvety Vanilla Custard (page 304) or Natural Live Coconut Yogurt (page 299)

Preheat the oven to 350°F (fan).

Put the rhubarb, strawberries, and cordial into a saucepan and place on medium heat. Add 3 tablespoons of water and the coconut sugar, then bring to a gentle simmer for 5 minutes until the rhubarb starts to soften.

Remove from the heat and transfer the fruit into a medium baking dish.

In a bowl, combine the oats, ground almonds, pecans, flaxseeds, chia seeds, hemp seeds, and mixed seeds.

Melt the coconut oil and stir in the honey. Mix into the crumble mixture and combine well.

Spread the crumble mixture over the fruit in an even layer, and finish with a sprinkle of flaked almonds (if using).

Bake for 20 minutes, until the topping is golden and crisp.

Serve hot or cold, with vanilla custard or coconut yogurt.

TOP TIP
For a lower-carb, grain-free option, swap the oats for more ground almonds and nuts.

NUTRITIONAL INFORMATION *(Per Serving)*

Calories 377Kcals ○ Net carbohydrates 29.3g ○ Fiber 6.7g ○ Fat 24.2g ○ Protein 10.7g

This is a family favorite that perfectly combines tangy sharpness from the rhubarb and natural sweetness from the strawberries with a crunchy oat and nut topping. The splash of elderflower elevates this hearty crumble into a delicate delight, while also packing in the health-boosting nutrients with plenty of antioxidants. Serve warm, with Velvety Vanilla Custard for the ultimate comfort food.

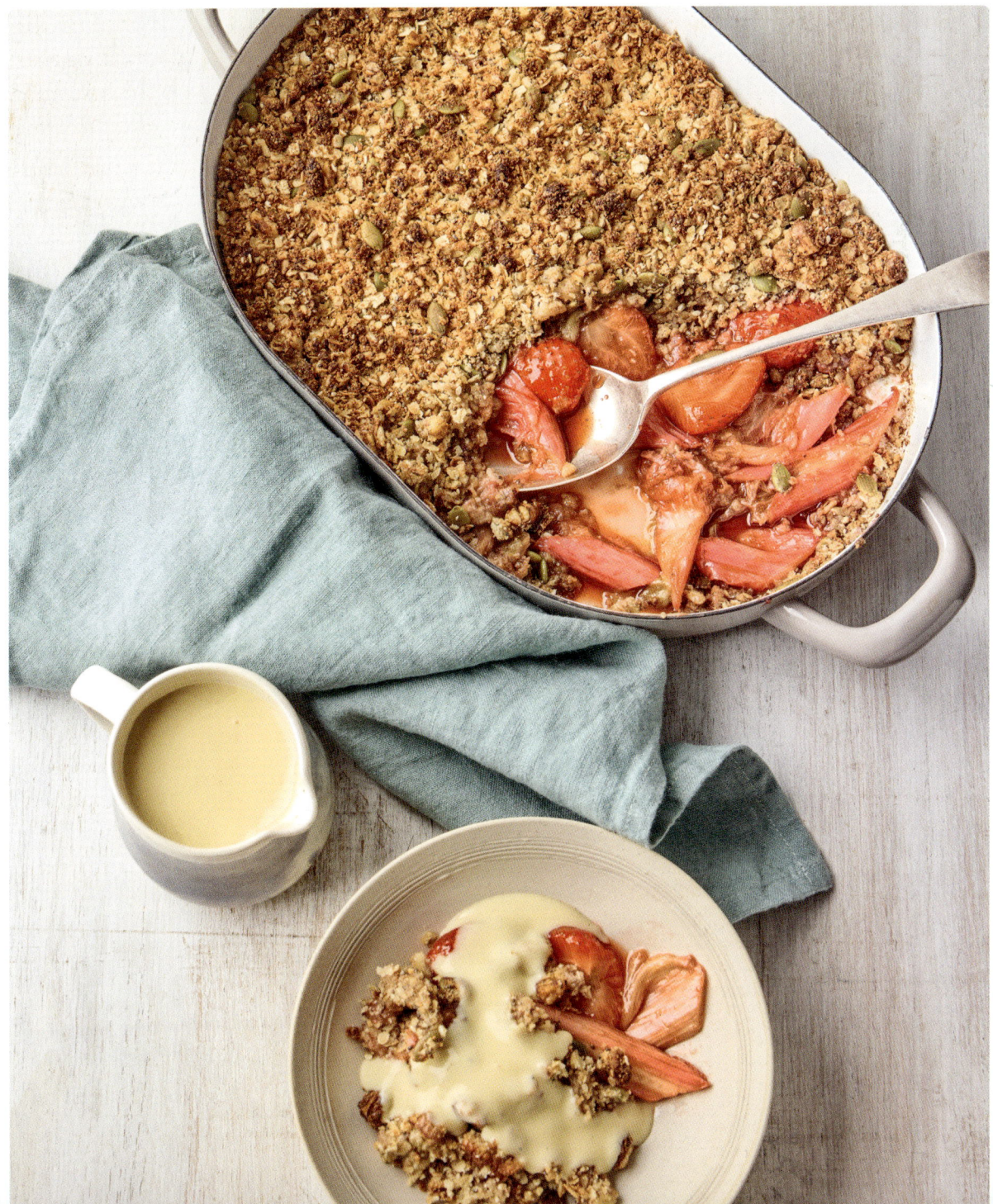

This panna cotta is to die for! With its creamy coconut base, hidden layer of juicy raspberries, and crunchy topping of pistachios and freeze-dried raspberries, it's the kind of dessert that looks like you've gone above and beyond, but with minimal effort! It's a magical, make-ahead-of-time dessert that's light, tasty, and just the right amount of fancy for a dinner party or weekend treat.

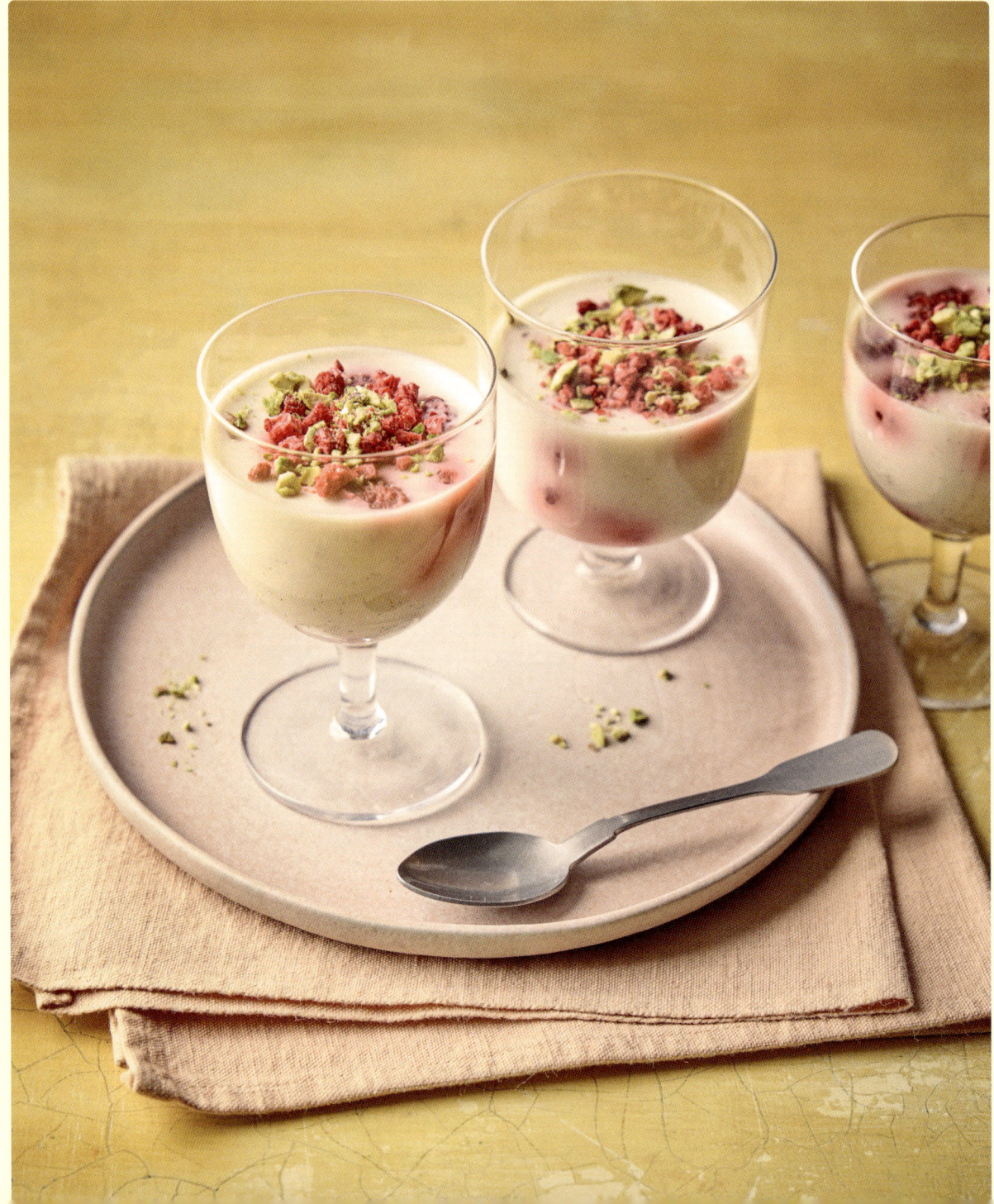

Raspberry & Pistachio Panna Cotta

SERVES 4 ○ DAIRY-FREE, GRAIN-FREE

INGREDIENTS

- ¾ cup/100g frozen raspberries
- 3 gelatin sheets (vegans can use 2–3 tbsp agar agar)
- 1½ cups/400ml full-fat coconut cream
- 2 tbsp plus 2 tsp/40ml maple syrup, or to taste
- 1 tsp vanilla paste
- 2 tbsp/20g shelled pistachios, finely chopped
- 1 tbsp freeze-dried raspberries, roughly crushed

Divide the frozen raspberries among 4 serving glasses, lightly crushing them at the bottom to help release their juice.

Place the gelatin sheets in a small bowl and top with cold water.

In a saucepan, combine the coconut cream, maple syrup, and vanilla paste, and heat gently until just below simmering.

Remove from the heat. Squeeze out the gelatin sheets and whisk them into the warm mixture until fully dissolved.

Very carefully, and slowly, pour the coconut mixture over the crushed raspberries, trying not to disturb the raspberries. Chill in the fridge for 3–4 hours, or until fully set.

Just before serving, top each panna cotta with a sprinkle of chopped pistachios and crushed freeze-dried raspberries.

TOP TIPS

These can be made a day ahead and stored chilled until ready to serve.

Serve with our Chocolate, Hazelnut & Orange Biscotti (page 281) for a more substantial dessert.

NUTRITIONAL INFORMATION *(Per Serving)*

Calories 329Kcals ○ Net carbohydrates 15g ○ Fiber 3.2g ○ Fat 24.9g ○ Protein 10.9g

No-Bake Vanilla Cheesecake

SERVES 8 ○ DAIRY-FREE, GRAIN-FREE, NATURALLY SWEETENED

INGREDIENTS

- 1½ cups/150g cashews
- 1 cup/100g pecans
- ½ cup/75g Medjool dates, pitted
- 1 tbsp coconut oil, melted
- 1¼ cups/300g silken tofu
- ¼ cup plus 1 tbsp/75ml maple syrup
- 1 tbsp vanilla paste
- Caramel Sauce (page 294) (optional)
- chopped hazelnuts (optional)

Place the cashews in a bowl and cover with water to soak. Soak overnight or, if you are in a hurry, soak in boiled water for at least 30 minutes.

Put the pecans, dates, and coconut oil into a food processor or blender and whiz until crumbly. Clean the blender before using again later.

Line a 7-inch loose-bottomed springform pan with parchment paper. Add the pecan mixture and press down well, using the back of a spoon. If the mixture sticks to the spoon, place a piece of parchment paper between the mixture and the spoon. Chill while you make the filling.

Drain the cashews and put them into your blender or food processor. Add the tofu, maple syrup, and vanilla and blend until completely smooth and creamy.

Pour this over the base and smooth the top. Cover and place in the fridge for at least 4 hours, or for a firmer texture, freeze for 1 hour before serving.

For added caramel flavor, if desired, top with Caramel Sauce and a sprinkle of chopped hazelnuts.

TOP TIPS

Add ⅓ cup plus 2 tbsp/100g of melted 85% dark chocolate to the mixture to create a fabulous chocolate cheesecake.

For a berry cheesecake, stir in ⅔ cup/100g of frozen raspberries or blueberries along with the zest of 1 lemon to help enhance the flavor.

Store in the fridge, covered, for 4 days, or freeze.

The cheesecake can be made as individual muffins.

NUTRITIONAL INFORMATION *(Per Serving)*

Calories 297Kcals ○ Net carbohydrates 18.5g ○ Fiber 2.9g ○ Fat 21.6g ○ Protein 7.7g

This creamy, no-bake cheesecake is made with soaked cashews and silken tofu, naturally sweetened with maple syrup. The nutty base adds just the right amount of chewy texture (while also adding healthy fats and fiber!). Chill and slice for an elegant, dairy-free dessert.

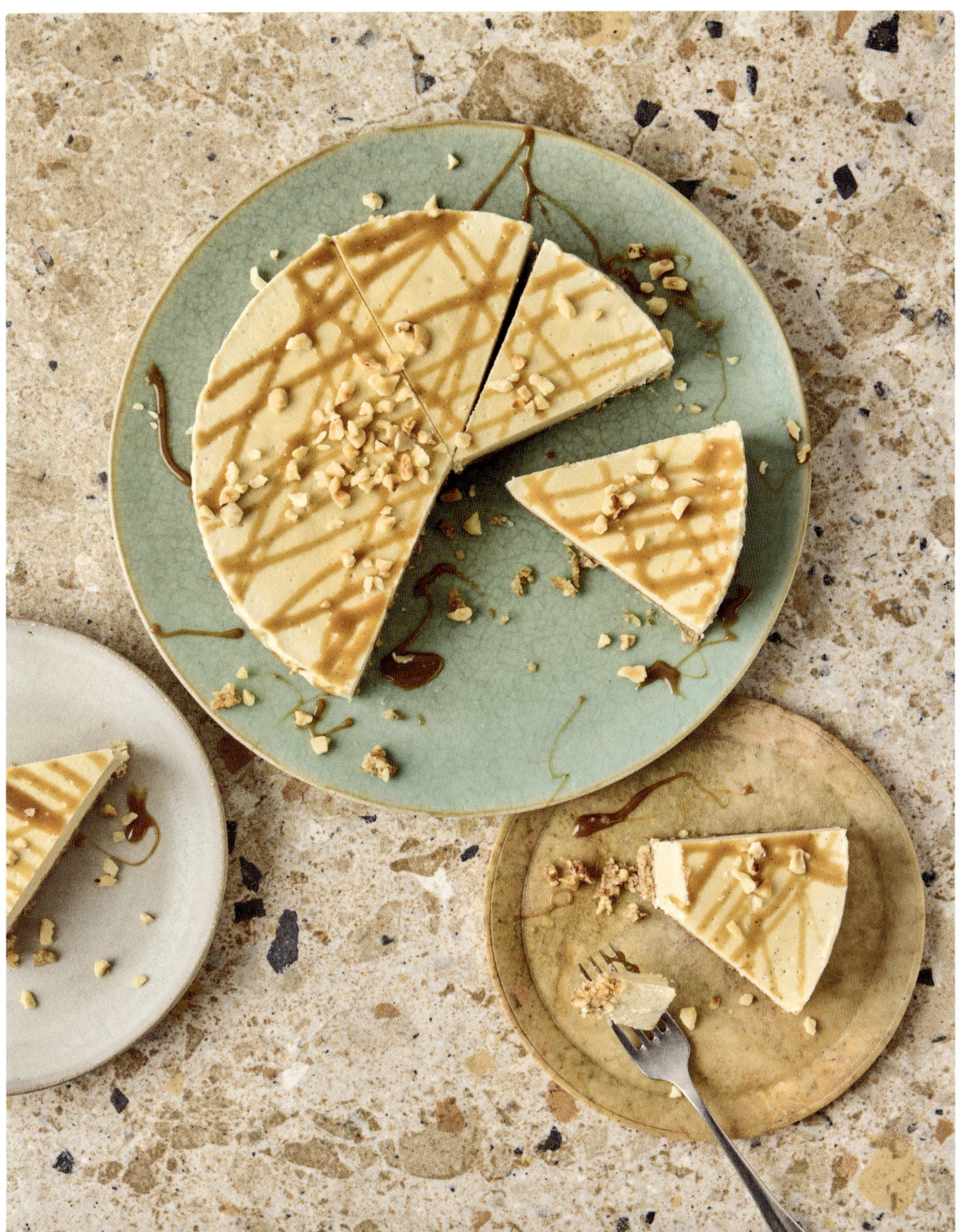

Indulgent chocolate goodness is absolutely still on the menu! This light, airy, and rich chocolate soufflé is a grain- and dairy-free option that's also high in protein. It's the perfect dessert that has a touch of decadence while being nutritious, too. I love mine fresh out of the oven for the best rise, topped with fresh berries and coconut cream for the ultimate finishing touch.

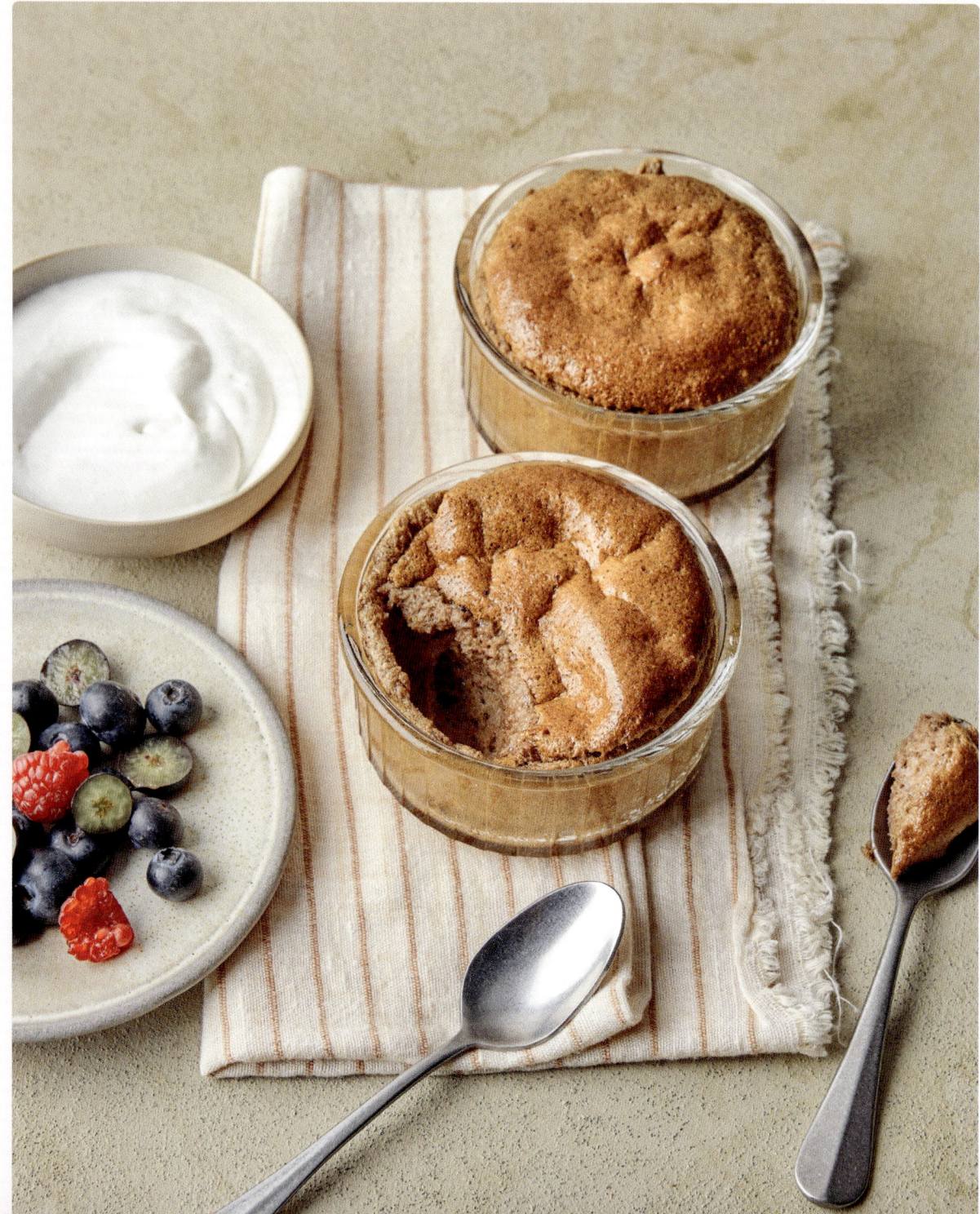

Chocolate Soufflés

SERVES 2   ○   GRAIN-FREE, NATURALLY SWEET

INGREDIENTS

coconut oil, for greasing
2 medium eggs
1 heaped tbsp cacao or cocoa powder
1 tbsp honey or maple syrup
a pinch of sea salt

To serve
berries and coconut cream

Preheat the oven to 350°F (fan). Grease two ramekin dishes thoroughly with coconut oil.

Separate the eggs, placing the whites in one bowl and the yolks in another.

Using an electric whisk, whisk the egg whites until stiff peaks form.

Move on to the egg yolks and whisk with the cacao, honey, and a pinch of sea salt until light and smooth.

Take 1 tbsp of the egg white and add it to the egg yolk mixture to help "slacken" it. Then, very carefully, fold the egg yolk mixture into the egg whites. Do this very gently to keep the air in and not deflate the egg whites too much. Do not overmix.

Pour the mixture into the ramekins. Place them on a baking sheet and pop them into the oven. Cook for 12–15 minutes. Be mindful that soufflés will naturally deflate shortly after being removed from the oven.

Serve immediately, with some berries and coconut cream.

NUTRITIONAL INFORMATION *(Per Serving)*

Calories 133Kcals   ○   Net carbohydrates 8.3g   ○   Fiber 2.1g   ○   Fat 6.8g   ○   Protein 8.8g

Mango & Lime Coconut Pots

SERVES 4   ○   NATURALLY SWEET, VEGAN

INGREDIENTS

- 1 large ripe mango, peeled and diced
- zest and juice of 1 lime
- 1½ tsp gelatin powder (or 3 sheets, soaked)
- 1 tbsp hot water
- 1 cup plus 1 tbsp/250ml coconut cream
- 2 tbsp maple syrup, or to taste
- 2 passion fruits
- juice of ½ a lime

Blend the mango with the lime juice and zest until smooth. Set aside.

In a small bowl, dissolve the gelatin powder in the hot water and let it bloom for 5 minutes. If you are using sheets, soak them in cold water for 5 minutes.

Gently heat the coconut cream in a pan over a low heat; do not boil. Whisk in the bloomed gelatin (or strained sheets) and maple syrup until fully dissolved.

Remove from the heat and stir in the mango purée.

Pour into small ramekins or glasses and chill in the fridge for at least 4 hours.

When ready to serve, place the pulp from the passion fruit in a bowl and add a little lime juice. Spoon this over the top of the set coconut-mango layer.

Serve immediately.

Delicious served with our Soft Coconut Macaroons with Dark Chocolate Drizzle (page 264) or Chocolate, Hazelnut & Orange Biscotti (page 281).

NUTRITIONAL INFORMATION *(Per Serving)*

Calories 210Kcals   ○   Net carbohydrates 7.2g   ○   Fiber 5g   ○   Fat 14g   ○   Protein 4g

These tropical coconut pots are sunshine in a glass . . . creamy, light, zesty, and naturally sweet from the mango, with a hint of lime. They're the perfect dessert that you can prepare well ahead of time, making them a refreshing finish to a spicy meal. They're made with zero refined sugar and a base of coconut milk and mango purée, topped with passion fruit—a dreamy, gut-friendly alternative to a traditional mousse or panna cotta.

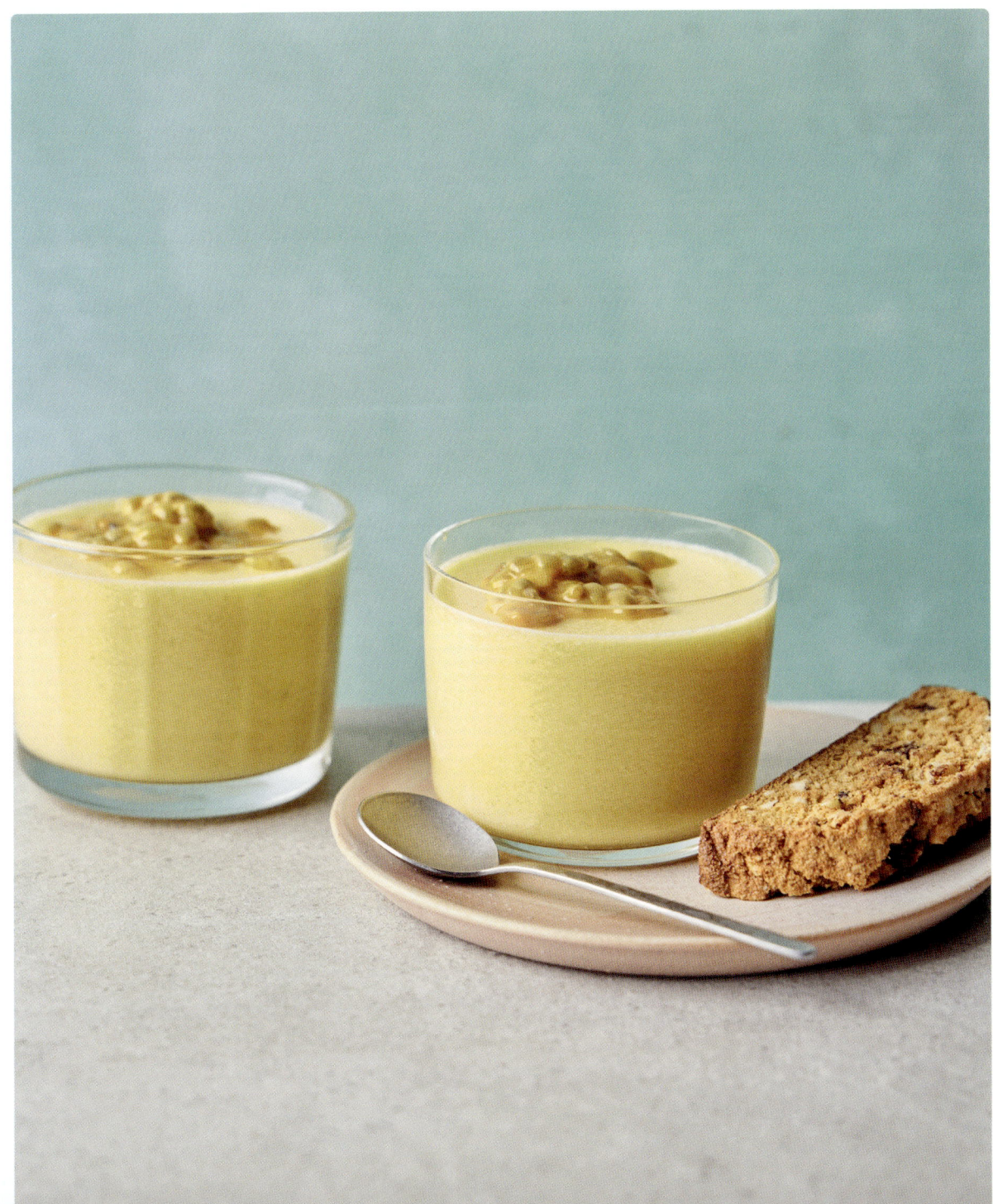

Rich, decadent, and incredibly indulgent, this No-Bake Chocolate Tart is my most requested recipe. It's pure chocolate heaven without the hassle, and the crunchy, nutty base pairs perfectly with the smooth silky chocolate ganache. It melts in your mouth and is naturally sweetened, while also being dairy-free. Whether you're treating yourself or a guest, this recipe really is a showstopper . . . and a personal favorite when I'm in my luteal phase!

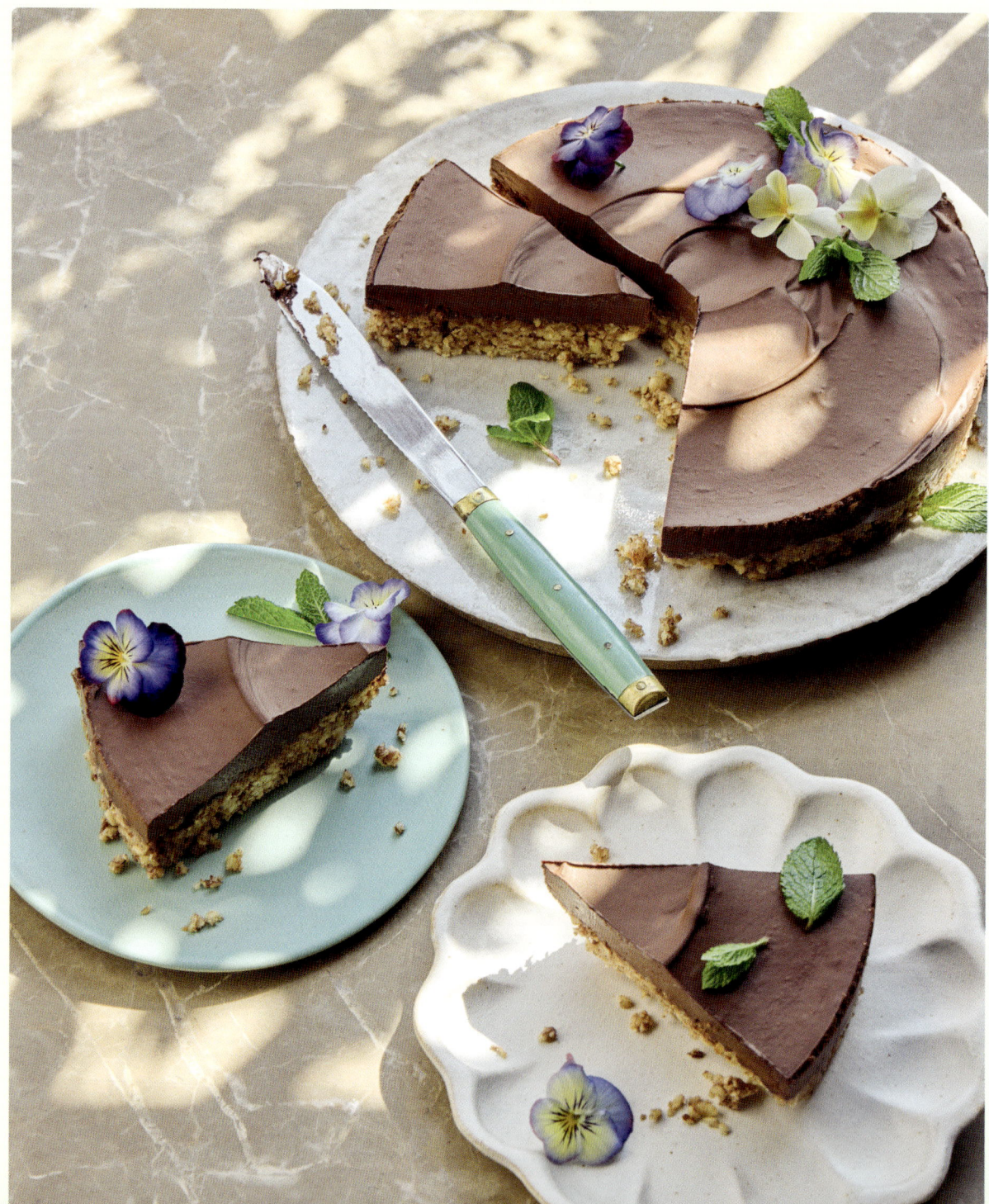

No-Bake Chocolate Tart

SERVES 10   ○   GRAIN-FREE, VEGAN, NATURALLY SWEET

INGREDIENTS

- 2 cups/200g pecans
- 1 cup/100g hazelnuts
- 2 tbsp coconut oil
- 2 tbsp smooth almond butter
- 1¼ cups/225g 85% dark chocolate
- ¾ cup/200g coconut cream
- cocoa powder (optional)
- mint leaves (optional)
- edible flowers (optional)

Place the nuts in a food processor and blend until they resemble breadcrumbs. If you don't have a food processor, place the nuts in a bag and bash gently with a rolling pin. Put them into a bowl.

Melt the coconut oil gently, then mix in the almond butter until it is smooth and lump-free. Add this to the nuts and combine well.

Grease an 8-inch loose-bottomed pan thoroughly with coconut oil. You can line the pan with parchment paper if you prefer.

Place the crumbled nuts in the pan and spread well until the base is evenly covered. Press down to form a solid base.

Place in the fridge to chill.

While the base is chilling, you can move on to the filling.

Chop the chocolate into small pieces and place in a heatproof bowl.

Place the coconut cream in a saucepan on medium heat and gently warm until it is hot but not boiling.

Remove from the heat and pour over the chocolate. Let it sit for a minute, then use a balloon whisk to mix until smooth and glossy. Stick with it; it will form a lovely, thick, glossy chocolate mixture.

Pour the mixture over the nut base and spread until smooth. Put it back into the fridge and leave it for 1–2 hours, until it sets.

Before serving, if desired, you can decorate with a sprinkle of cocoa or some mint leaves and edible flowers.

TOP TIPS

Base swaps: You can use almonds, walnuts, macadamias, pecans, or hazelnuts in any combination, up to 3 cups/300g total weight.

Are you a fan of chocolate orange or chocolate mint flavors? Add a few drops (to taste) of your favorite extract to the ganache mixture.

NUTRITIONAL INFORMATION *(Per Serving)*

Calories 423Kcals   ○   Net carbohydrates 7.9g   ○   Fiber 2.4g   ○   Fat 39.5g   ○   Protein 7.1g

Sav
snac

ory
ks

Kale Crisps

SERVES 4* ◦ VEGAN, GLUTEN-FREE, HIGH IN FIBER

These kale crisps are the perfect snack or side dish—they have the most satisfying crunch and are full of flavor, too. They're nutrient dense, rich in antioxidants and fiber, and can easily be customized with different seasonings to suit your taste. I love them with just sea salt and olive oil, but if you prefer spice or a cheesy taste, jazz them up in any way you like!

INGREDIENTS

- 3 to 4 cups/100g curly kale
- ½ tbsp olive oil or melted coconut oil
- a pinch of sea salt
- a pinch of freshly ground black pepper
- ½ tsp garlic powder
- ¼ tsp chili powder (optional)
- ½ tbsp nutritional yeast (optional, for a cheesy flavor)

(snack size)

** (this is dried weight, as they become dehydrated from 100g total weight to around 20–30g)

image on page 256

Preheat the oven to 250°F (fan). Line a baking sheet with parchment paper.

Wash the kale. Make sure you dry it thoroughly, as moisture can prevent crisping. Remove tough stems and tear the leaves into bite-size pieces.

In a large bowl, toss the kale with the olive oil and all the seasonings. Massage gently to ensure even coating.

Spread the kale in a single layer on the baking sheet and bake for 20–25 minutes, turning halfway through, until crisp.

Turn off the oven, leaving the kale inside for another 5–10 minutes to dry further.

Once cooled, store in an airtight container for 2–4 days.

TOP TIPS

For extra crispness, use a dehydrator instead of the oven.

Avoid sogginess: Make sure the kale is completely dry before seasoning.

Flavor variations: Try turmeric, cumin, or za'atar for different twists.

SERVING OPTIONS

Enjoy as a snack on its own.

Sprinkle over soups and salads for added crunch.

Serve with dips such as guacamole or hummus.

NUTRITIONAL INFORMATION *(Per 5-7 Serving)***

Calories 30Kcals ◦ Net carbohydrates 1.5g ◦ Fiber 1.1g ◦ Fat 1.9g ◦ Protein 1.4g

Roasted Chickpeas

SERVES 4 ○ VEGAN, GRAIN-FREE

If you've never tried roasted chickpeas, you're in for a treat. These make a deliciously crunchy snack but are also perfect for adding to salads or bowls—like my Marinated Salmon Bowl (page 182).

INGREDIENTS

- two 14oz/400g cans of chickpeas
- 1 tsp smoked paprika
- ½ tsp cayenne pepper
- 1 tsp chili powder
- 1 tsp tamari
- 1 tbsp olive oil

image on page 256

Preheat your oven to 350°F (fan).

Drain and rinse the chickpeas, then pat them dry with a clean tea towel or paper towel. The drier they are, the crispier they'll get.

When dry, place the chickpeas in a bowl and add the spices and tamari. Add a little olive oil at a time and toss to coat thoroughly.

Place on a baking sheet and spread them out evenly; don't overcrowd them.

Place in the oven and cook for 20 minutes. Shake or stir the chickpeas around the baking sheet before returning them to the oven for another 10–15 minutes, or until dry and crunchy.

TOP TIPS

For the crunchiest texture, allow the chickpeas to cool completely before storing.

If they soften after a day or two, simply reheat in the oven for 5–8 minutes to crisp them up again.

SPICE COMBINATIONS

Switch up the flavors with these fun twists:

Smoky BBQ: *1 tsp smoked paprika, ½ tsp garlic powder, ½ tsp onion powder, a pinch of cinnamon.*

Za'atar & Lemon: *1 tbsp za'atar, ½ tsp sumac, zest of ½ a lemon.*

Mexican Fiesta: *1 tsp chipotle powder, ½ tsp ground coriander, ½ tsp ground cumin, 1 tsp lime juice after roasting.*

Maple & Cinnamon (sweet): *1 tbsp maple syrup, ½ tsp ground cinnamon, pinch of sea salt (add syrup for the final 5 minutes).*

NUTRITIONAL INFORMATION *(Per Serving)*

Calories 91Kcals ○ Net carbohydrates 22.3g ○ Fiber 9g ○ Fat 7.2g ○ Protein 10.4g

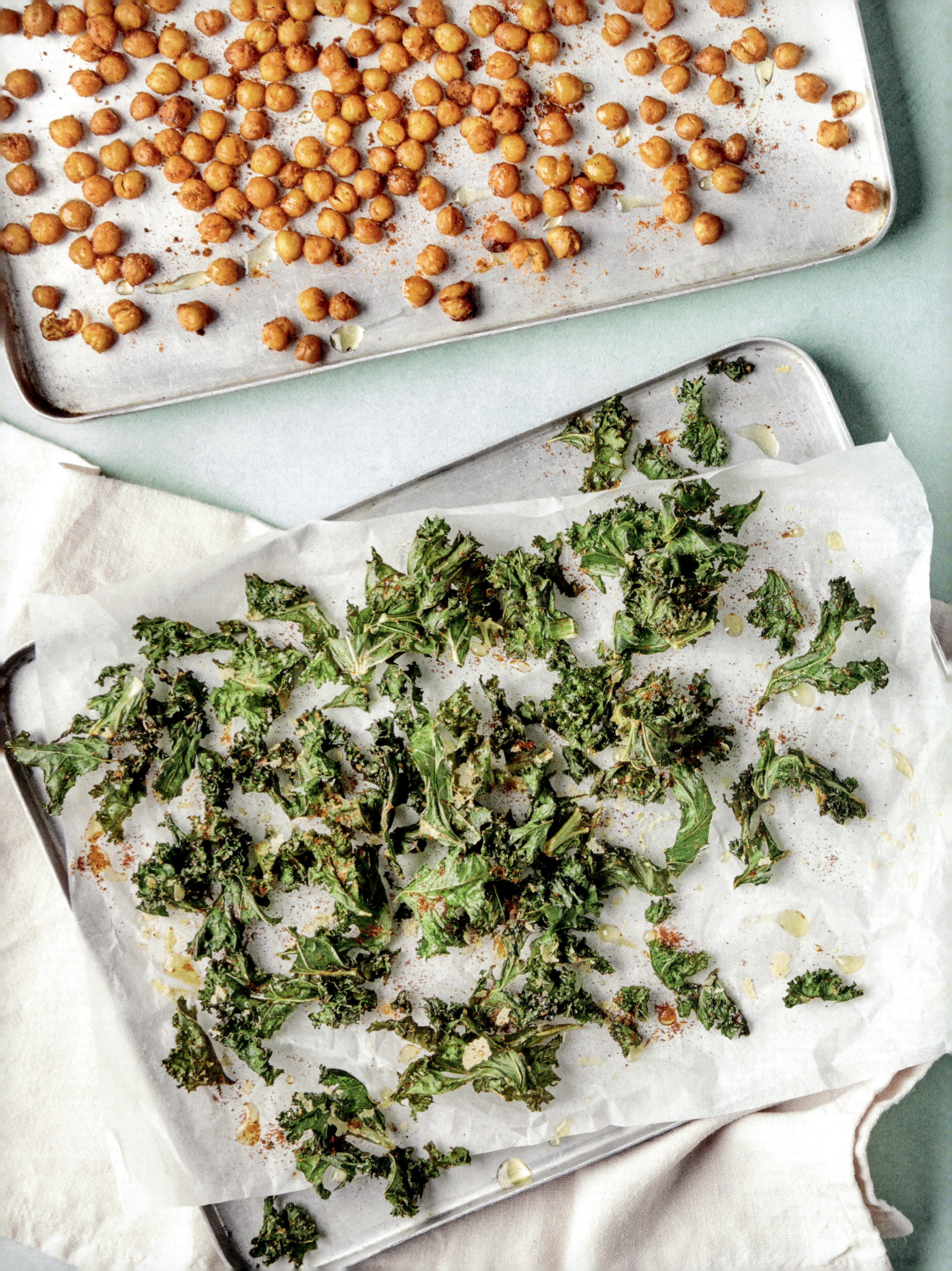

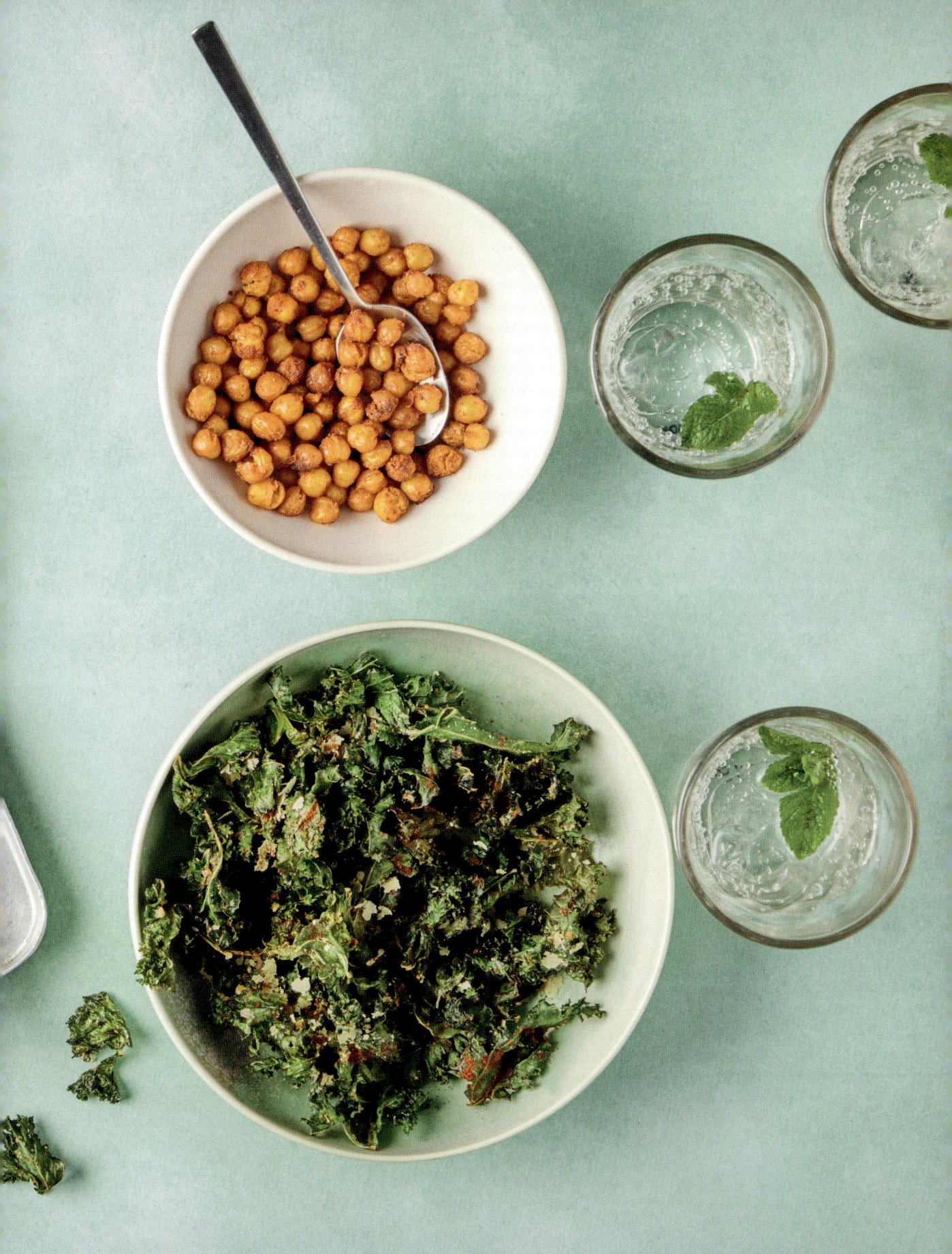

Grain-Free Seeded Bread

MAKES 1LB LOAF*   ○   VEGAN, GRAIN-FREE, HIGH FIBER

Bread is STILL on the menu, so we can all breathe! This grain-free seeded bread is gut-friendly, easily digestible, and has a nutty flavor similar to dark rye bread. It's dense, perfect for spreads, and packed full of healthy fats, fiber, and protein, making it the ideal alternative to supermarket processed breads. It's also incredibly versatile, so you can enjoy it toasted with your favorite toppings or as a base for a delicious sandwich. If you're craving some chocolate spread on toast, combine this recipe with the Healthy Chocolate Spread on page 295 and you will be obsessed.

INGREDIENTS

- 2 tbsp coconut oil
- 8 eggs
- 6 tbsp water
- 1½ cups/240g ground flaxseeds
- 1 cup/120g ground almonds or almond flour (alternatives: coconut flour or chestnut flour)
- 2 tsp baking powder
- 2 tsp cream of tartar
- ½ tsp sea salt
- 4 to 5 tbsp/60g mixed seeds (e.g. sunflower, pumpkin, sesame, chia, flaxseeds, or hemp seeds)
- 6 tbsp/60g ground chia seeds
- 3 tbsp/40g additional mixed seeds for topping (optional, for extra crunch)

* (approx. 10 slices)

image on page 260

Preheat the oven to 350°F (fan) and line a 1lb loaf pan with parchment paper.

Melt the coconut oil and put it into a bowl. Leave to cool.

Add the eggs and water, then beat well until thoroughly combined.

Stir in the ground flaxseeds, ground almonds, baking powder, cream of tartar, salt, mixed seeds, and ground chia seeds. Mix thoroughly to form a thick batter.

Pour the batter into the prepared loaf pan and smooth the top. Sprinkle with additional mixed seeds, if using.

Bake for 30–40 minutes, or until golden and firm to the touch.

Remove from the oven and allow to cool on a wire rack before slicing.

TOP TIP

If you don't eat much bread, slice it once cooled and freeze the individual slices. When you need a piece, simply toast it or allow it to defrost for a sandwich.

NUTRITIONAL INFORMATION *(Per Serving)*

Calories 82Kcals   ○   Net carbohydrates 2.1g   ○   Fiber 5.5g   ○   Fat 14.8g   ○   Protein 8.1g

Flax & Chia Crackers

SERVES 4   ○   VEGAN, GRAIN-FREE, HIGH FIBER

If unprocessed nutty goodness is what you're after, you'll go "crackers" for these (sorry, I had to!). These delicious, fiber-fueled crackers are super simple to make and can easily be batch cooked and saved for a quick snack on the go. Try them paired with a delicious avocado or hummus dip!

INGREDIENTS

- 2½ cups/250g milled flaxseeds
- ½ cup/50g milled chia seeds
- ½ cup/50g milled hemp seeds (or you can use a total of 350g of a milled brand of your choice, such as Linwoods' flax, hemp, and chia)
- ½ tbsp psyllium husk
- ¼ tsp sea salt
- ¼ tsp onion powder
- ¼ tsp garlic powder
- ¼ tsp dried oregano
- ½ tsp melted coconut oil
- ¼ cup to ½ cup/50–100ml boiling water

Place all the dry ingredients in a bowl and add the melted coconut oil. Season to taste.

Boil your kettle and add a little of the boiled water at a time until the flax forms a dough. Leave to sit for 10 minutes.

Preheat the oven to 350°F (fan).

Put the dough into a lined baking sheet roughly 9 x 13-inches, and flatten it until it is thin and fills the baking sheet.

Bake for 25 minutes, until golden and crispy. Leave to cool in the baking tray.

Once cool, snap into crackers.

Serve with your favorite dip.

image on page 261

NUTRITIONAL INFORMATION *(Per Serving)*

Calories 433Kcals   ○   Net carbohydrates 2.4g   ○   Fiber 27.9g   ○   Fat 32.2g   ○   Protein 19.6g

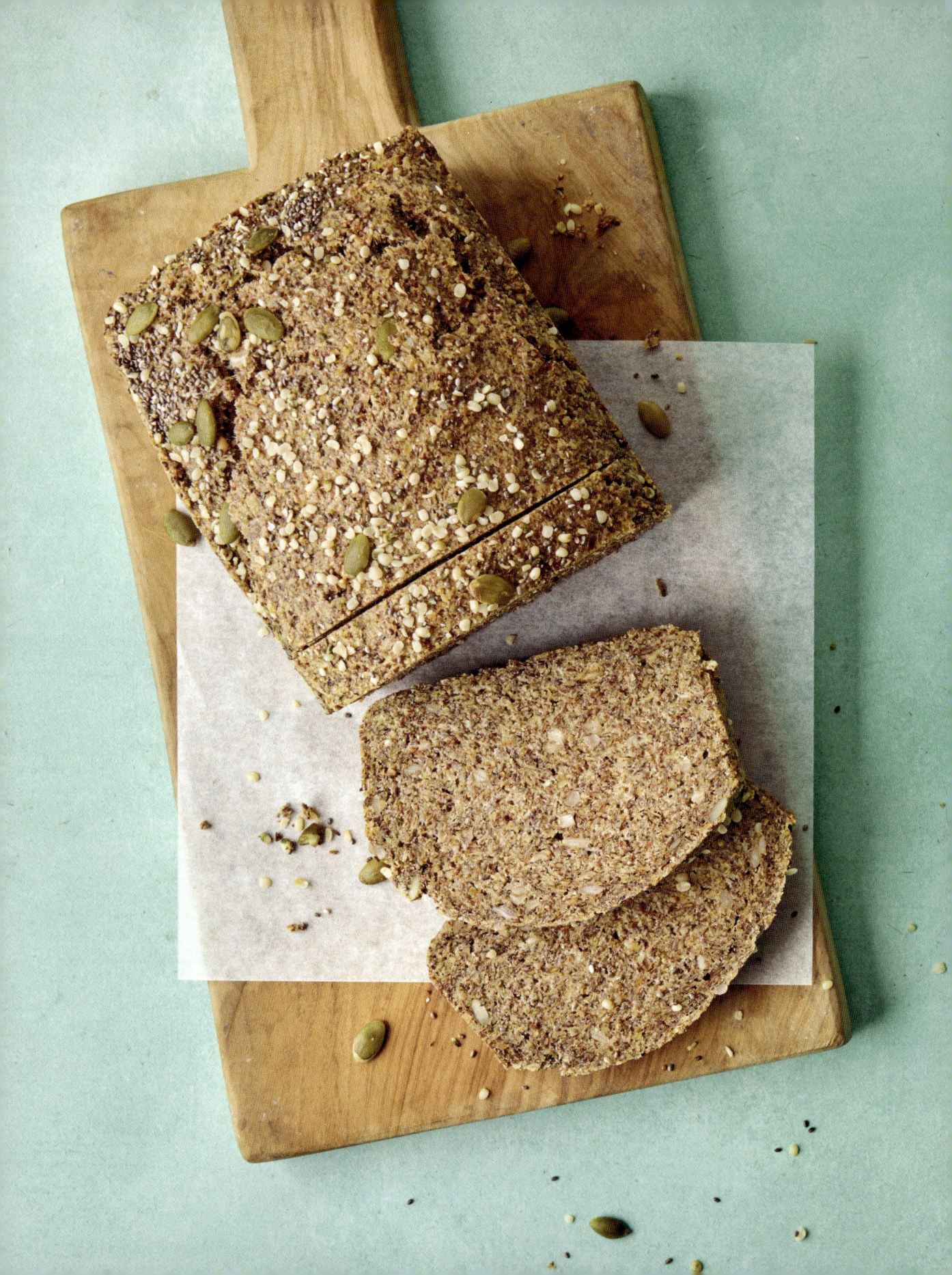

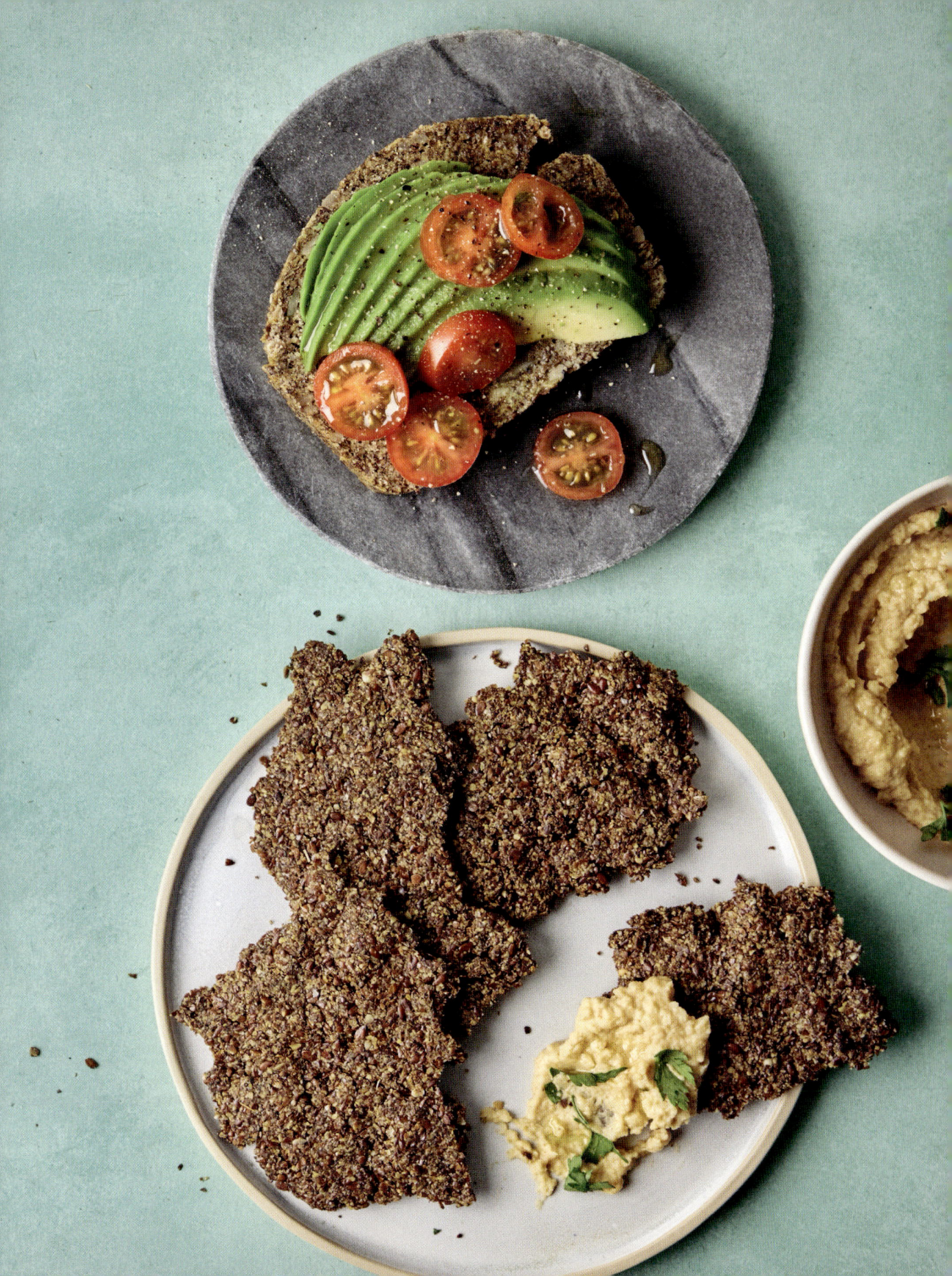

Swe
snac

et
ks

Soft Coconut Macaroons
with Dark Chocolate Drizzle

MAKES 30 SMALL* ○ GRAIN-FREE, DAIRY-FREE

These soft, chewy coconut macaroons are naturally sweetened with maple syrup and have the extra indulgent touch of a spoonful of coconut cream. They're moist inside with a golden edge, and a drizzle of dark chocolate and pinch of sea salt gives them the perfect finish.

INGREDIENTS

- 4 egg whites
- 3 cups/250g desiccated coconut
- 3 tbsp/50g coconut cream
- 3 tbsp/60g maple syrup
- 1 tsp vanilla paste
- ¼ cup/50g dark chocolate (melted, for drizzle)

* (or 12 large)

image on page 267

Preheat the oven to 325°F (fan) and line a baking sheet with parchment paper.

In a large bowl, whisk the egg whites until light and frothy (no need for stiff peaks).

Add the desiccated coconut, coconut cream, maple syrup, and vanilla, and mix until fully combined.

For mini macaroons, use a tablespoon to scoop and drop on to the sheet—they'll bake up to approx. 1½- to 2-inch diameter. For larger macaroons, shape by hand into mounds using around 2½ tablespoons of mixture.

Bake for 10–15 minutes, or until lightly golden around the edges. Keep a close eye on them toward the end, to avoid overbaking.

Cool on a wire rack. Once fully cooled, drizzle with melted dark chocolate. Allow to set before serving.

TOP TIPS

These store well in an airtight container for up to 5 days.

For a flavor variation, stir in 2 cups/50g of freeze-dried raspberries (crushed).

NUTRITIONAL INFORMATION *(Per mini macaroon)*

Calories 75Kcals ○ Net carbohydrates 2.5g ○ Fiber 1.8g ○ Fat 6.8g ○ Protein 1.4g

Coconut Macaroon Thumbprints

with Raspberry & Chia Seed Jam

MAKES 12 LARGE ○ VEGAN, GRAIN-FREE

These were my favorites growing up, so I knew I had to make a healthy version of these jammy coconut thumbprint macaroons (my niece and nephews love them, too!). The raspberry and chia jam brings a nice pop of fruitiness while also feeding your gut with fiber, and the coconut gives that satisfying chew we all love. A drizzle or dip of dark chocolate makes them even more special.

INGREDIENTS

- Soft Coconut Macaroons (as opposite)
- ⅓ cup/100g Easy Sugar-Free Raspberry & Chia Seed Jam (page 303)
- dark chocolate, melted (optional)

image on page 266

Follow the main recipe on the previous page, shaping the mixture into 12 large mounds.

Using your thumb or the back of a teaspoon, press a shallow indent into the center of each macaroon.

Fill each hollow with around ½ teaspoon of the raspberry & chia jam.

Bake as directed (10–15 minutes) until golden around the edges.

Allow to cool completely on a wire rack.

Optional: once cooled, drizzle with melted dark chocolate or dip the base into chocolate and allow to set on a sheet of parchment paper.

TOP TIP

You can freeze these (undecorated) and add the jam after thawing if preferred. They make lovely gifts or lunch box treats.

NUTRITIONAL INFORMATION *(Per Serving)*

Calories 83Kcals ○ Net carbohydrates 3.2g ○ Fiber 2.5g ○ Fat 7g ○ Protein 1.6g

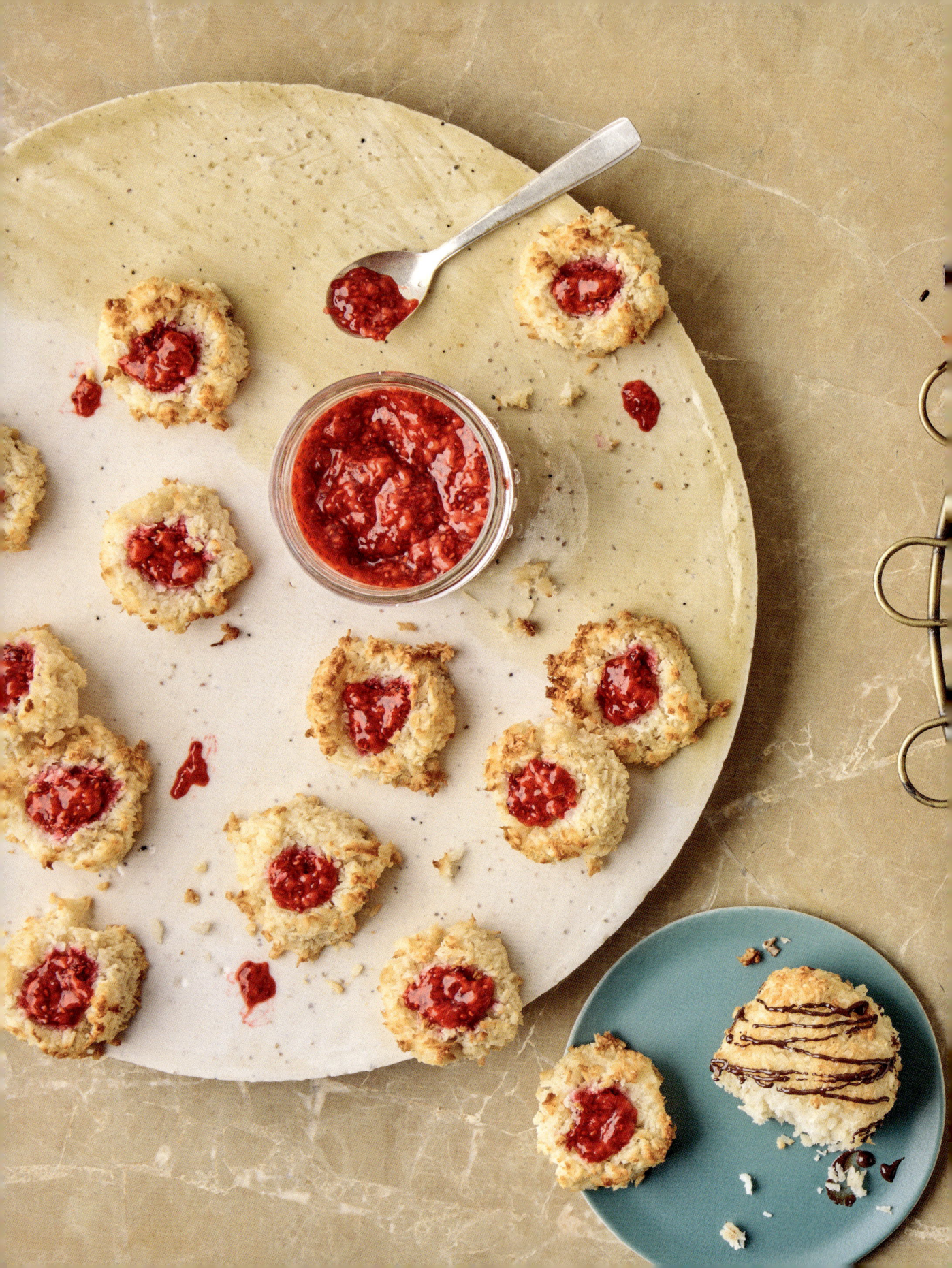

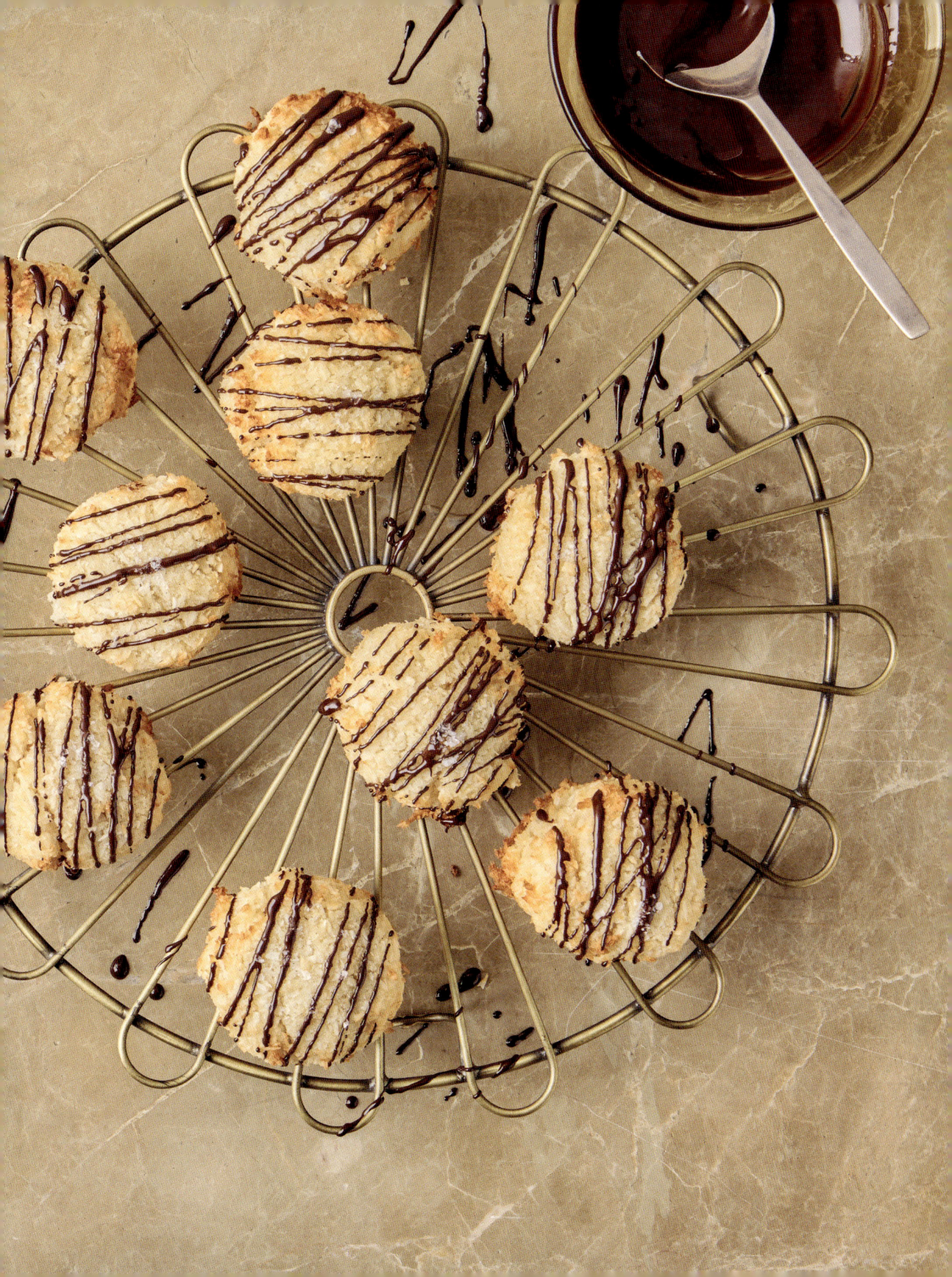

Breakfast bars were a staple in my diet, but when I found out the store-bought ones were loaded with butter, syrup, and enough sugar to crash an elephant . . . I knew my breakfast-bar obsession could be the cause of some of my inflammation. These anti-inflammatory breakfast bars have had a healthy makeover. They are packed full of fiber, are naturally sweetened, and are perfect to snack on, use as a pre-workout boost, or pack in your lunch box—trust me, you're going to love them.

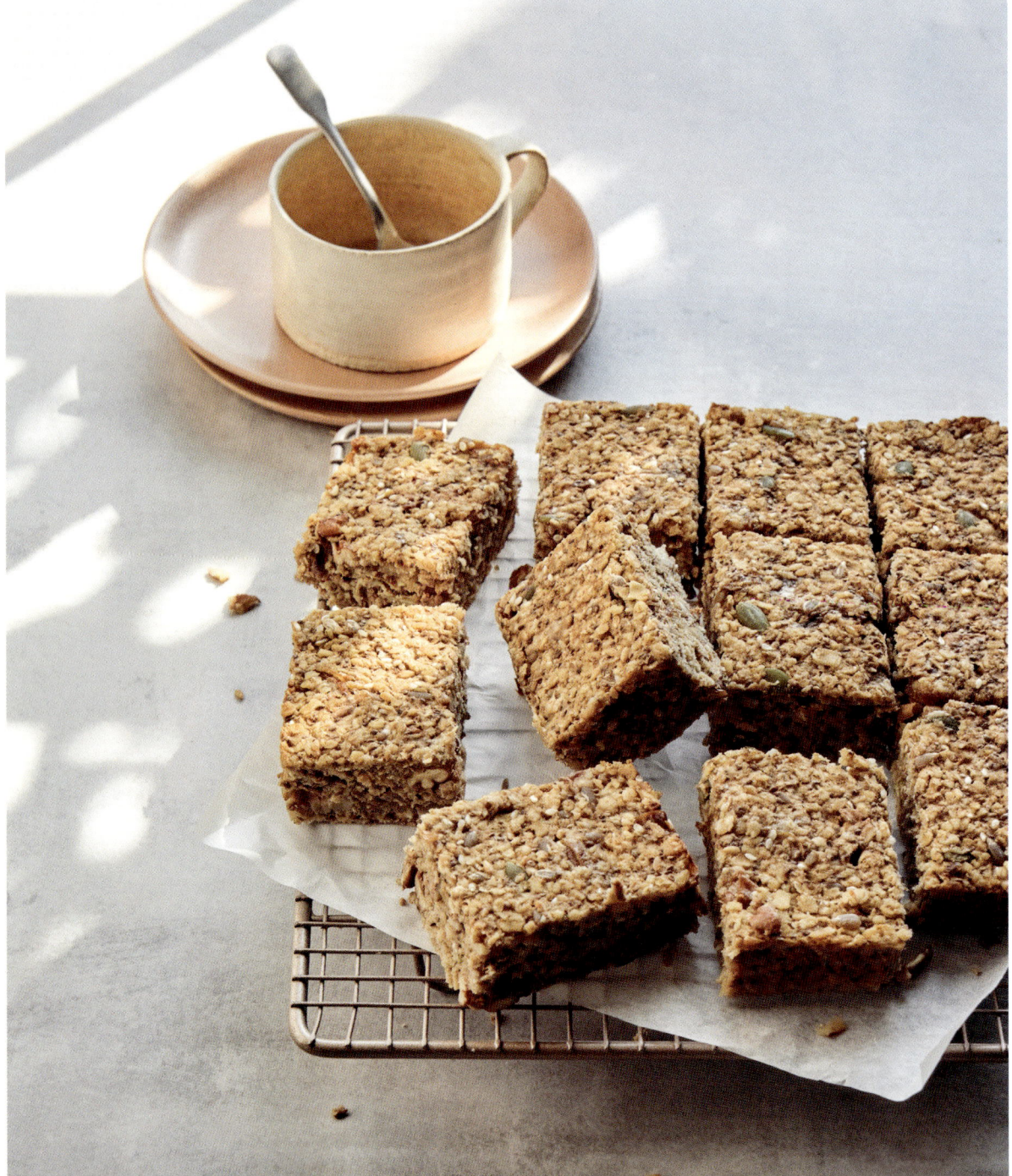

Fruit & Nut Breakfast Bars

MAKES 12   ○   HIGH FIBER, NATURALLY SWEETENED

INGREDIENTS

2 tbsp chia seeds
2½ cups/200g gluten-free oats
¾ cup/75g pecans, chopped
50g mixed seeds
1½ tsp ground cinnamon
a pinch of sea salt
2 ripe bananas
½ cup/100g stewed apple (or 2 fresh apples, cored and blended)
2 tbsp almond butter
½ tsp vanilla extract
2 tbsp coconut oil, melted
3 Medjool dates, pits removed, finely chopped

Preheat the oven to 350°F (fan) and line a 8-inch square baking pan with parchment paper.

Put the chia seeds into a small bowl and add 5 tbsp of water. Leave to soak.

Mix the oats, pecans, mixed seeds, cinnamon, and salt in a large bowl.

Put the bananas into a bowl and mash well. Add the stewed (or blended) apple, almond butter, vanilla, and coconut oil. Stir well until all is combined. Add the chia seeds and dates and combine again, ensuring the dates are evenly spread out, as they can tend to stick together. It may not look great, but believe in the process!

Stir the wet mixture into the dry ingredients until well combined.

Press the mixture very firmly into the lined pan and smooth the surface with the back of a spoon.

Bake for 20–25 minutes, or until golden brown.

Remove from the oven and lightly score into rectangles, making it easier to cut when they are cool. Leave until cool before cutting completely and removing from the pan.

Store in an airtight container for 3–4 days.

OPTIONS

For chocoholics, add ¼ cup/50g of 85% dark chocolate chips to the mixture. Alternatively, when cut and cooled, drizzle with melted dark chocolate.

For coconut lovers, add ½ cup/40g of desiccated coconut to give the dish a delicious yet sweet new flavor.

NUTRITIONAL INFORMATION *(Per Serving)*

Calories 217Kcals   ○   Net carbohydrates 22.3g   ○   Fiber 4.4g   ○   Fat 12.7g   ○   Protein 4.8g

The 2-Minute Craving Crusher

SERVES 1 ○ VEGAN, GRAIN-FREE

INGREDIENTS

- 1 apple (Pink Lady for sweetness, Granny Smith for a tangy kick)
- 2 tbsp almond butter
- ½ tsp ground cinnamon
- 1 tbsp/10g dark chocolate chips (85% cocoa or higher)

Core the apple using an apple corer and slice it into thick rings.

Spread each ring with almond butter.

Finish with a sprinkle of cinnamon and some dark chocolate chips.

PROTEIN HITS

Prosciutto & almond butter: Wrap a thin slice of prosciutto around the apple ring and top with almond butter. The sweet-salty contrast is amazing!

Smoked salmon & creamy tahini: Spread with a little tahini or cashew butter, then top with smoked salmon and a sprinkle of sesame seeds.

Tuna & avocado smash: Mash an avocado with lemon juice and a drained 110g can of tuna, then spread over the apple slice for a fresh, protein-rich twist.

SERVING OPTIONS & VARIATIONS

Nut butter choices: Try cashew butter, peanut butter, or tahini for a twist.

Savory hit: Spread with tahini or hummus and top with cucumber, sun-dried tomatoes, or olives.

Crunch factor: Add crushed walnuts, pecans, or a sprinkle of cacao nibs.

Extra sweetness: Drizzle with maple syrup or top with a few chopped Medjool dates.

Gut-friendly additions: Add ground flaxseeds or chia seeds for extra fiber and omega-3.

NUTRITIONAL INFORMATION *(Per Serving)*

Calories 288Kcals ○ Net carbohydrates 17.2g ○ Fiber 7.3g ○ Fat 21.2g ○ Protein 7.9g

We **ALL** have those moments where we need something sweet ASAP, and this quick snack is a lifesaver—it completely satisfies our sweet tooth, while also keeping us full. It's packed with protein, healthy fats, and fiber, so it's the perfect way to curb our cravings in minutes. Super simple, and delicious!

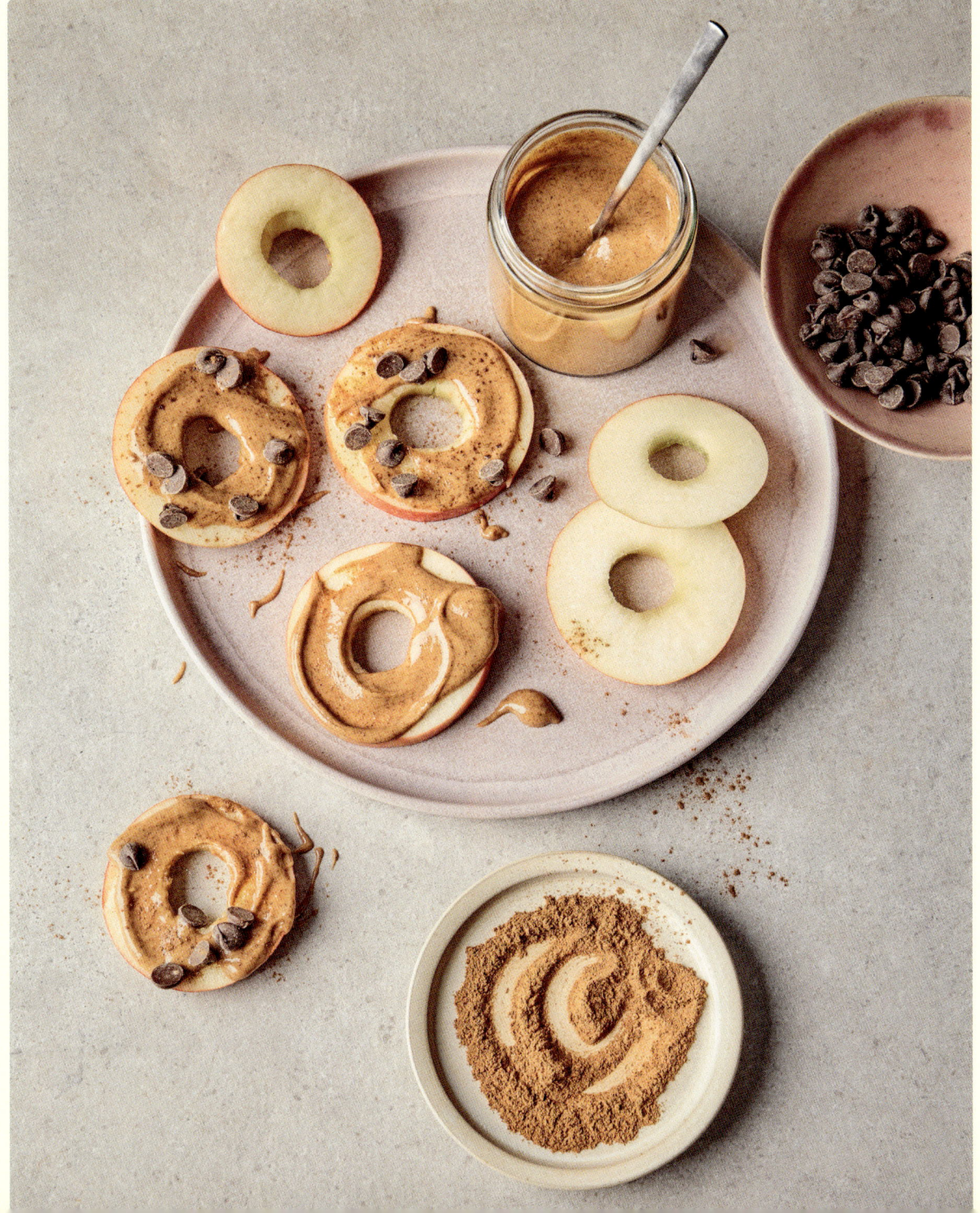

Cookies on an anti-inflammatory reset? Yes, please! These chewy, nutty, and deliciously indulgent cookies are everything you'd expect from a regular cookie, and more. The combination of macadamia nuts, coconut, and dark chocolate chips makes the most incredibly rich and satisfying flavor, all while being completely gluten- and dairy-free. They're naturally sweetened, taste incredible, and are the perfect snack no matter what time of day it is. These are a MUST-make recipe!

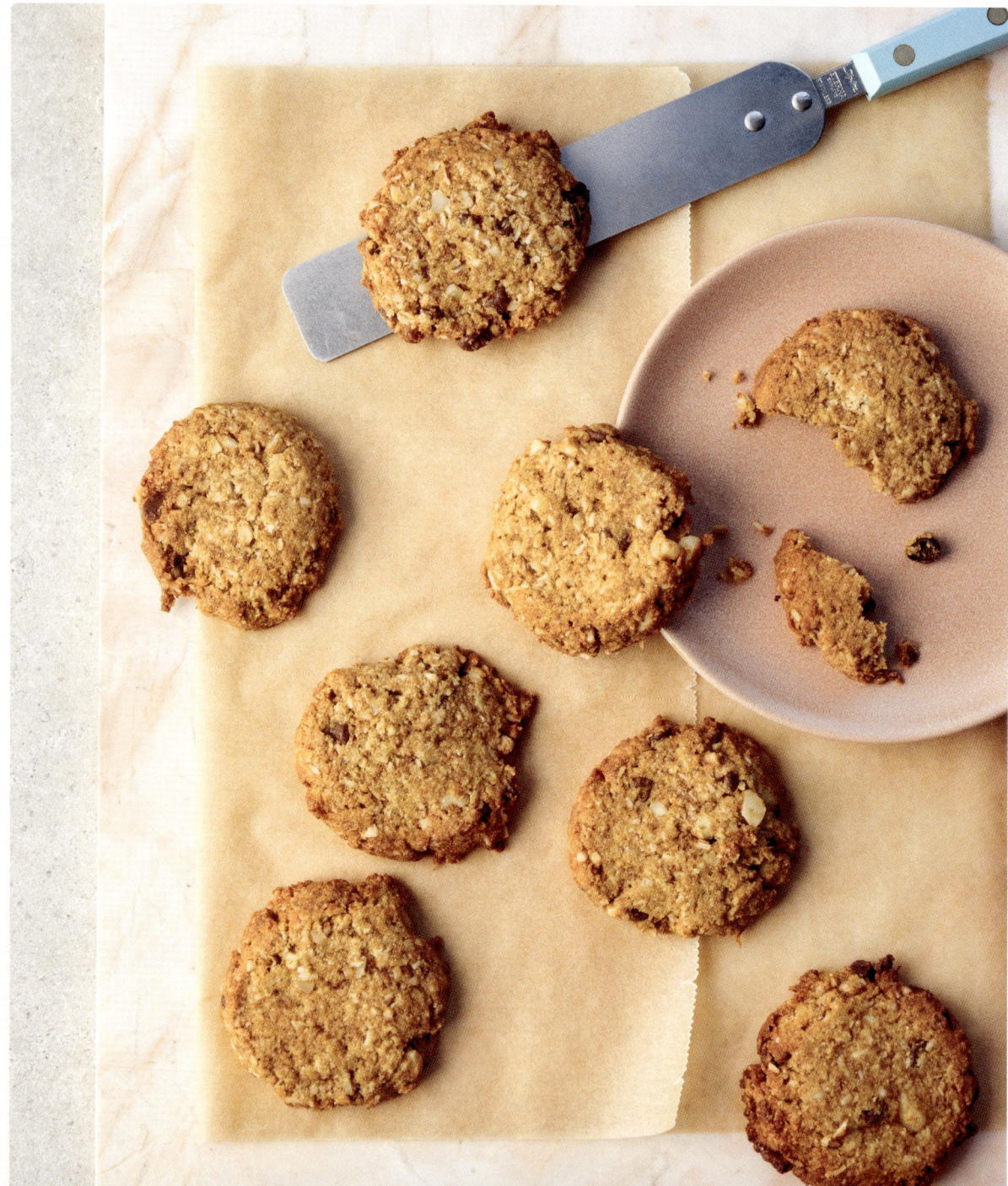

Coconut, Chocolate Chip & Macadamia Cookies

MAKES 14 ○ VEGETARIAN, GRAIN-FREE

INGREDIENTS

7 tbsp/100g coconut oil
2 medium eggs
½ tsp vanilla paste
¾ cup/100g coconut sugar
¼ tsp sea salt
⅔ cup/50g desiccated coconut
½ cup/75g macadamia nuts, chopped/crushed
¼ cup/50g 85% dark chocolate chips
⅔ cup/75g almond flour
⅓ cup/30g coconut flour

Preheat the oven to 325°F (fan) and line a baking sheet with parchment paper.

Melt the coconut oil and allow it to cool slightly.

Whisk together the eggs, vanilla paste, and melted coconut oil in a mixing bowl until well combined.

In a separate bowl, combine the coconut sugar, salt, desiccated coconut, macadamia nuts, dark chocolate chips, almond flour, and coconut flour.

Gradually add the wet ingredients to the dry mixture, stirring well to ensure even distribution.

Allow the dough to rest for a few minutes to let the coconut flour absorb the moisture.

Take 1 dessertspoon-sized portion of the mix. Place on the lined baking sheet and press flat, to approximately 2½ inches in diameter.

Repeat with the rest of the mixture, leaving small gaps between the cookies to allow for a slight spread as they cook.

Bake for 12–15 minutes, or until lightly golden.

Allow the cookies to cool completely before removing them from the sheet.

Store in an airtight container for freshness.

NUTRITIONAL INFORMATION *(Per Serving)*

Calories 227Kcals ○ Net carbohydrates 9.1g ○ Fiber 2.3g ○ Fat 19.3g ○ Protein 3.6g

Salted Caramel Swirl Brownies

MAKES 9 ○ RICH, INDULGENT, VEGETARIAN, AND GRAIN-FREE

INGREDIENTS

- ¾ cup/150g 85% dark chocolate
- 7 tbsp/100g coconut oil
- ¾ cup/100g coconut sugar
- 2 medium eggs
- 1 tsp vanilla paste
- ½ cup/65g almond flour
- ¼ cup/30g cocoa powder
- ½ tsp gluten-free baking powder
- ½ tsp sea salt, plus extra for garnish
- 2–3 tsp Caramel Sauce (page 294)

Preheat the oven to 350°F (fan) and line an 8-inch square baking pan with parchment paper.

Melt the dark chocolate and coconut oil together in a heatproof bowl over simmering water (or microwave in short bursts). Stir until smooth.

In a separate bowl, whisk together the coconut sugar, eggs, and vanilla until light and fluffy.

Once the coconut oil and chocolate are melted, stir into the egg mixture until fully combined.

Sift in the almond flour, cocoa powder, baking powder, and sea salt, and fold gently until just combined.

Pour into your lined pan and smooth the surface until it is evenly spread.

Drizzle the Caramel Sauce in little dollops randomly over the cake batter, then use a knife or skewer to swirl the sauce into the batter.

Sprinkle with extra sea salt flakes for an added salty kick.

Bake for 18–22 minutes. It is best if it has a very slight wobble in the center, so you get a gooey brownie.

Allow to cool for at least 15 minutes (unless you like to eat it hot) before slicing into 9 pieces.

Store in an airtight container for 3–4 days, or in the fridge for a fudgier texture.

SERVING OPTIONS

Serve hot or cold. If hot, they are delicious with a dollop of coconut yogurt and a drizzle of Caramel Sauce.

NUTRITIONAL INFORMATION *(Per Serving)*

Calories 328Kcals ○ Net carbohydrates 12.5g ○ Fiber 3.9g ○ Fat 29.73g ○ Protein 5.8g

These are the BEST brownies you will ever taste, so stop what you're doing and get cooking immediately! These fudgy, chocolatey brownies are a perfect balance of dark chocolate richness and salted caramel sweetness. The swirls of homemade caramel add a gooey texture that pairs perfectly with the deep, intense cocoa flavor. Incredible for dessert lovers looking for a grain-free treat without sacrificing on taste or texture.

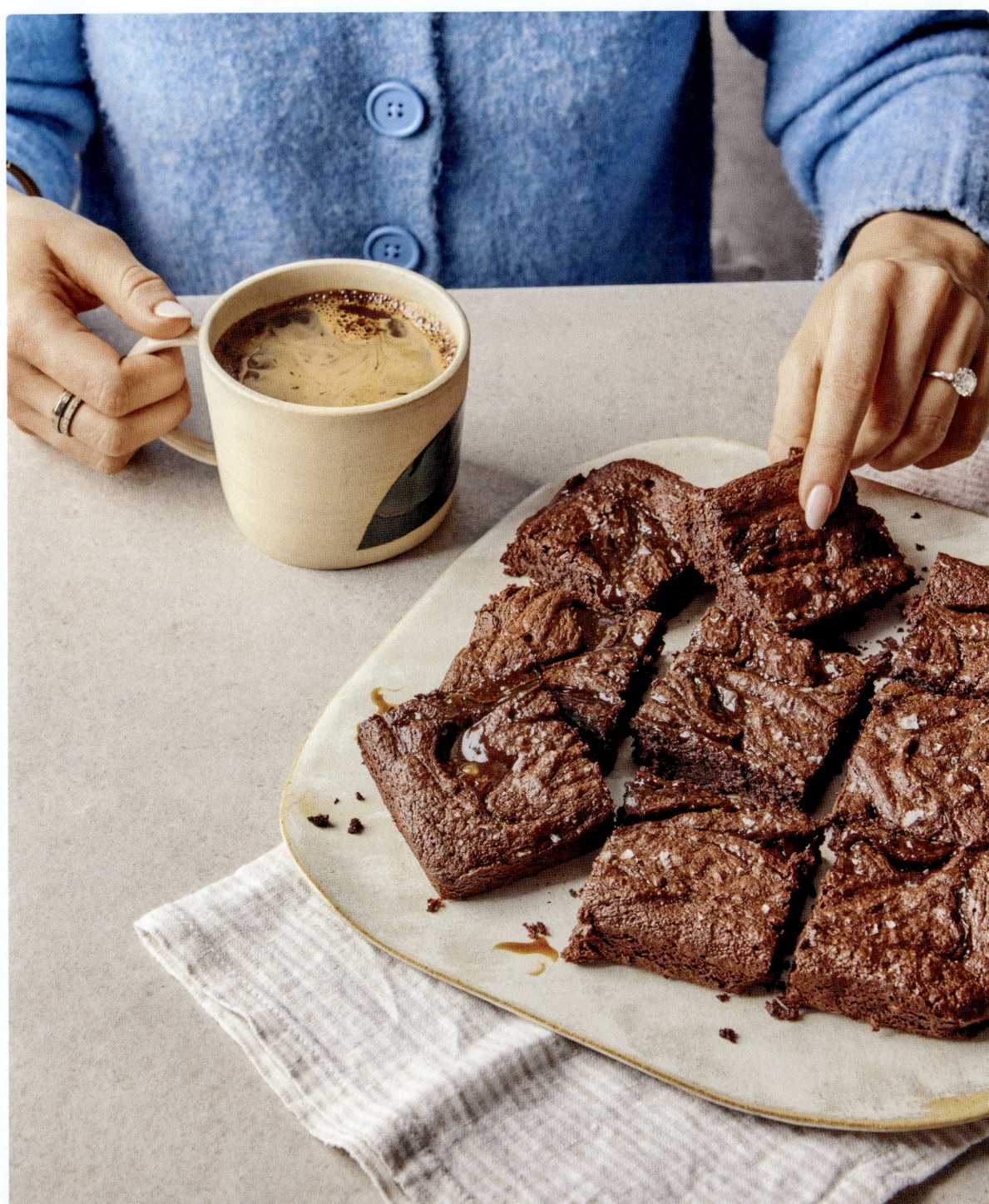

This most indulgent, moist, and tasty spiced apple cake will win over anyone with a sweet tooth, while also being packed with fiber, protein, and healthy fats—so it's a nourishing twist on the classic apple loaf. With warm spices, chunks of Bramley apple, and a natural sweetness from banana, dates, and maple syrup, it's ideal for cozy afternoons or a wholesome breakfast slice. Serve it on its own, or—my personal favorite—with a big spoon of Natural Live Coconut Yogurt (page 299).

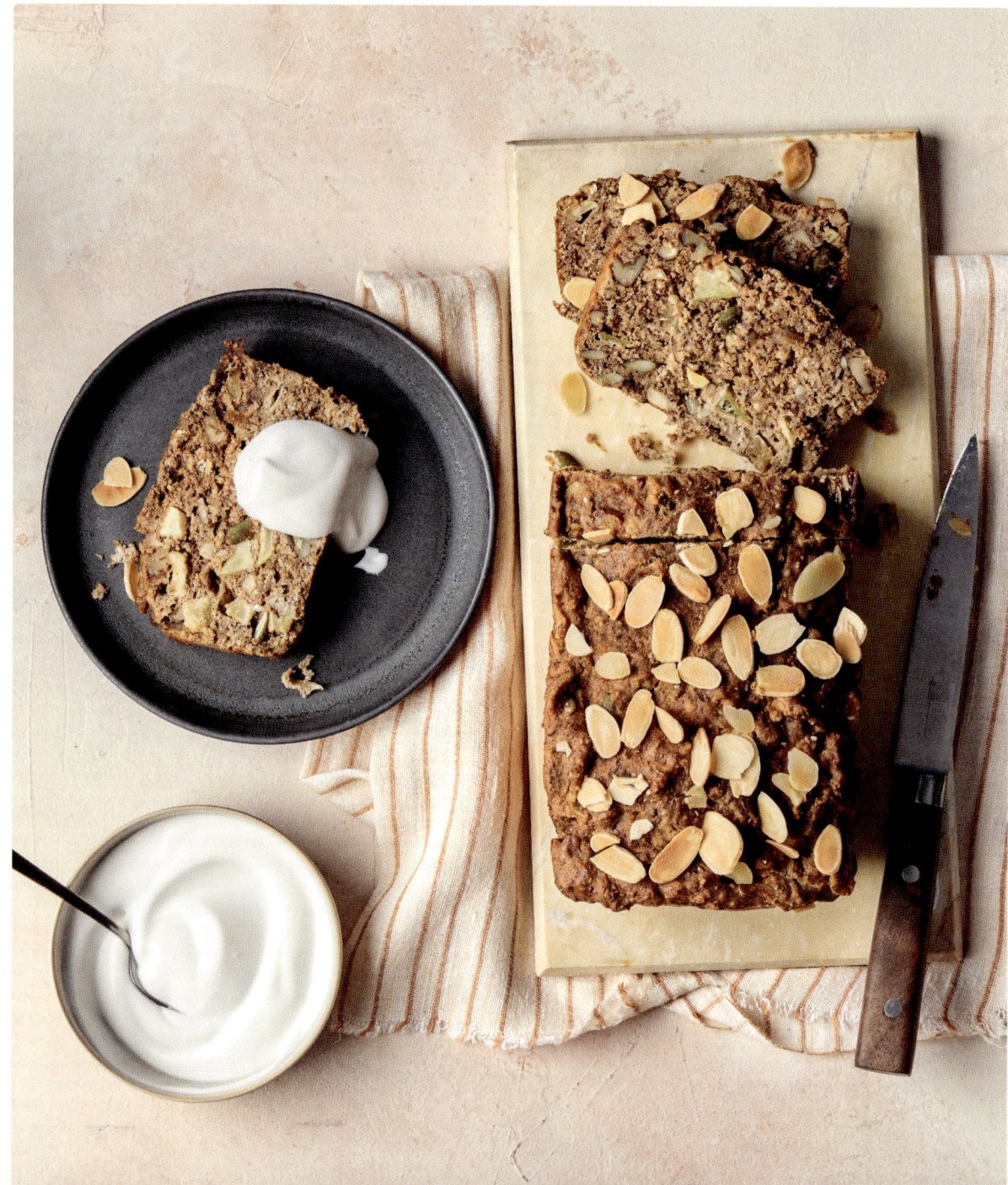

Loaded Apple Tea Cake

SERVES 8-10 ○ HIGH FIBER, NATURALLY SWEETENED

INGREDIENTS

- 1 cup/120g oat flour or buckwheat flour
- ½ cup/50g ground almonds
- ½ cup/50g gluten-free oats
- 1 tsp baking powder
- 2 tsp ground cinnamon
- ½ tsp ground cardamom
- ½ tsp ground ginger
- a pinch of sea salt
- ¼ cup/40g chopped walnuts
- 2 tbsp pumpkin seeds
- 1 tbsp chia seeds
- 1 tbsp milled flaxseeds
- 3 medium eggs
- ¼ cup/50ml olive oil
- 1 tsp vanilla extract
- 2 tbsp maple syrup
- ½ cup/100ml unsweetened almond milk
- 1 ripe banana, mashed
- 3 Medjool dates, pitted and finely chopped
- 1 Bramley cooking apple, cored and diced
- 1 tbsp sliced almonds

Preheat the oven to 350°F (fan) and line a 2lb/900g loaf pan with parchment paper or a cake liner.

Place all the dry ingredients in a bowl, including the nuts and seeds, and combine well.

Put the eggs into a jug with the olive oil, vanilla extract, maple syrup, and almond milk, and combine well.

Pour the wet ingredients into the dry ingredients, then add the banana, dates, and apple and combine well.

Place the cake batter in your loaf pan and sprinkle with the almonds.

Bake for 40–45 minutes, until the cake is firm to the touch. Insert a knife or skewer into the center of the cake; when cooked, it should come out clean.

Remove the cake from the oven. Cool in the pan for 10 minutes, then transfer to a wire rack to cool completely.

Once cooled, store in an airtight container.

TOP TIPS

For a sweeter cake, add an extra 2 tbsp of maple syrup.

Oat flour creates a softer, moister crumb, while buckwheat flour gives a slightly earthier, denser texture. Both work beautifully—choose based on your preference.

Bake in muffin pans to make breakfast muffins. Adjust the timing to 18–22 minutes.

Can be frozen.

Add 3 tbsp/30g of golden raisins for more sweetness.

For a crusty topping, mix 1 tsp of coconut sugar with 1 tsp of ground cinnamon and sprinkle over the batter before baking.

Cut into slices and spread with almond butter.

NUTRITIONAL INFORMATION *(Per Serving)*

Calories 264Kcals ○ Net carbohydrates 24.2g ○ Fiber 4.6g ○ Fat 15.9g ○ Protein 7.5g

Oaty Cookies

MAKES 15 COOKIES ◦ VEGAN

INGREDIENTS

- 1¾ cups/150g gluten-free oats
- ⅔ cup/30g oat fiber (see Note below)
- ½ tsp baking powder
- ½ tsp sea salt
- 1 tsp ground cinnamon
- ¼ cup/50g coconut sugar
- ¼ cup plus 1 tbsp/75ml maple or date syrup
- 5½ tbsp/80g coconut oil
- 1 tsp vanilla extract
- 2 medium eggs

Preheat the oven to 350°F (fan) and line a baking sheet with parchment paper.

In a bowl, combine the oats, oat fiber, baking powder, salt, and cinnamon. Add the coconut sugar.

Put the syrup, coconut oil, and vanilla into a saucepan and heat gently over a medium heat until they are thoroughly combined.

Pour the syrup and the eggs into the dry ingredients and combine well.

Shape the cookies into small balls about the size of a walnut. Place them on your lined baking sheet and flatten them to about ³⁄₁₆-inch/5mm thick.

Bake for 12–15 minutes, until golden.

Remove from the oven and allow to cool.

Store in an airtight container for 4–5 days.

SERVING OPTION

Chocolate lovers can coat the cookies in dark chocolate.

Note: Not all oat fibers are the same. Some are more like oat bran and look like flour. This recipe uses Oat Fiber from Groovy Keto, which is incredibly light oat fiber—it looks like fluff. It is much finer and fluffier than typical oat fiber and creates lovely light results. If you use a different brand of oat fiber, you may need to add a little more, up to around ½ cup/ 50g; if it is a denser oat fiber and add another egg if it is too dry.

NUTRITIONAL INFORMATION *(Per Serving)*

Calories 122Kcals ◦ Net carbohydrates 13.7g ◦ Fiber 2.8g ◦ Fat 6.8g ◦ Protein 2g

A spin on the classic oat cookie, these are a softer, chewier version—so if you love texture, this one's for you! Made with wholesome oats, with a touch of natural sweetness, and a warm cinnamon hit—they're ridiculously easy to make. Want to go the extra mile? Dip them in dark chocolate, because let's face it, everything's better with chocolate, right?

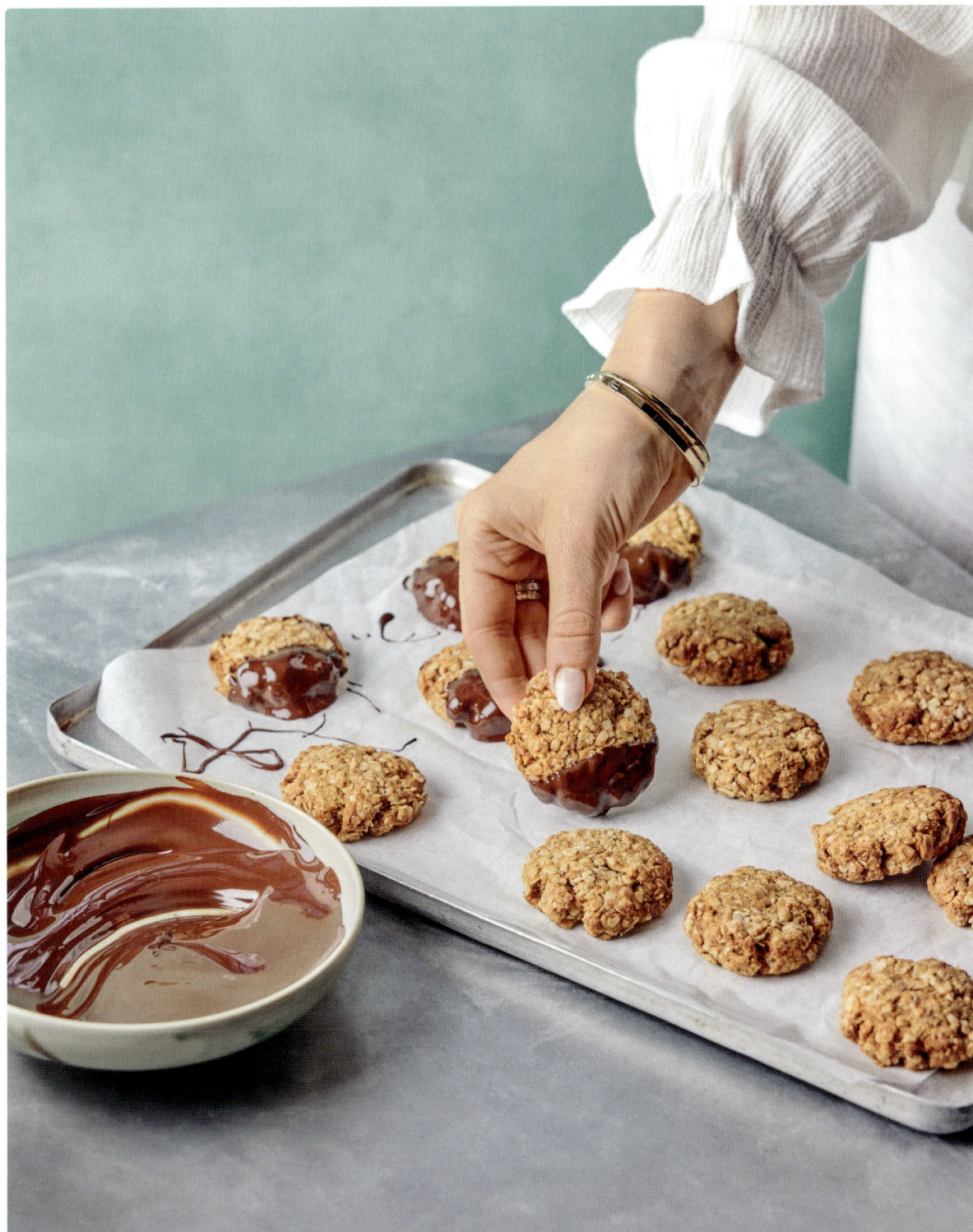

These mouth-watering chocolatey twice-baked biscotti are a gorgeous blend of dark chocolate, toasted hazelnuts, and zesty orange. They're naturally sweetened with coconut sugar and are made without grains . . . so they're perfect for anyone with a sweet tooth who's struggling with digestion! I love dipping these into coffee, batch cooking them for friends or, if you're feeling *extra,* pair them with creamy desserts like my Rich & Creamy Chocolate Mousse (page 239).

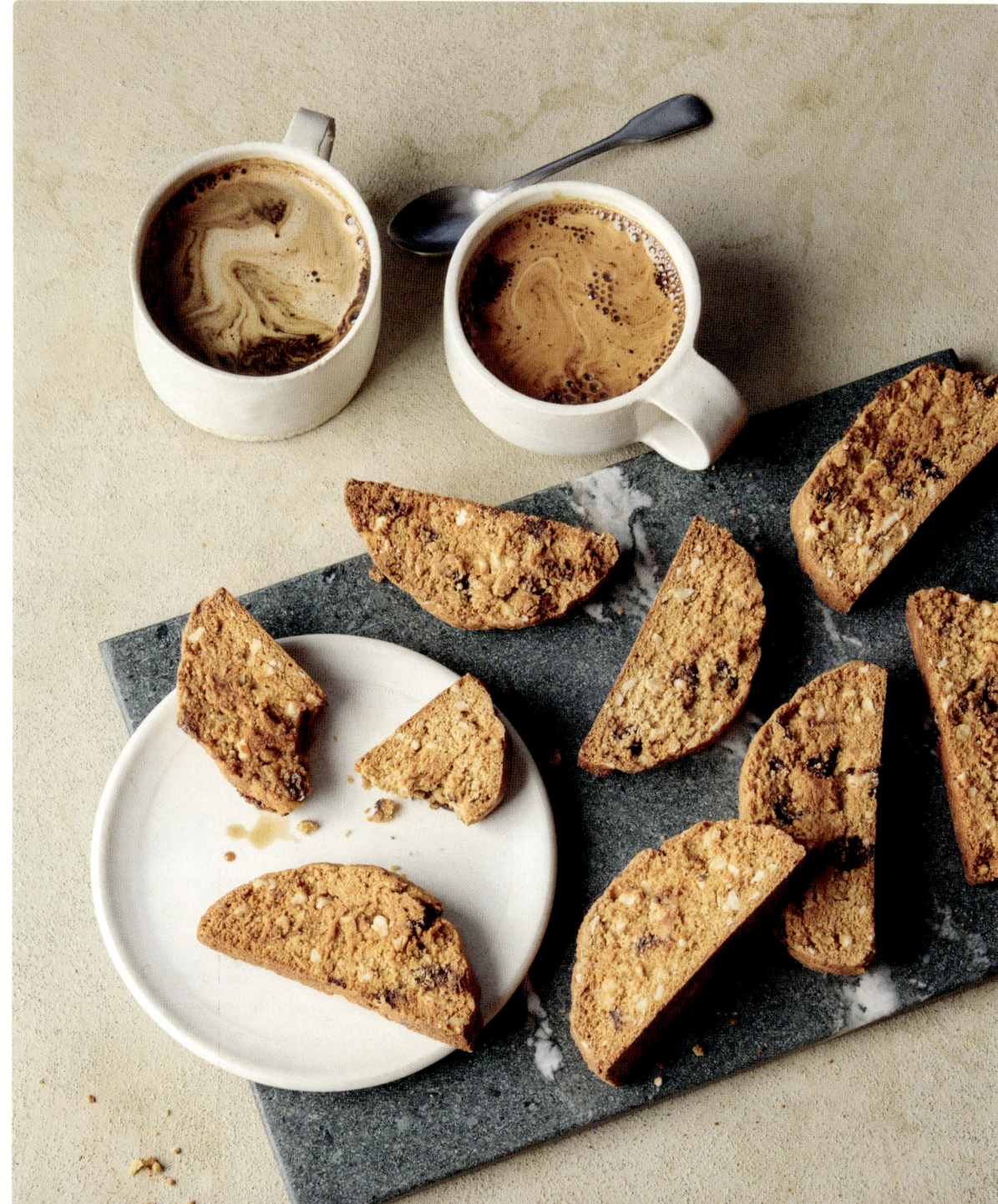

Chocolate, Hazelnut & Orange Biscotti

MAKES 12 BISCOTTI ○ GRAIN-FREE, DAIRY-FREE

INGREDIENTS

- 2 cups/240g ground almonds
- 1 tsp baking powder
- a pinch of sea salt
- 2 medium eggs
- ½ cup/60g coconut sugar
- zest of 1 orange
- 1 tsp vanilla extract
- 3 tbsp/40g 85% dark chocolate chips
- ½ cup/60g chopped hazelnuts

Preheat the oven to 325°F (fan) and line a baking sheet with parchment paper.

In a large bowl, mix the almonds, baking powder, and salt.

In a separate bowl, whisk the eggs with the coconut sugar, orange zest, and vanilla.

Combine the wet and dry ingredients, then fold in the chocolate chips and hazelnuts. The dough will be sticky but firm. Shape into a domed log (approx. 9½ inches long, 2½ inches wide) and place on the baking sheet. Flatten slightly.

Bake for 20–25 minutes, until firm to touch. Remove and cool for at least 10 minutes.

Reduce the oven temperature to 284°F (fan). Using a sharp knife, slice the log into ¾-inch biscotti. When the bake is still warm, you may find this gets a bit messy with the melted chocolate chips, but use a sharp knife with a firm cut, or allow the bake to get completely cold before slicing.

Lay the slices flat on the sheet and bake for another 10–15 minutes, flipping halfway through to crisp and dry out the biscotti.

Remove from the oven and cool completely, then store in an airtight container for up to 2 weeks.

TOP TIPS

As these are made grain-free with nut flour, they can get soft over a few days, so you may want to do an extra dry-out to crisp them up.

For an edible gift, dip them in melted 85% chocolate and sprinkle with crushed hazelnuts or orange zest before setting.

For a deeper chocolate flavor, add 2 tbsp/20g of cocoa powder to the dough and reduce the ground almonds by the same amount.

NUTRITIONAL INFORMATION *(Per Serving)*

Calories 212Kcals ○ Net carbohydrates 7.3g ○ Fiber 2.1g ○ Fat 16.8g ○ Protein 7.1g

No-Bake Nut & Seed Bars

MAKES 12 BARS ○ HIGH FIBER, NATURALLY SWEET

INGREDIENTS

- ½ cup/100g 85% dark chocolate
- ⅔ cup/75g almonds, roughly chopped
- ⅔ cup/75g cashews, roughly chopped
- ⅓ cup/40g pecans, roughly chopped
- 3 tbsp/30g pumpkin seeds
- 3 tbsp/30g sunflower seeds
- 2 tbsp flaxseeds
- 1 tbsp chia seeds
- ½ tsp ground cinnamon
- ¼–½ tsp sea salt
- ½ cup/120ml honey
- 5 tbsp/75g maple syrup
- 1 tsp vanilla extract

Line an 8-inch square baking sheet with parchment paper, leaving the paper hanging over the edge for easy removal.

Melt the chocolate in a bowl over a pan of boiling water on low heat.

Pour half of the melted dark chocolate into your baking sheet, spreading it to form a thin coat over the base. Place the sheet in the freezer to set quickly.

Leave the remaining chocolate on low heat until you are ready to use it.

Toast the nuts, pumpkin seeds, and sunflower seeds lightly in a dry pan for 3 minutes. Put them in a large bowl with the flaxseeds, chia seeds, cinnamon, and sea salt and combine well.

In a small pan, heat the honey, maple syrup, and vanilla. Stir until well combined, then bring to the boil until the syrup reaches 257°F. Use a candy thermometer to test this. It will be very hot, so do not be tempted to touch it. Once it reaches temperature, pour the syrup immediately over the nut and seed mixture and combine well until everything is sticky. This step is key for holding the bars together—don't skip the thermometer!

Remove the sheet from the freezer and press the nut mixture firmly into your lined sheet, smoothing the top. To avoid getting your hands sticky, place a sheet of parchment paper over the mixture and use it to press down firmly.

Drizzle the melted chocolate over the nut base.

Place in the fridge for at least 2 hours. Once set, lift out using the parchment paper and cut into bars, using a very sharp knife.

Store in an airtight container, ideally in the fridge for up to 10 days, but they can be kept at room temperature for 3–4 days.

TOP TIP

If these are going into a packed lunch, wrap them in a piece of parchment paper, which can be held together with string.

NUTRITIONAL INFORMATION *(Per Serving)*

Calories 224Kcals ○ Net carbohydrates 16.1g ○ Fiber 4g ○ Fat 15.3g ○ Protein 5.1g

These bars are the perfect blend of crunchy nuts, chewy sweetness, and a hint of indulgent dark chocolate. Unlike traditional store-bought bars, they're naturally sweetened, loaded with fiber, and packed with healthy fats to keep you full and energized. Plus, a no-bake recipe means no fuss, too—it's a win-win!

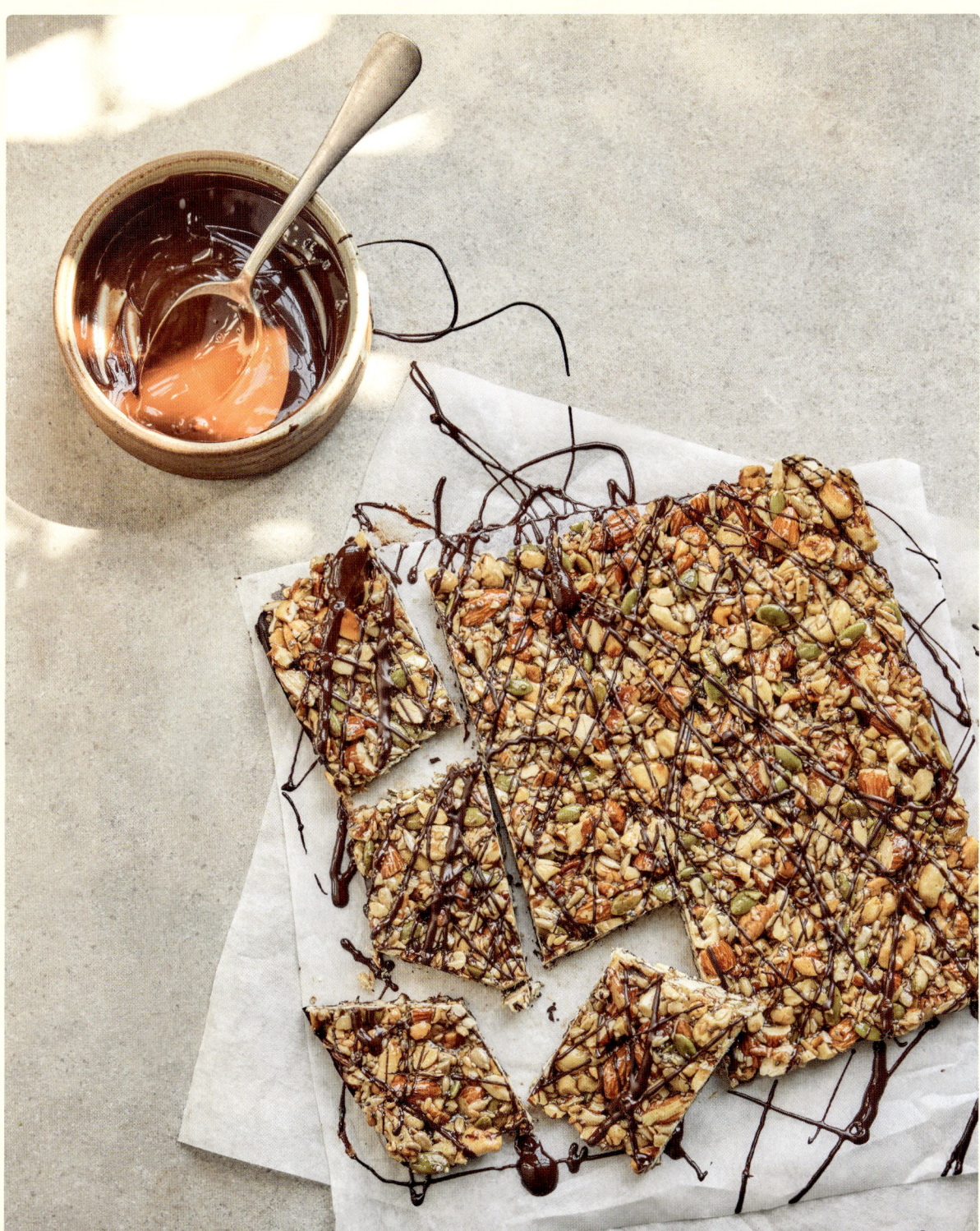

This decadent, fudgy chocolate sandwich cake is completely dairy-free but just as rich and satisfying as a traditional chocolate cake. Made with olive oil, dark chocolate, and plant yogurt, it's indulgent enough for a celebration but is made with ingredients that tick all the right nutritional boxes. The smooth ganache filling takes it to the next level.

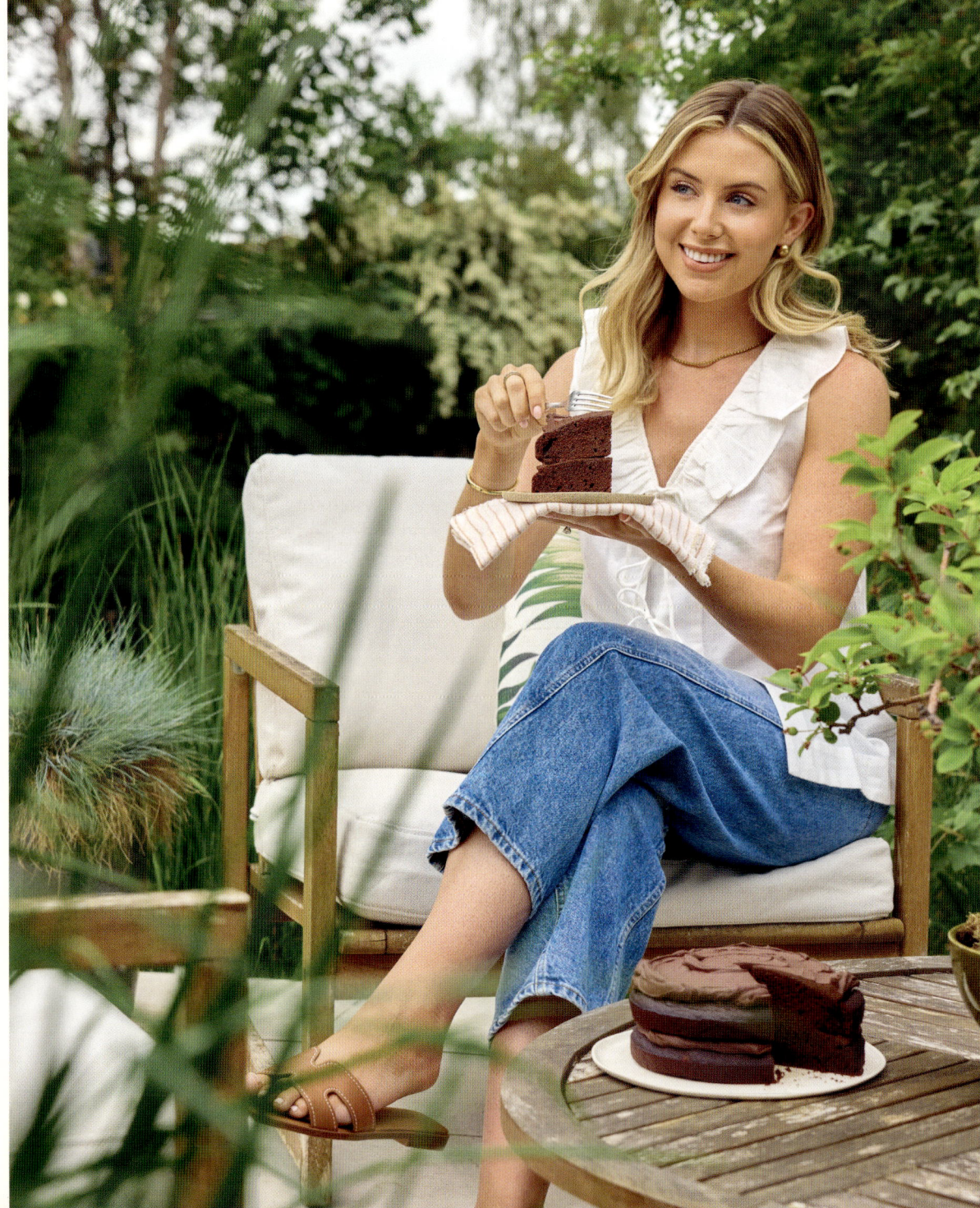

Rich Chocolate Cake
with Ganache Filling

SERVES 10 ○ GLUTEN-FREE, DAIRY-FREE

INGREDIENTS

- 1¼ cups/150g ground almonds
- ½ cup/60g oat flour or buckwheat flour
- ½ cup/60g unsweetened cocoa powder
- 2 tsp baking powder
- a pinch of sea salt
- 4 medium eggs
- ⅔ cup/150g Natural Live Coconut Yogurt (page 299) or plant-based yogurt
- ½ cup/120ml olive oil
- 150g coconut sugar
- ⅔ cup/150ml freshly brewed coffee, cooled
- ⅓ cup/75g 85% dark chocolate, melted
- 1½ tsp vanilla extract

For the ganache
- ¾ cup/150g 85% dark chocolate, finely chopped
- ½ cup plus 1 tbsp/150g coconut cream

Preheat the oven to 350°F (fan). Grease and line two 8-inch cake pans.

In a large bowl, mix together almonds, oat or buckwheat flour, cocoa powder, baking powder, and salt.

In another bowl, beat the eggs with the yogurt, olive oil, and coconut sugar until light and well combined. Add the coffee, melted chocolate, and vanilla to the wet mix and combine well.

Add the dry mixture and fold gently until combined. Divide the mixture equally between the two pans, spreading to cover the base and create a smooth, level top.

Bake for 20–25 minutes, until the sponge bounces back when touched and a skewer comes out clean. Remove from the oven and allow the cakes to cool in the pans for 5 minutes, then transfer them to a wire rack.

While the cakes are cooling, prepare the ganache. Place the chocolate pieces in a bowl. Heat the coconut cream in a small pan until steaming. Pour this over the chocolate and let it sit for 1 minute, then stir until thick and glossy. This can take several minutes. Chill for 10–15 minutes to thicken slightly.

Once the cakes are completely cold, use half the ganache to sandwich the cakes together. Spread the top with the remaining ganache.

Store in an airtight container. If kept in the fridge, it will last 4–5 days, but bring to room temperature before serving.

CARB BUSTER

To reduce the carb content of this cake (to under 8g per slice):

Replace the ½ cup/60g of oat/buckwheat flour with an additional ¾ cup/100g of ground almonds (making a total of 2 cups/250g of ground almonds).

Add ⅓ cup/30g of coconut flour to support the structure and absorb excess moisture.

Swap the coconut sugar for a sweetener such as erythritol, monk fruit, or stevia blend—adjust quantity to taste, as sweetness varies.

NUTRITIONAL INFORMATION *(Per Serving)*

Calories 508Kcals ○ Net carbohydrates 29.5g ○ Fiber 7.6g ○ Fat 37.8g ○ Protein 10.9g

Cocoa & Almond Energy Bars

MAKES 8 BARS ○ VEGAN, GRAIN-FREE, NATURALLY SWEET

INGREDIENTS

- 1 cup/200g Medjool dates, pitted
- 1 cup/100g almonds
- ¼ cup/30g cashews
- 2 tbsp/20g cocoa powder
- 1 tsp vanilla extract
- a pinch of sea salt

Berry Bliss Bars

- 1 cup/200g Medjool dates, pitted
- ¼ cup/40g dried cranberries or freeze-dried raspberries
- 1 cup/120g cashews
- 2½ tbsp/20g almonds
- zest of ½ a lemon
- ½ tsp vanilla extract
- a pinch of sea salt

Peanut Cocoa Fudge Bars

- 1 cup/200g Medjool dates, pitted
- 1 cup/120g roasted peanuts
- 2 tbsp/20g cocoa powder
- 1 tsp vanilla extract
- a pinch of sea salt

Cashew Cookie Dough Bars

- 1 cup/200g Medjool dates, pitted
- 1 cup/120g cashews
- 1 tsp vanilla extract
- a pinch of sea salt

Line a small loaf pan with parchment paper.

If your dates are dry, soak them in warm water for 10 minutes and drain well.

In a food processor, blitz the almonds and cashews until coarsely ground.

Add the dates, cocoa, vanilla, and salt, and blend until the mixture clumps together into a sticky dough.

Press the mixture firmly into your lined pan, smoothing the top. To avoid getting your hands sticky, place a sheet of parchment paper over the mixture and use it to press down firmly.

Chill in the fridge for 1–2 hours, then slice into 8 bars. Store chilled in an airtight container for up to 1 week.

TOP TIPS

For extra chewiness, pulse in 1 tbsp of nut butter or 1 tbsp of coconut oil.

Roll into balls instead of bars for date truffles.

Freeze for up to 3 months.

FLAVOR VARIATIONS

Try the base recipe as is, or explore the flavor variations on the left for different combinations of nuts, fruits, and spices. In each case, blitz the nuts as in the base recipe.

NUTRITIONAL INFORMATION *(Per Serving)*

Calories 170Kcals ○ Net carbohydrates 20.5g ○ Fiber 4.2g ○ Fat 8.6g ○ Protein 4.3g

These chewy Cocoa & Almond Energy Bars are made with just a handful of whole-food ingredients and with **NO** baking required—so it's easy-peasy! Naturally sweetened with dates and packed with nuts, they're perfect for a quick snack, packed lunch, or pre-workout hit. A healthy, unprocessed, on-the-go treat.

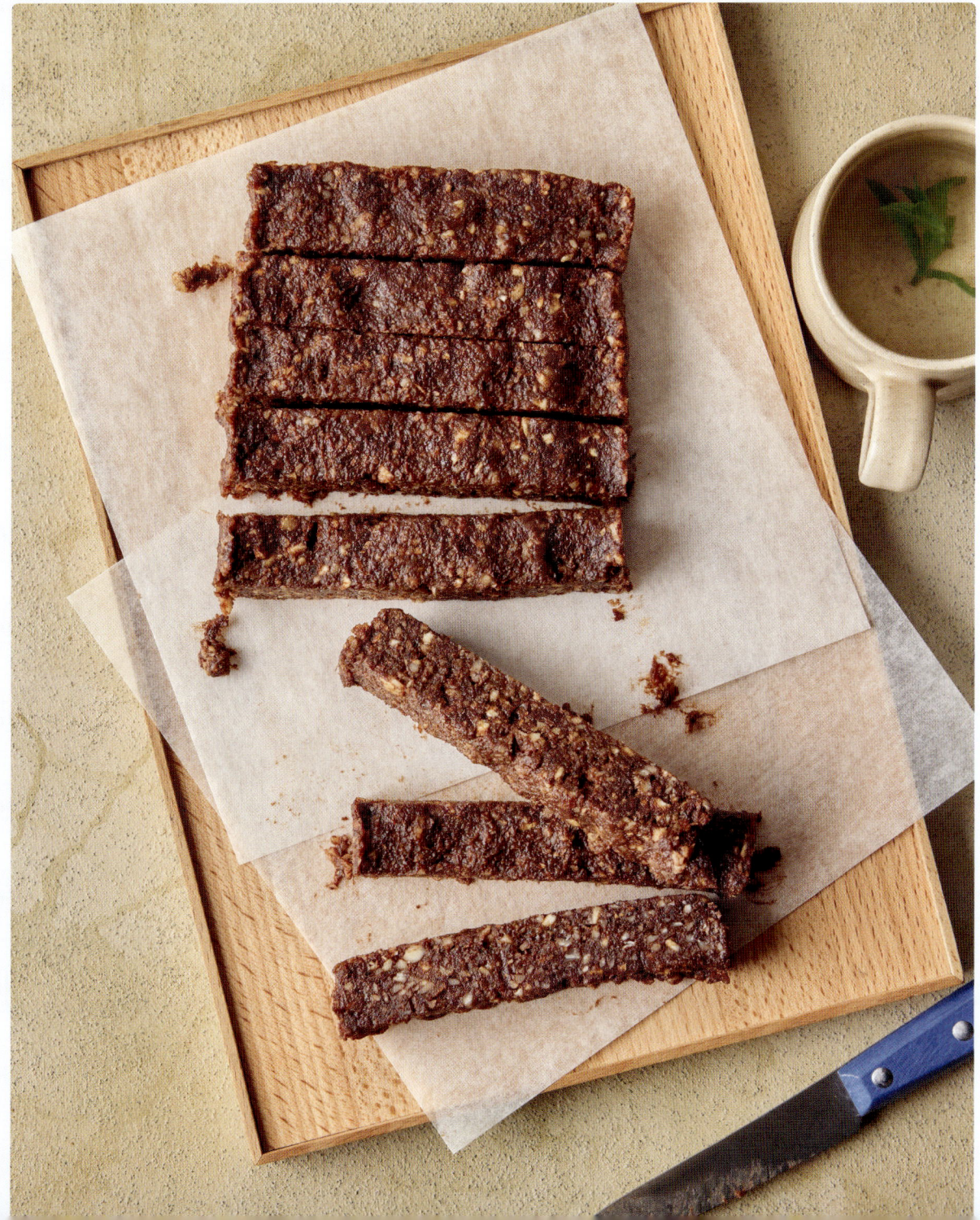

Pant

ry

This is a gut-boosting, must-make recipe. It's a vibrant, gut-loving fermented mix, full of fiber, antioxidants, and natural probiotics (remember, food is medicine, too!). It's the perfect side dish or topping to support digestion, microbiome health, and it tastes great, too.

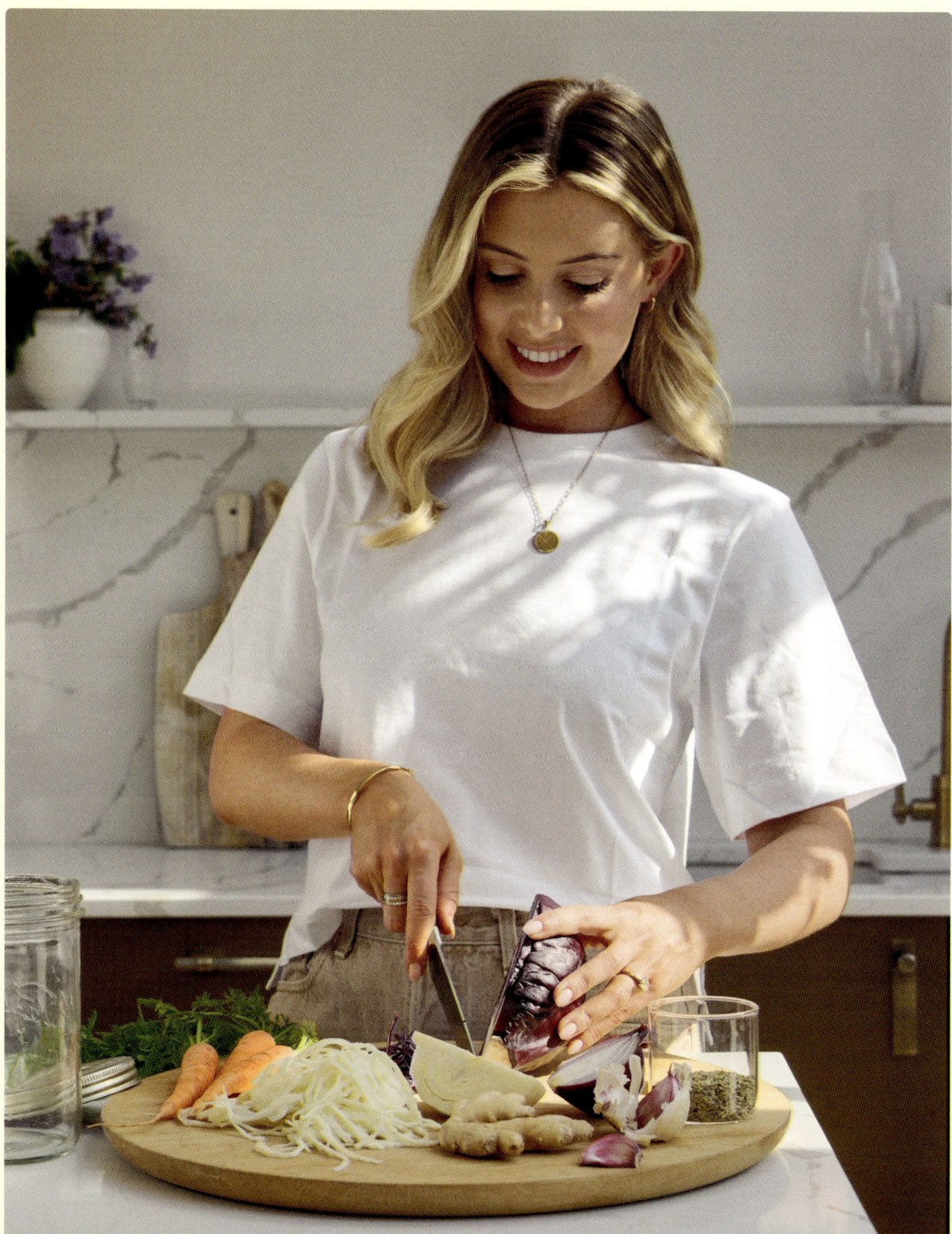

Fermented Rainbow Kraut

MAKES ONE 1-LITER JAR* ○ GUT-FRIENDLY

INGREDIENTS

- ½ a small red cabbage (approx. 3¼ cups/400g), finely shredded
- ½ a small green cabbage (approx. 3¼ cups/400g), finely shredded
- 1 medium carrot, grated
- ½ a small red onion, finely sliced
- 1 tbsp fresh ginger, peeled and grated
- 1 clove of garlic, finely grated (optional)
- 1½ tsp fine sea salt (non-iodized)
- 1 tsp caraway seeds or fennel seeds (optional)

(ferments for 5–7 days, depending on temperature)

Combine all the ingredients in a large mixing bowl. Massage well with your hands for 5–10 minutes, until the liquid begins to be released and the cabbage softens. You're creating the brine through this process.

Pack the mixture tightly into a clean 1-liter glass jar, pressing down as you go so that the brine rises to cover the vegetables.

Leave a little headspace at the top (about ¾ inch). Weigh down with a clean cabbage leaf and a fermentation weight or small sterilized glass to keep the kraut submerged.

Seal loosely with a lid or use a breathable fermenting lid.

Leave to ferment at room temperature, out of direct sunlight, for 5–7 days. Check daily, pressing down if needed to keep submerged.

Taste after 5 days. Once tangy enough, seal fully and move to the fridge, where it will keep for several months.

TOP TIPS

If scum forms on the top, skim it off—this is harmless and part of the natural fermentation.

For a more earthy kraut, add a grated raw beet. For heat, a little fresh chile works brilliantly.

Use as a side dish, in wraps, over avocado toast, or stirred through salads.

NUTRITIONAL INFORMATION *(Per 150g Serving)*

Calories 22Kcals ○ Net carbohydrates 2.7g ○ Fiber 1.9g ○ Fat 0.1g ○ Protein 0.7g

Chimichurri Sauce

MAKES APPROX. ½ CUP/100ML   ○   VEGAN

INGREDIENTS

¼ cup/60ml extra virgin olive oil
juice of ½ a lemon
2 tbsp red wine vinegar
3 cloves of garlic, crushed
1 small jalapeño, finely chopped (optional for spice)
1 cup/30g flat-leaf parsley, finely chopped
⅓ cup/10g fresh cilantro, finely chopped
½ tsp dried oregano
½ tsp smoked paprika
sea salt and freshly ground black pepper, to taste

Prepare the chimichurri in a bowl by combining the olive oil, lemon juice, red wine vinegar, garlic, jalapeño, parsley, cilantro, oregano, smoked paprika, salt, and black pepper.

Stir well and set aside for at least 10 minutes to let the flavors infuse.

Store in the fridge until ready to serve.

NUTRITIONAL INFORMATION *(Per 1 tbsp/15ml Serving)*

Calories 79Kcals   ○   Net carbohydrates 0.2g   ○   Fiber 0.2g   ○   Fat 8.8g   ○   Protein 0.1g

I will ALWAYS have a big jar of chimichurri sauce in my fridge, because it goes with everything. Meat, fish, salads, you name it and I'm putting chimichurri on it. It's exactly why I've made it a staple in a few of the recipes (Chimichurri Steak on page 220 and Grilled Chimichurri Chicken Salad on page 173). Quick, easy, refreshing, and full of flavor.

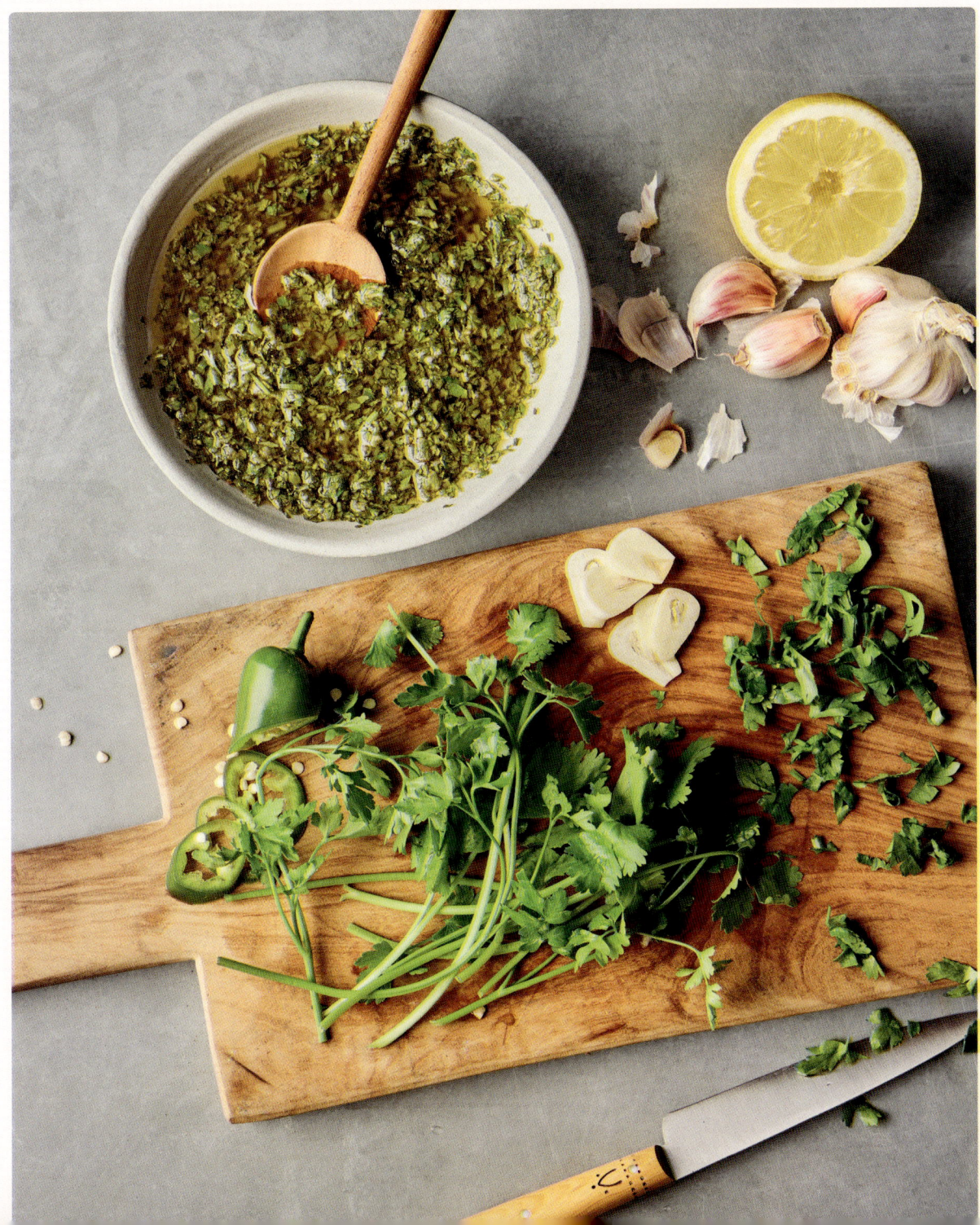

Caramel Sauce

MAKES APPROX. ⅔ CUP/150G ○ VEGAN, FREE FROM REFINED SUGARS

This velvety, thick, dairy-free caramel sauce is truly divine. It's the perfect accessory to your healthy desserts, made with just a few natural ingredients. The coconut cream and natural sweetness combine to give a rich, deep caramel flavor, with none of the ultra-processed ingredients you'll find in the supermarket alternatives (it tastes much better, too!). Drizzle it over your favorite dairy-free ice cream, swirl it into yogurt . . . oh, and of course you **MUST** use this on the Salted Caramel Swirl Brownies (page 274) for the perfect treat. The sauce sets to a soft consistency in the fridge, but don't worry—it will loosen back to liquid when gently heated.

INGREDIENTS

- ½ cup/100ml coconut cream
- ¼ cup/50g coconut sugar
- 1 tbsp maple syrup or date syrup
- ½ tsp sea salt
- ½ tsp vanilla paste

image on page 296

Heat the coconut cream, coconut sugar, maple syrup, and sea salt in a small saucepan over low/medium heat.

Stirring continuously to prevent it sticking or burning, let it simmer gently on low-medium heat for 5–7 minutes until it starts to thicken.

Remove from the heat and stir in the vanilla paste. Let it cool slightly.

Pour into a bowl or jar and place in the fridge, ideally for at least 2–3 hours to allow it to set to a soft consistency.

The sauce can be stored in the fridge for up to 1 week.

NUTRITIONAL INFORMATION *(Per 15g Serving)*

Calories 56Kcals ○ Net carbohydrates 6.5g ○ Fiber 0.2g ○ Fat 3.5g ○ Protein 0.4g

Healthy Chocolate Spread

MAKES APPROX. 1½ CUPS/350G   ○   HIGH IN OMEGAS AND POLYPHENOLS

This divine, velvety nutty chocolate spread is a game changer! It's rich, chocolatey, and packed with nourishing fats from the hazelnuts and can be used in so many ways. I love dolloping it onto apple slices, toast, and of course straight off the spoon... don't judge, you'll be doing it too once you've tried it! Naturally free from dairy, refined sugar, and gluten, too—what a dream.

INGREDIENTS

- 1 cup/100g blanched hazelnuts
- 1 cup/100g pumpkin seeds
- ½ cup/100g 85% dark chocolate
- 1 tbsp date syrup or honey
- ½ tsp vanilla extract
- a pinch of sea salt

image on page 296

Preheat the oven to 350°F (fan) and line a baking sheet with parchment paper. Spread the hazelnuts and pumpkin seeds in a single layer and roast for 8–10 minutes, until golden and fragrant. Keep an eye on them, as they can burn quickly.

Break the chocolate into pieces and melt in a heatproof bowl set over a pan of gently simmering water, making sure the bowl doesn't touch the water. Stir until smooth.

Transfer the toasted nuts and seeds to a food processor and blitz for 6–8 minutes, until smooth and buttery, scraping down the sides as needed.

Add the melted chocolate, date syrup or honey, vanilla, and sea salt. Blitz again until fully combined.

Spoon into a clean jar and store in the fridge for up to 2 weeks.

TOP TIPS

Add a pinch of cinnamon or espresso powder for a deeper chocolate hit.

Swirl through coconut yogurt for an indulgent treat.

Delicious served with sliced banana or apple, or dolloped on to pancakes.

NUTRITIONAL INFORMATION *(Per 20g Serving)*

Calories 112Kcals   ○   Net carbohydrates 2.8g   ○   Fiber 1.8g   ○   Fat 8.8g   ○   Protein 4.4g

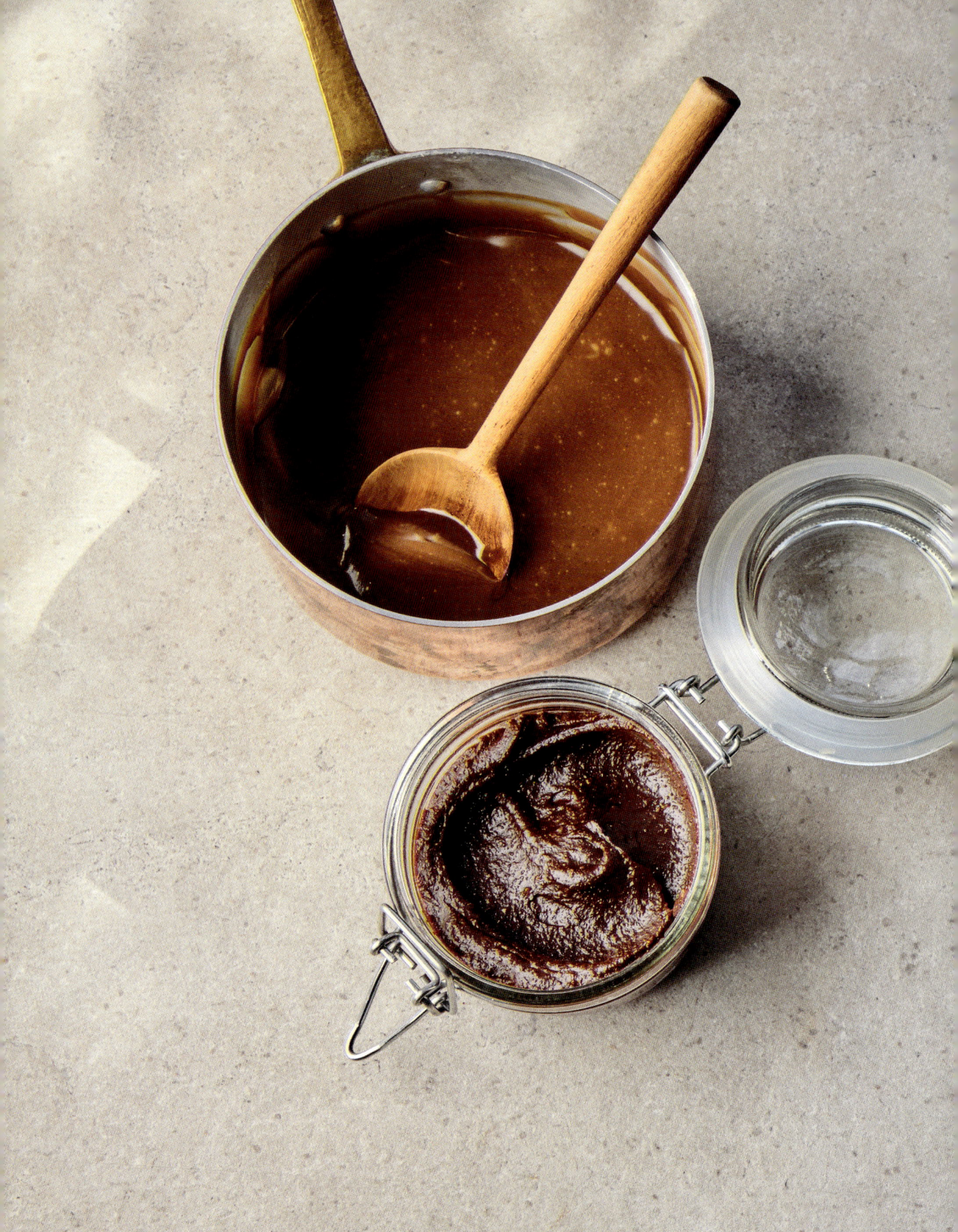

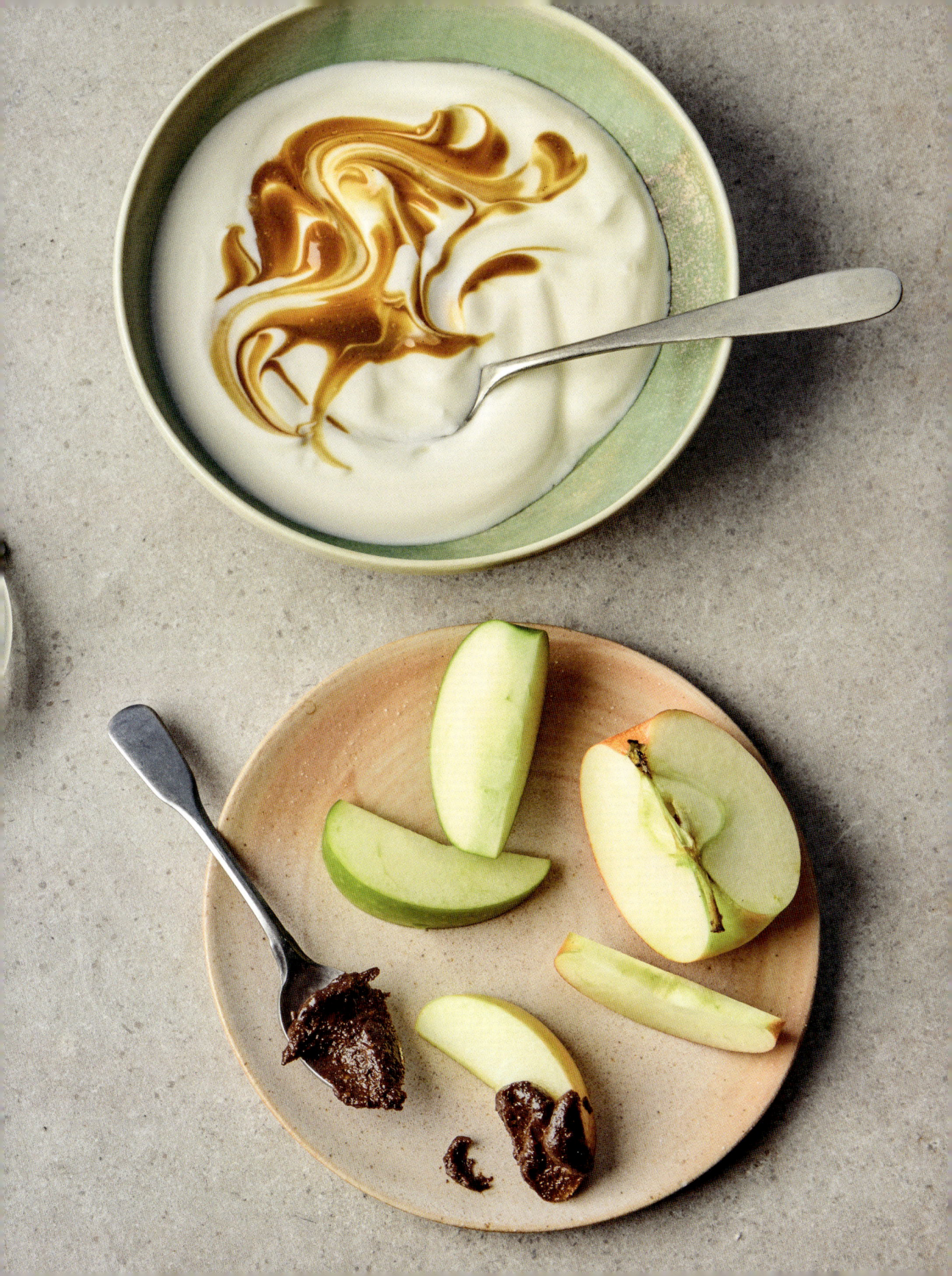

Homemade coconut yogurt is ridiculously simple and this recipe has a natural gut booster, too! It's rich, creamy, and naturally dairy-free, with all the gut-loving benefits of live cultures but none of the ultra-processed nasties. This recipe uses just a couple of ingredients and can be customized to whatever you fancy on the day—whether it's vanilla, berries, or a caramel twist, the choice is yours. It's perfect for dolloping on to granola, swirling into soups, or using in cakes and dressings. Once you've made your first batch, you'll never go back to store-bought!

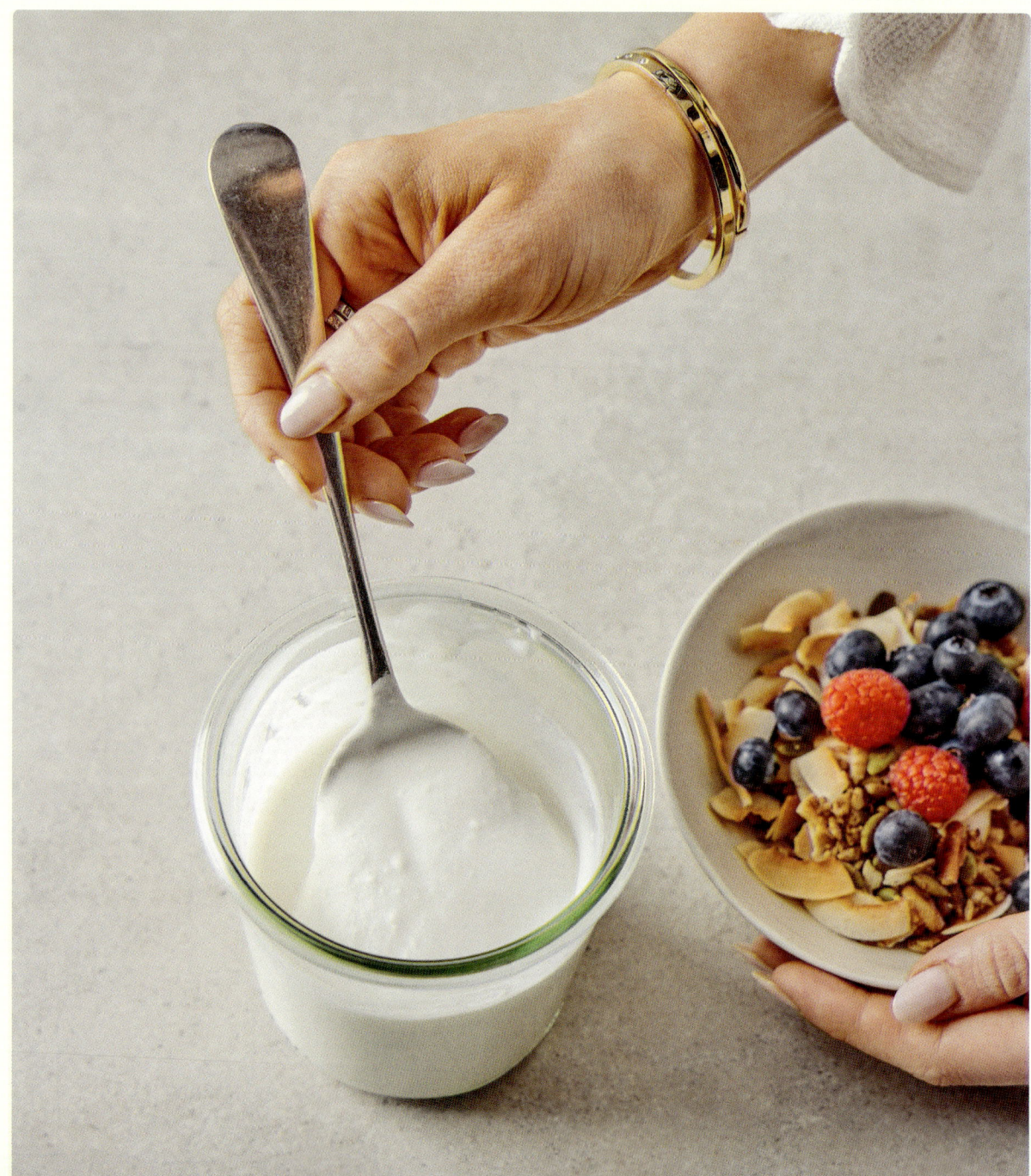

Natural Live Coconut Yogurt

MAKES APPROX. 2 CUPS PLUS 2 TBSP/500ML   ○   DAIRY-FREE, VEGAN, GUT-FRIENDLY

INGREDIENTS

- 1½ cups/400ml full-fat coconut milk
- 2 tbsp coconut cream
- 1 live probiotic capsule (or 2 tbsp plain live coconut yogurt as a starter)
- 1 tsp maple syrup or inulin (prebiotic to feed the bacteria) (optional)

In a bowl or a jug, whisk together the coconut milk and coconut cream until smooth. Open the probiotic capsule and stir the powder into the milk. If using a yogurt starter, mix it in well. Add the maple syrup or inulin if desired.

Pour into a sterilized jar. Cover loosely with a lid or clean muslin secured with an elastic band and leave in a warm place (ideally 70–85°F) for 12–24 hours, or until it thickens and tastes tangy.

Once fermented, stir gently and transfer to the fridge for at least 6 hours to fully set. The yogurt will thicken as it chills.

TROUBLESHOOTING

My yogurt has separated: Simply stir to recombine. For a more stable result, use a thicker coconut milk or add ½ tsp of tapioca starch before fermenting.

It's too runny: Some coconut milks don't contain enough fat to create a thick yogurt. Try using one with 60–70% coconut extract or stir in a little coconut cream. Chill it fully to let it firm up, or thicken with a natural setting agent like agar-agar or tapioca.

It smells or tastes too sour: It may have fermented for too long. Reduce the fermentation time next batch—12–16 hours is usually ideal, depending on room temperature.

There's no tang or very little thickening: The probiotic may be inactive or the room may be too cold. Make sure you're using a fresh, high-quality probiotic (multi-strain is ideal) and try placing in the oven with the light on to keep things warm.

There's mold or a strange color: Unfortunately, this batch needs to be discarded. This usually happens if equipment wasn't properly sterilized or if it was left too long in a warm environment. Always start with clean utensils and jars.

NUTRITIONAL INFORMATION *(Per 100g Serving)*

Calories 179Kcals   ○   Net carbohydrates 2.3g   ○   Fiber 1g   ○   Fat 18.6g   ○   Protein 1.4g

Savory Soft Crumble

SERVES 10 ○ VEGAN, GRAIN-FREE

INGREDIENTS

- 1 cup/100g pumpkin seeds
- ½ cup/50g sunflower seeds
- ⅓ cup/50g sesame seeds
- ¼ cup/50g hemp seeds
- ¼ cup/50g cooked Puy lentils (or canned lentils, drained)
- ⅓ cup/40g walnuts, roughly chopped
- ¼ cup/30g blanched almonds, chopped
- 1 tsp dried rosemary
- 1 tsp dried thyme
- ½ tsp garlic granules
- ¼ tsp smoked paprika (optional)
- ½ tsp sea salt
- 1 tbsp ground flaxseed
- 1 tbsp psyllium husk
- 1 tbsp nutritional yeast (adds umami and B_{12} boost—optional)
- 1 tbsp olive oil
- 2 tbsp tahini
- 2 tbsp water

Preheat the oven to 325°F (fan) and line a baking sheet with parchment paper.

In a large bowl, mix all the seeds, lentils, nuts, herbs, spices, flaxseed, psyllium, and nutritional yeast.

In a small bowl, whisk together the olive oil, tahini, and water until smooth. Pour this into the dry mixture and stir well to combine—it should clump slightly but not be overly wet.

Spread the mixture on the baking sheet in a rustic layer—aim for a crumble texture rather than one large slab.

Bake for 15–20 minutes, stirring once halfway through. It should feel set and just be turning golden, but should still be soft in parts.

Allow to cool on the baking sheet—it will firm up slightly more as it cools.

TOP TIPS

For a crunchier finish, spread the mixture out more thinly and bake for an additional 10–15 minutes at 275°F (fan), keeping a close eye to avoid burning. Allow it to cool completely on the baking sheet—it will crisp up further as it cools. You can pop it back in the oven for 5 minutes before serving to re-crisp, if needed. It also works well in a dehydrator.

The crumble can be stored in an airtight container for up to 2 weeks.

Spoon over soups, salads, or roasted vegetables.

Use as a crunchy topping for baked sweet potatoes.

Add to lunch boxes for a nutritious nibble.

NUTRITIONAL INFORMATION *(Per Serving)*

Calories 165Kcals ○ Net carbohydrates 2.9g ○ Fiber 4.1g ○ Fat 13.4g ○ Protein 6.4g

A fiber-rich, gut-friendly topping that also doubles up as a snack mix? Yes please! It's perfect for soups, salads, roasted veg, or even stirred into porridge. There's genuinely nothing you can't do with this savory soft crumble, so cook up a big batch and enjoy.

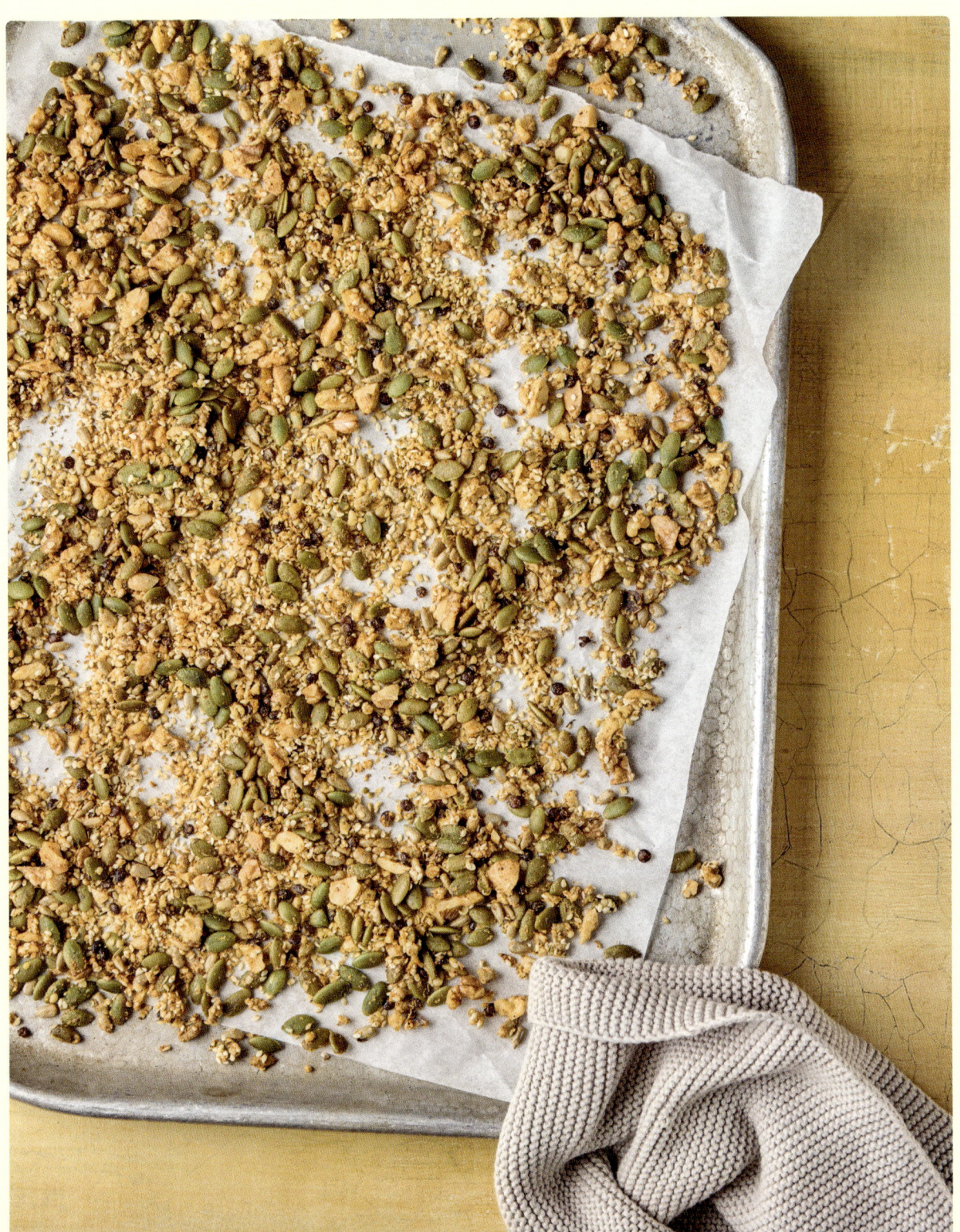

If sweet treats and healthy eating were crammed into a jar, this would be it. It's full of color, flavor, and anti-inflammatory omega goodness, as well as being refined sugar free, making it a breakfast staple. Quick to make, bursting with berry goodness and naturally thickened with chia seeds (which your digestion will love, by the way!). Ideal for toast, pancakes, yogurt . . . or, if you're like me, straight off the spoon.

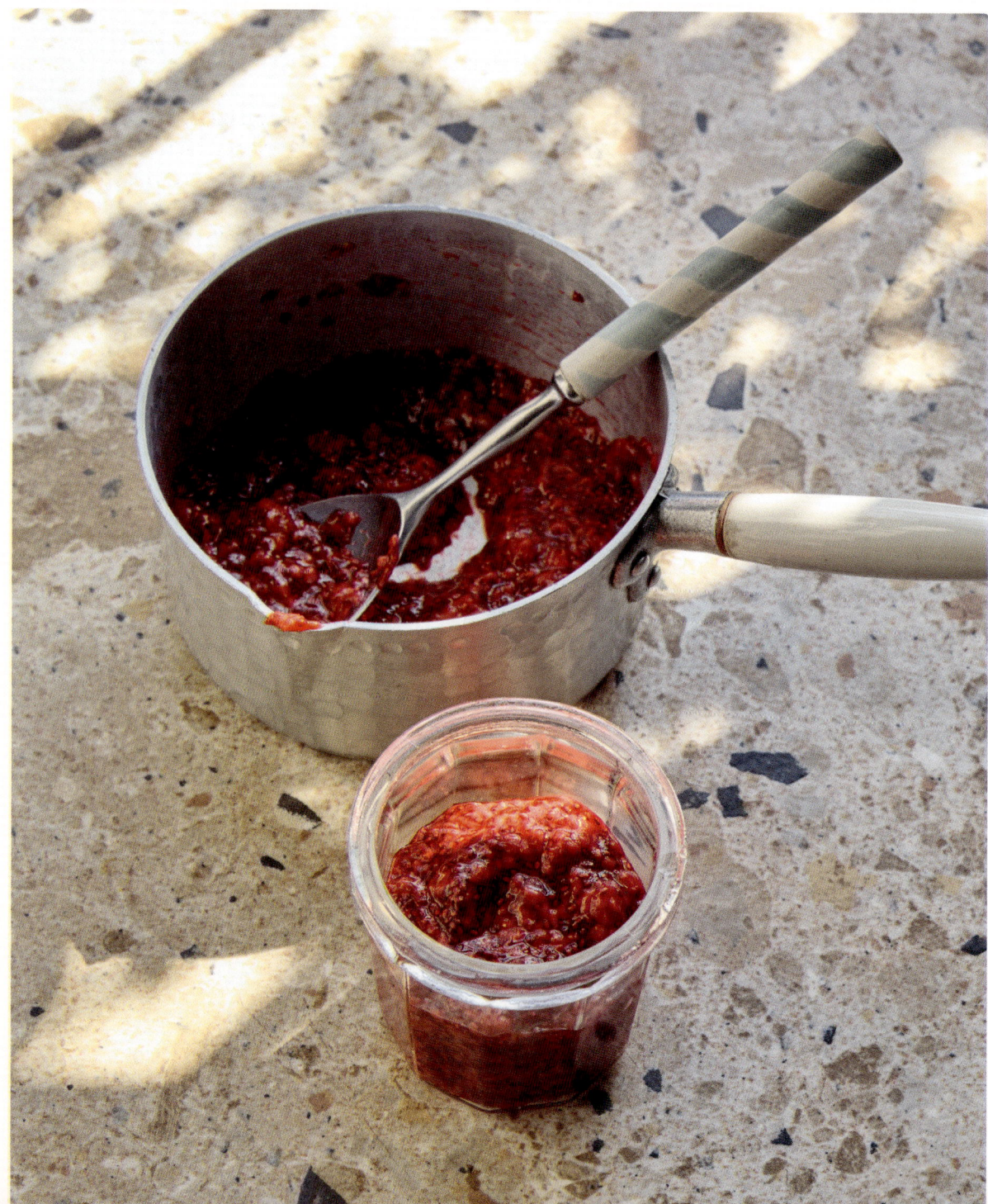

Easy Sugar-Free Raspberry & Chia Seed Jam

MAKES ABOUT 2 CUPS/350G ○ GRAIN-FREE

INGREDIENTS

- 2 tbsp chia seeds
- 4 tbsp water
- 2 cups/350g frozen raspberries
- juice and zest of ½ a lemon
- 1 tbsp honey or date syrup (or to taste)

Place the chia seeds in a bowl and add the water. Leave to one side.

Place the raspberries in a saucepan and heat gently, stirring regularly until the berries have melted and released their juice.

Add the lemon juice and zest. Add the chia seeds and honey and continue to cook on a low simmer for 5 minutes, until it thickens. Adjust the sweetness if needed.

Pour into a sterilized jar. It will set a little more once cooled.

Keep in the fridge for up to 2 weeks.

TOP TIPS

Try this with blueberries or a mix of berries for variation.

Freeze in ice-cube trays for instant berry hits to stir into yogurt or porridge.

PROTEIN BOOSTER

Stir in 1-2 tbsp of collagen powder before pouring into sterilized jars to enhance the protein.

FLAVOR TWIST

Strawberry, Raspberry & Elderflower Jam: Use 1 cup/175g of strawberries and 1¼ cups/175g of raspberries and stir in 2 tablespoons of elderflower cordial. You may wish to adjust the sweetener to taste.

NUTRITIONAL INFORMATION *(Per 20g Serving)*

Calories 23Kcals ○ Net carbohydrates 2.3g ○ Fiber 2.1g ○ Fat 0.6g ○ Protein 0.6g

Velvety Vanilla Custard

MAKES 1½ CUPS/400ML   ○   DAIRY-FREE

INGREDIENTS

- 1½ cups/400ml full-fat coconut milk
- 2 tsp vanilla paste
- 3 egg yolks
- 2 tbsp maple syrup, or to taste
- 1 tbsp arrowroot

In a small saucepan, whisk together the coconut milk and vanilla. Gently heat over low-medium heat until steaming but not boiling.

In a bowl, whisk the egg yolks, maple syrup, and arrowroot until smooth.

Slowly pour the warm milk into the egg mixture while whisking constantly, to temper the eggs.

Pour the mixture back into the saucepan and stir continuously over low heat until it thickens enough to coat the back of a spoon (don't let it boil).

Remove from the heat and continue stirring for 1 minute to prevent curdling.

Pour the custard into a jug and cover the surface with parchment paper or plastic wrap to prevent a skin from forming. Chill or serve warm.

TOP TIPS

For a deeper flavor, infuse a split vanilla pod in the milk first, and remove before thickening.

Keep in the fridge for 3–4 days, or freeze in portions.

NUTRITIONAL INFORMATION *(Per 100g Serving)*

Calories 313Kcals   ○   Net carbohydrates 11.7g   ○   Fiber 0.1g   ○   Fat 27g   ○   Protein 3.8g

This glossy vanilla custard is pure comfort—rich, creamy, and loaded with real vanilla flavor (not like the artificial ones you'll find in the shops!). It's the perfect pour-over for crumbles, tarts, and warm baked puddings, and it's made with coconut milk, free from dairy, and contains zero refined sugar. Once you've tasted this, you'll never buy store-bought custard again!

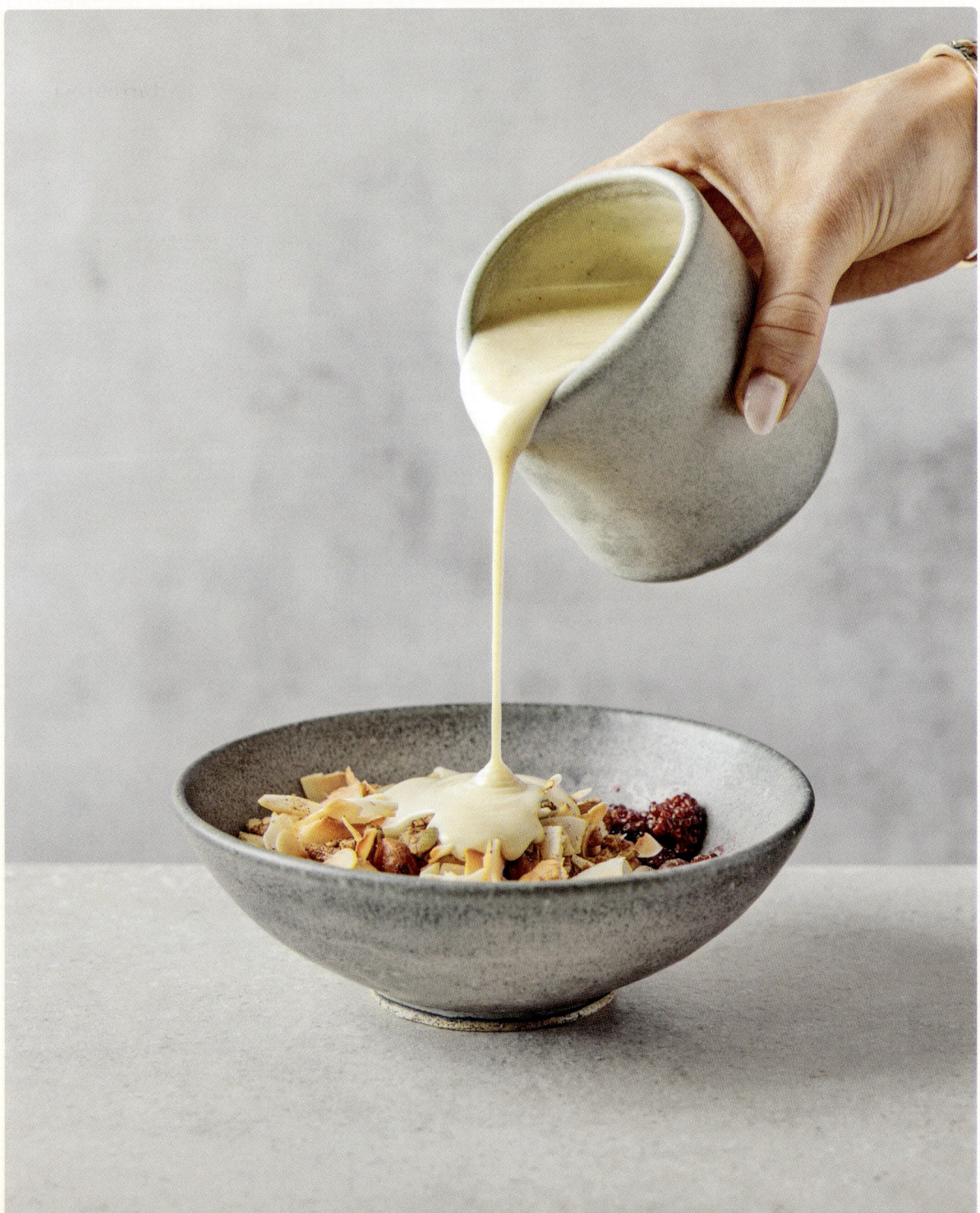

Drin

ks

These ginger shots went VIRAL for a reason! They're quick and easy to make, they don't require a juicer (just chuck everything in a blender), and they're the perfect anti-inflammatory start to your day. The entire mixture will cost you less than a single ginger shot in the supermarket—so this isn't just a tasty, healthy, anti-inflammatory hack, it'll help you save money, too. Leaving the pulp in will help with balancing blood sugar, so it's actually advised to just blend, rather than using a juicer and losing all that wonderful fiber!

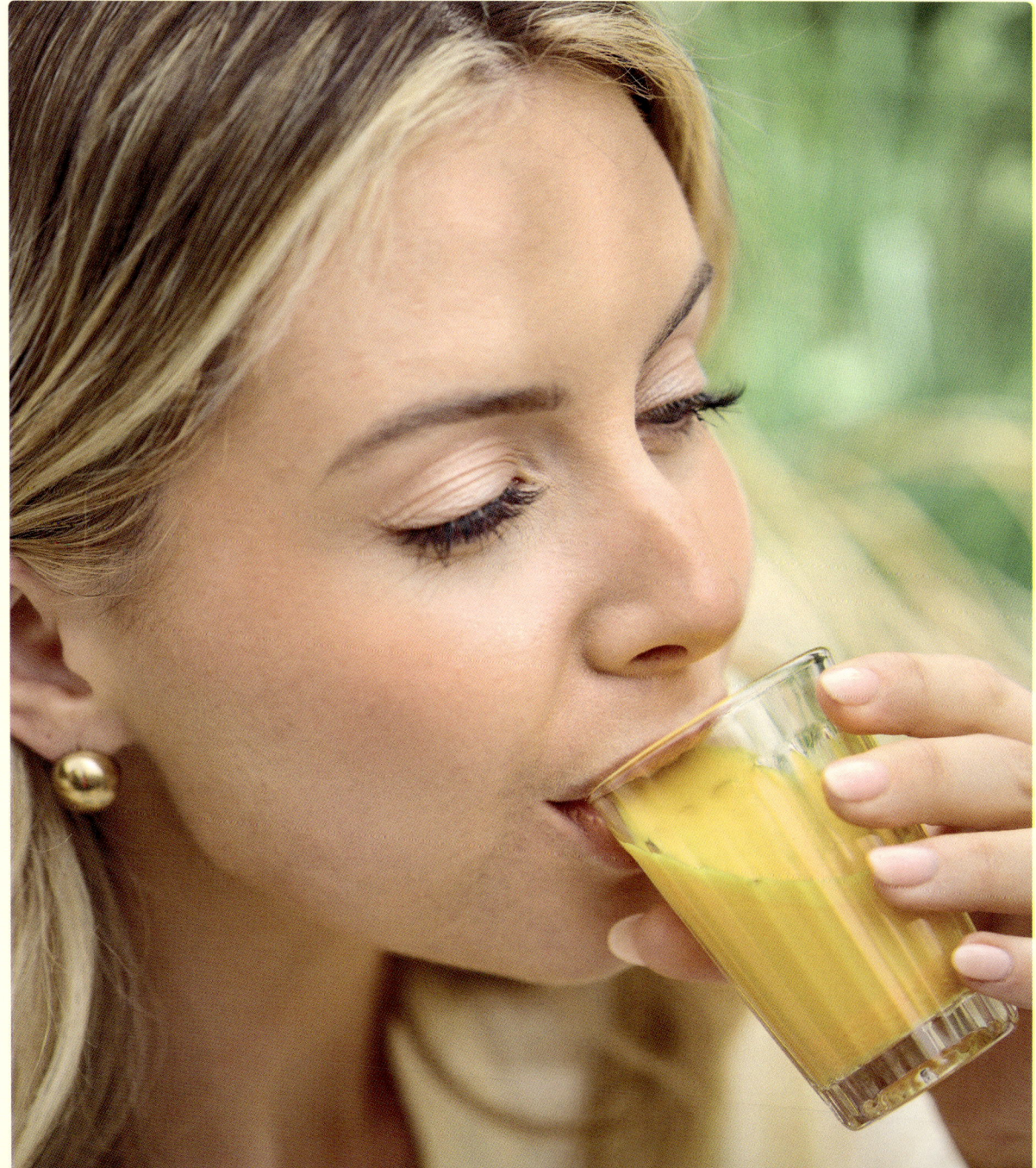

Ginger Shots

MAKES 7 SHOTS   GUT-FRIENDLY

INGREDIENTS

½ an organic lemon
1 organic orange
1 piece of ginger (approx. 1 tbsp/14g)
1 tbsp fresh turmeric, peeled and finely chopped, approx. 20g (can be replaced with 1 tbsp ground turmeric)
½ tsp freshly ground black pepper
½ tbsp olive oil
1½ cups/350ml filtered water (enough to achieve your desired consistency)

Blend all the ingredients together, serve in a small shot glass, and enjoy.

TOP TIPS

These can be kept in the fridge for 3–4 days.

Peel the orange and lemon if they are not organic. Same with the ginger and turmeric.

Freeze in ice-cube trays for a quick and easy pick-me-up whenever you need it.

NUTRITIONAL INFORMATION *(Per Serving)*

Calories 19Kcals ◦ Net carbohydrates 2.3g ◦ Fiber 0.4g ◦ Fat 1.1g ◦ Protein 0.3g

Ginger-Lime Electrolyte Cooler

SERVES 1 ○ VEGAN, GRAIN-FREE

This zingy, naturally hydrating drink is the ultimate mineral booster, full of essential nutrients and anti-inflammatory properties. The ginger adds a fiery kick, which is balanced perfectly with a dash of citrusy goodness and the sweetness from the honey.

INGREDIENTS

juice of 1 lime or lemon
¾-inch piece of ginger, or to taste
1 cup plus 1 tbsp/250ml coconut water
1 tsp honey or maple syrup, or to taste
a pinch of Himalayan or Celtic sea salt
a handful of ice cubes

To garnish (optional)
fresh mint

Blend all the ingredients except for the mint in a high-speed blender until smooth.

Pour into a glass and serve chilled.

Optional: top with fresh mint.

---

image on page 312

NUTRITIONAL INFORMATION *(Per Serving)*

Calories 81Kcals ○ Net carbohydrates 17.6g ○ Fiber 3g ○ Fat 0.6g ○ Protein 2.1g

Quick & Easy Homemade Lemonade

SERVES 2   ◦   NATURALLY SWEET, HYDRATING

When life gives you lemons, you make a healthy, hydrating lemonade, with a subtle sweetness and a pinch of mineral rich salt! The extra splash of apple cider vinegar makes this a great gut-and blood-sugar friendly alternative to the store-bought version.

INGREDIENTS

- juice of 2 large lemons (add more if you like a strong citrus kick)
- 1 tbsp honey or maple syrup (or to taste)
- a pinch of Himalayan or Celtic sea salt
- 1 tsp apple cider vinegar (with mother)
- 2 cups plus 2 tbsp/500ml filtered water or sparkling water
- a handful of ice cubes

To garnish
mint leaves (optional)
lemon slices

image on page 313

Mix the lemon juice, honey, salt, and apple cider vinegar in a jug.

Add the water and stir to combine.

Serve over ice, with a garnish of mint leaves (if desired) and a slice of lemon.

TOP TIPS

Add the juice from a 1-inch piece of fresh ginger for a spicy immune-boosting kick.

Make more and store in a bottle in the fridge until needed for up to 3 days.

Great as a healthy mixer.

NUTRITIONAL INFORMATION *(Per Serving)*

Calories 30Kcals   ◦   Net carbohydrates 8g   ◦   Fiber 0.1g   ◦   Fat 0g   ◦   Protein 0.1g

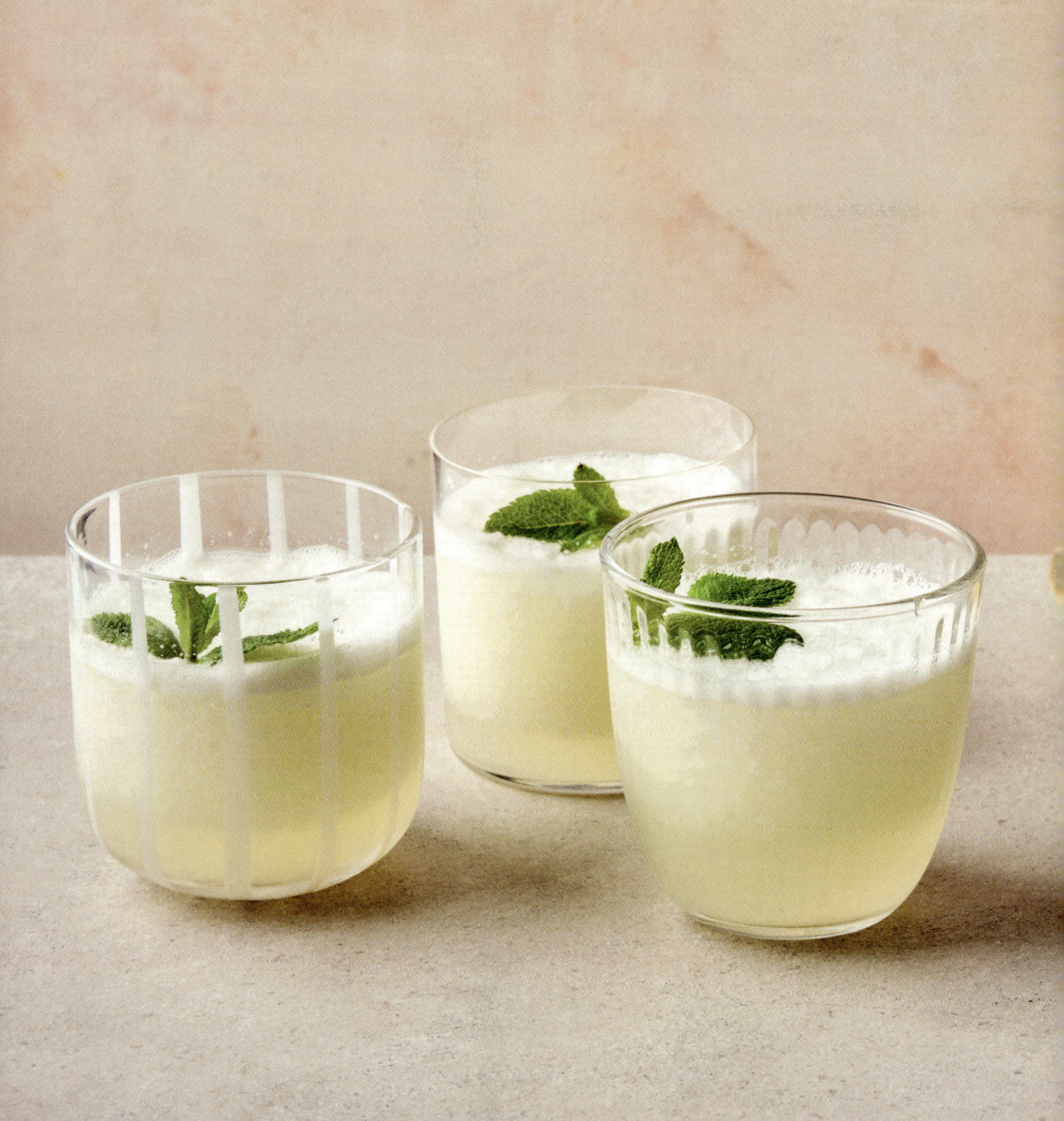

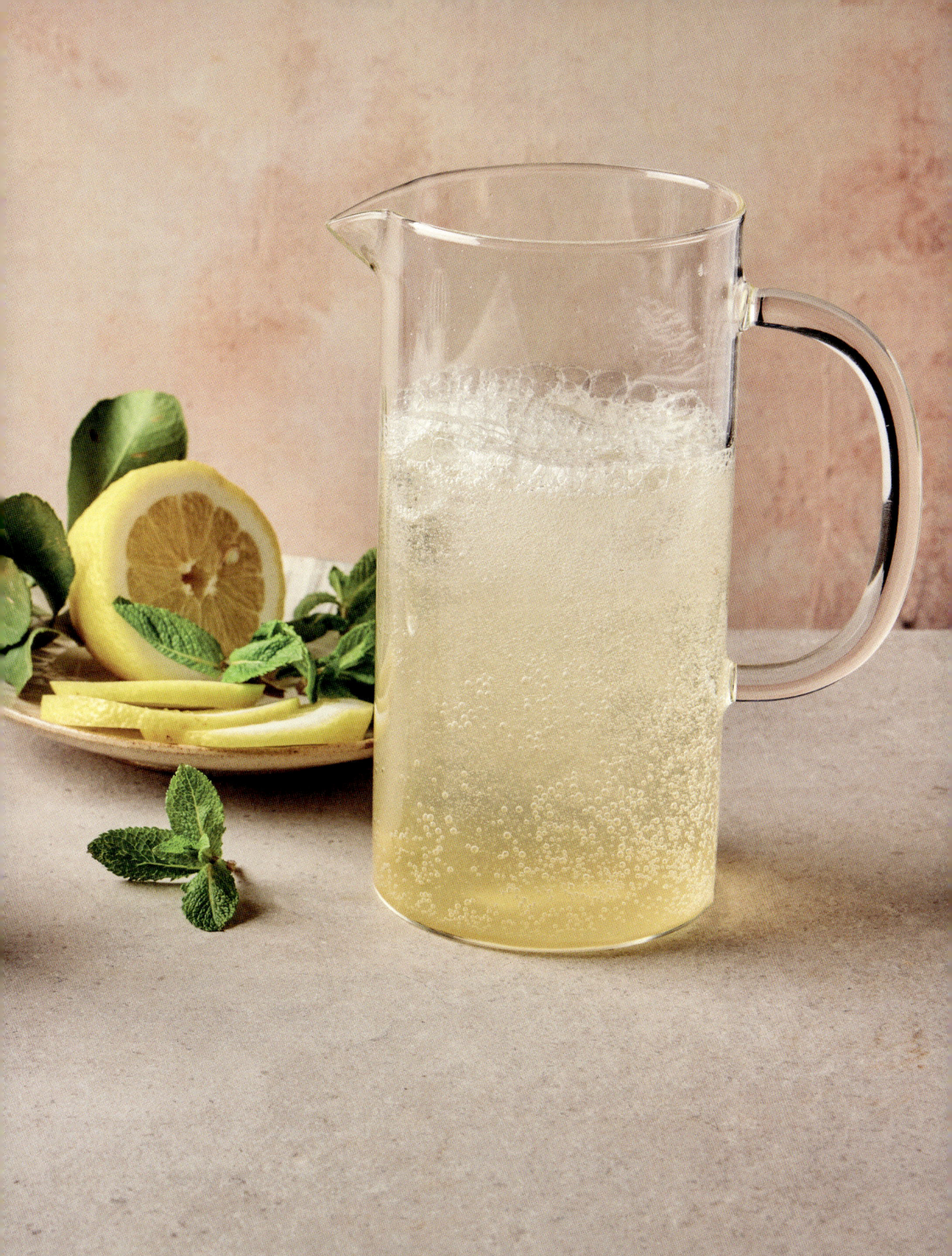

Avocado-Matcha Smoothie

SERVES 1 ○ VEGAN, GRAIN-FREE, HIGH-PROTEIN

INGREDIENTS

- ½ a ripe avocado
- 1 banana
- 1 tsp matcha powder
- ¾ cup/200ml unsweetened almond milk
- 1 tbsp chia seeds plus more for garnish (optional)
- 2 tbsp/20g unflavored protein powder
- 1 tsp vanilla extract (optional)

Put all the ingredients into a high-speed blender.

Blend until smooth and creamy, adding more almond milk if necessary to adjust the consistency.

Serve immediately, with a few extra chia seeds sprinkled on top.

TOP TIP

Swap the banana for mango, for a tropical twist.

I love!
Ancient & Brave Matcha & Collagen powder combines matcha with good-quality collagen peptides for skin, joints, and hormone support.

NUTRITIONAL INFORMATION *(Per Serving)*

Calories 433Kcals ○ Net carbohydrates 30.9g ○ Fiber 10.2g ○ Fat 2.9g ○ Protein 26.5g

We love a matcha moment, right? This creamy green smoothie gives you a hit of antioxidants from the matcha and an omega-rich boost from the chia, all perfectly balanced with healthy fats from the avocado. It's a fantastic post-workout option or quick breakfast-on-the-go, with protein powder to keep you fuller for longer.

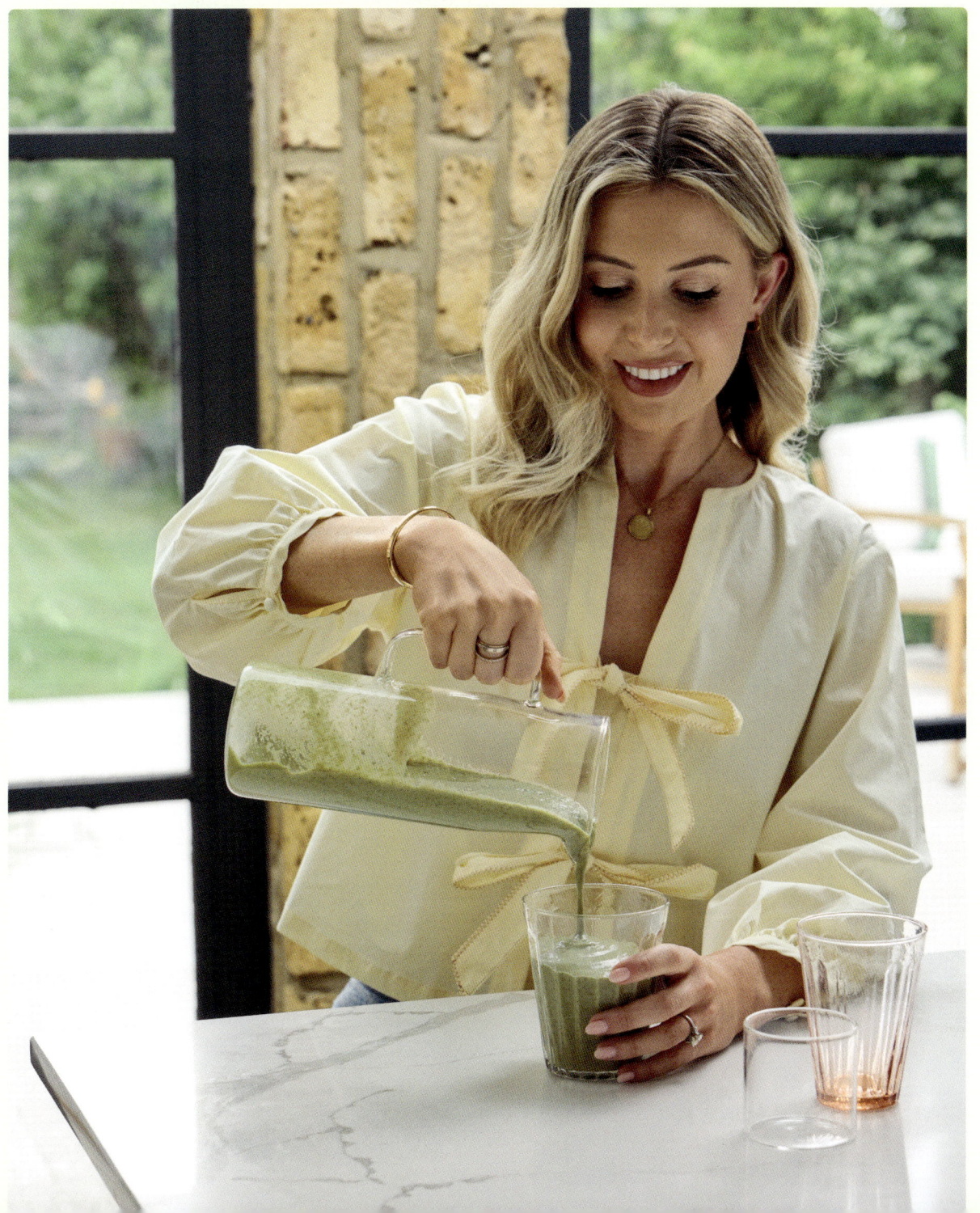

A super-refreshing frappé, low in sugar and full of fruit! It's rich in antioxidants and fiber—perfect for a mid-afternoon pick-me-up or a light breakfast on warmer days.

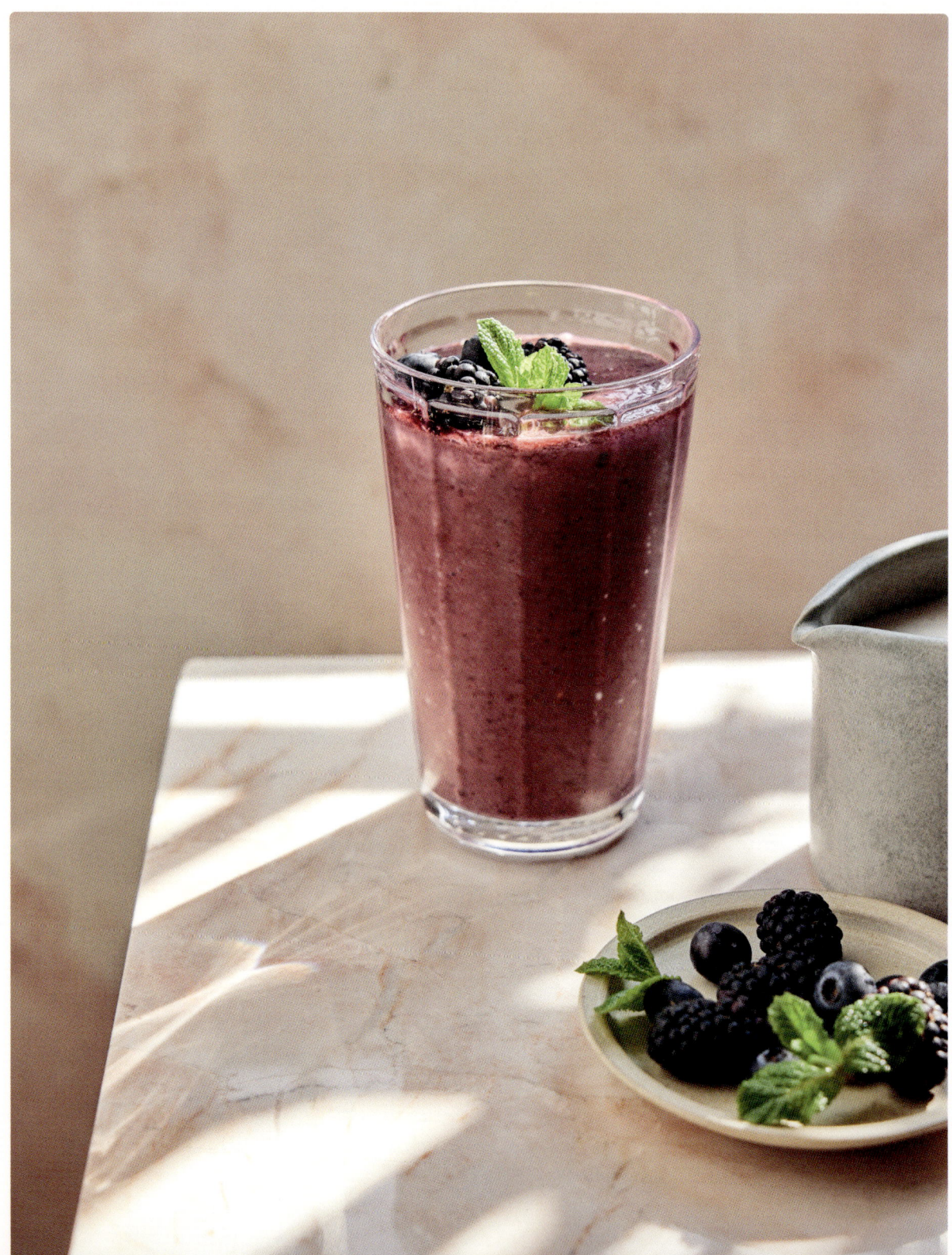

Berry Antioxidant Frappé

SERVES 1   ○   VEGAN, HIGH PROTEIN, GRAIN-FREE

INGREDIENTS

¾ cup/100g frozen mixed berries
1 tsp acai powder
¾ cup/200ml unsweetened oat or almond milk
1 tsp flaxseeds
½ banana or 1 Medjool date (for sweetness)
1 scoop of unflavored protein powder

To garnish (optional)
fresh mint
berries

(6.2g without powder)

Blend all the ingredients in a high-speed blender until smooth. Adjust with more oat or almond milk if needed.

Pour into a glass and serve chilled.

Optional: top with fresh mint and a few whole berries.

TOP TIPS

Add 1 tsp of beet powder to enhance blood flow and workout recovery.

Add a squeeze of lemon for a zingy finish.

NUTRITIONAL INFORMATION *(Per Serving)*

Calories 318Kcals   ○   Net carbohydrates 21.7g   ○   Fiber 8.6g   ○   Fat 12.4g   ○   Protein 25.4g*

Gut-Friendly Lemon, Turmeric & Ginger Switchel

MAKES 1 PINT ○ GUT-FRIENDLY

INGREDIENTS

- 1½ cups/400ml filtered water
- 2 tbsp apple cider vinegar (with mother)
- juice of 2 large lemons
- 2-inch piece of fresh ginger, peeled and grated
- 2–3 pieces of turmeric root, peeled and grated
- 1–2 tbsp honey, or to taste
- a pinch of sea salt

Place all the ingredients in a jug or jar and stir well to combine.

Cover and leave to sit at room temperature for 12–24 hours, to allow the flavors to infuse and prebiotic fermentation to begin.

Strain if desired and store in the fridge. Serve chilled as a shot or diluted with filtered or sparkling water over ice.

PROTEIN BOOSTERS

Keeps for 5–7 days when stored in the fridge.

Adjust the sweetness to taste. If preferred, you can use a little maple syrup or coconut sugar instead of honey.

NUTRITIONAL INFORMATION *(Per 20ml Serving)*

Calories 5Kcals ○ Net carbohydrates 1.1g ○ Fiber 0.1g ○ Fat 0g ○ Protein 0.1g

We know how important the gut is by now—and this refreshing, tangy tonic that aids hydration is the perfect way to help digestion and support your gut health. It's naturally sweetened, packed with electrolytes and prebiotics, and ideal as a post-exercise rehydrator or daily digestive tonic.

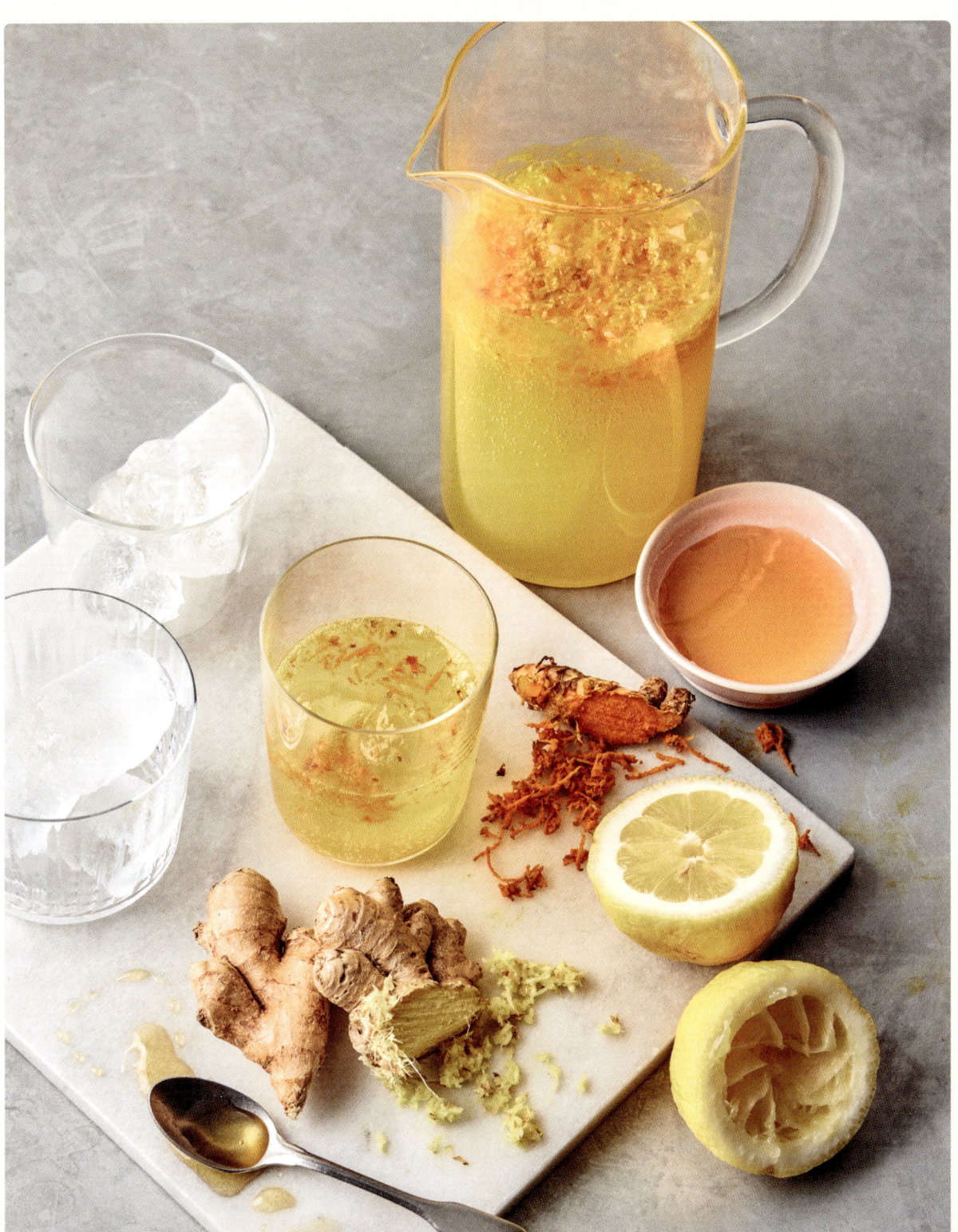

Healthy Hot Chocolate

SERVES 1   ○   VEGAN, HIGH PROTEIN

We all want a chocolatey hug-in-a-mug sometimes, and now you can have it while ticking off your health goals, too! It's got just enough sweetness from the syrup, and the raw cacao is naturally rich in magnesium and antioxidants... which are incredible for supporting energy and hormone balance. A healthy way to satisfy your chocolate cravings, especially around the mid-afternoon dip or evening wind-down.

INGREDIENTS

- ¾ cup/200ml unsweetened almond or coconut milk
- 1 tbsp raw cacao or cocoa powder, plus more for garnish
- 1 scoop of collagen peptides or chocolate collagen
- ¼ tsp ground cinnamon, plus more for garnish
- ½ tsp vanilla extract
- 1 tsp maple syrup or date syrup
- a pinch of sea salt

image on page 322

Warm the milk gently in a saucepan (do not boil).

Whisk in the cacao, collagen, cinnamon, vanilla, syrup, and salt until smooth. You can use a milk frother or a small whisk to help blend the cacao fully and create frothy milk.

Pour into a mug, top with a sprinkle of cacao or cinnamon, and serve warm.

TOP TIPS

Use ½ cup/100ml of coconut cream and ½ cup/100ml of almond or coconut milk for a creamier version.

Add 1 tsp of smooth almond butter for a nourishing boost, or a dash of cayenne or chili powder for a kick of heat.

Add a serving of ashwagandha powder for extra hormone support.

Blend after heating for a frothy café-style drink.

ADD-ONS I LOVE!

Ancient & Brave Cacao + Reishi (contains hops, ashwagandha, and reishi to aid relaxation and sleep).

Freja Foods Chocolate Bone Broth Shake.

Hunter & Gather Cacao Collagen Creamer.

NUTRITIONAL INFORMATION *(Per Serving)*

Calories 179Kcals   ○   Net carbohydrates 8g   ○   Fiber 6.4g   ○   Fat 7.6g   ○   Protein 16.6g

Spiced Golden Latte

SERVES 1   ○   HIGH PROTEIN, ANTI-INFLAMMATORY

A warming anti-inflammatory blend of turmeric, ginger, cinnamon, and creamy coconut milk. Perfect for winding down in the evening or as a comforting caffeine-free boost. I love adding protein powder or collagen for extra nourishment, but this is optional!

INGREDIENTS

- ¾ cup/200ml unsweetened almond milk
- 1 tsp ground turmeric
- ¼ tsp ground ginger
- ½ tsp ground cinnamon
- a pinch of freshly ground black pepper
- 1 tsp honey or maple syrup, or to taste
- 1 scoop of bovine collagen (optional)

image on page 322

Warm the milk in a saucepan over low-medium heat.

Add the spices, black pepper, and honey or maple syrup, and stir well to combine.

Add the collagen (if desired).

Whisk until frothy and golden. Do not boil.

Pour into a mug and enjoy warm.

TOP TIPS

Use ½ cup/100ml of coconut cream and ½ cup/100ml of almond or coconut milk for a creamier version.

You can use a velvetizer or a milk frother instead of a saucepan.

Ideal before bed or as a mid-morning anti-inflammatory boost.

NUTRITIONAL INFORMATION *(Per Serving)*

Calories 141Kcals   ○   Net carbohydrates 11g   ○   Fiber 2.4g   ○   Fat 4.6g   ○   Protein 14g

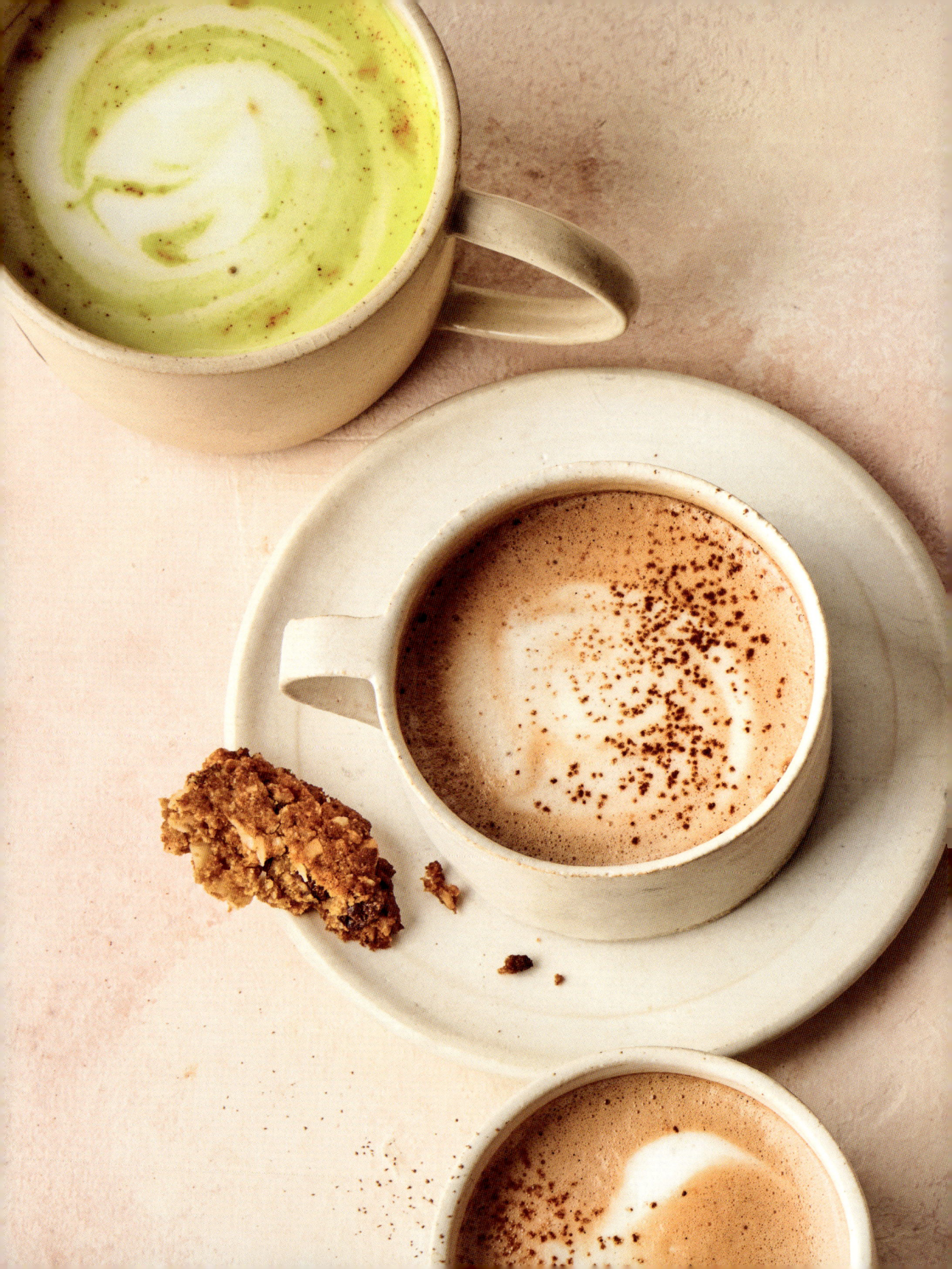

Universal Conversion Chart

OVEN TEMPERATURE EQUIVALENTS

250°F = 120°C   350°F = 180°C   450°F = 230°C
275°F = 135°C   375°F = 190°C   475°F = 240°C
300°F = 150°C   400°F = 200°C   500°F = 260°C
325°F = 160°C   425°F = 220°C

MEASUREMENT EQUIVALENTS

Measurements should always be level unless directed otherwise.

⅛ teaspoon = 0.5 mL   ½ teaspoon = 2 mL
¼ teaspoon = 1 mL   1 teaspoon = 5 mL
1 tablespoon = 3 teaspoons = ½ fluid ounce = 15 mL
2 tablespoons = ⅛ cup = 1 fluid ounce = 30 mL
4 tablespoons = ¼ cup = 2 fluid ounces = 60 mL
5⅓ tablespoons = ⅓ cup = 3 fluid ounces = 80 mL
8 tablespoons = ½ cup = 4 fluid ounces = 120 mL
10⅔ tablespoons = ⅔ cup = 5 fluid ounces = 160 mL
12 tablespoons = ¾ cup = 6 fluid ounces = 180 mL
16 tablespoons = 1 cup = 8 fluid ounces = 240 mL

References

Inflammation

1. Inflammation definition—Anna L. Kiss, "Inflammation in Focus: The Beginning and the End," *Pathology and Oncology Research*, 27-2021 (2022), Abstract.

Hormones

1. Perspectives on Menopause—Danah Gutierrez, "Vagina Talks: The Japanese Guide to Embracing Menopause With Grace," www.abs-cbn.com, (28 February 2025).
2. Perspectives on Menopause—Jennifer Chandler, "Menopause Around the World," https://www.mindsethealth.com/matter/menopause-around-the-world . (15 October 2021)

Pillar 1: Food Is More Than Fuel

1. https://dutchtest.com/dutch-complete

Pillar 2: Gut Health

1. Megan Rossi's Super Six—*Eat More, Live Well* by (2021) Dr. Megan Rossi
2. Gut microbiome in endometriosis: a cohort study on 1000 individuals—Pérez-Prieto, I., Vargas, E., Salas-Espejo, E. et al, BMC Med 22, 294, https://doi.org/10.1186/s12916-024-03503-y, (18 July 2024)
3. Gut microbiome-wide association study of depressive symptoms. *Nat Commun* 13, 7128—Radjabzadeh, D., Bosch, J.A., Uitterlinden, A.G. et al, https://doi.org/10.1038/s41467-022-34502-3, (06 December 2022)
4. The critical role of gut microbiota in obesity. Front. Endocrinol. 13:1025706. doi: 10.3389/fendo.2022.1025706—Cheng Z, Zhang L, Yang L and Chu H, https://www.frontiersin.org/journals/endocrinology/articles/10.3389/fendo.2022.1025706/full?utm, (20 October 2022)

Pillar 3: Detoxification

1. Cytochrome P450 Enzymes and Drug Metabolism in Humans. Int J Mol Sci—Zhao M, Ma J, Li M, Zhang Y, Jiang B, Zhao X, Huai C, Shen L, Zhang N, He L, Qin S, https://pmc.ncbi.nlm.nih.gov/articles/PMC8657965/, (26 November 2021)

Pillar 4: Sleep

1. Sleep disorders and the development of insulin resistance and obesity. Endocrinol Metab Clin North Am, Mesarwi O, Polak J, Jun J, Polotsky VY, https://pmc.ncbi.nlm.nih.gov/articles/PMC3767932/, (September 2013)
2. Chronic Diseases and Sleep, https://www.amwa-doc.org/our-work/initiatives/sleep/the-impact-of-sleep-on-chronic-disease/, American Medical Women's Association
3. Role of sleep deprivation in immune-related disease risk and outcomes. Commun Biol—Garbarino S, Lanteri P, Bragazzi NL, Magnavita N, Scoditti E, https://pmc.ncbi.nlm.nih.gov/articles/PMC8602722/#:~:text=At%20the%20molecular%20levels%2C%20sleep,and%20TLR%20signaling)%2C%20oxidative%20stress, (18 November 2021)
4. Women, Are Your Hormones Keeping You Up at Night?—Jennifer Chen, https://www.yalemedicine.org/news/women-are-your-hormones-keeping-you-up-at-night, Yale Medicine, (10 July 2017)
5. Huberman's tools for better sleep—Andrew Huberman, "Toolkit for Sleep," www.hubermanlab.com, (20 September 2021)

6. NSDR (Non-Sleep Deep Rest) with Dr. Andrew Huberman, https://www.youtube.com/watch?v=AKGrmY8OSHM, YouTube, (11 September 2022)

7. Huberman's tools for better sleep—Andrew Huberman, "Toolkit for Sleep," www.hubermanlab.com, (20 September 2021)

Pillar 5: Stress

1. A once-Olympic hopeful who said her body broke down after working with a Nike coach had a disturbingly common condition—Gabby Landsverk, https://www.businessinsider.com/nike-runner-mary-cain-female-athlete-triad-reds-2019-11?utm, Business Insider, (08 November 2019)

2. A Comprehensive Study of Therapeutic Applications of Chamomile—Sah, A.; Naseef, P.P.; Kuruniyan, M.S.; Jain, G.K.; Zakir, F.; Aggarwal, G, https://doi.org/10.3390/ph15101284, Pharmaceuticals, (19 October 2022)

3. Effectiveness of chamomile tea on glycemic control and serum lipid profile in patients with type 2 diabetes. J Endocrinol Invest—Rafraf M, Zemestani M, Asghari-Jafarabadi M, https://pubmed.ncbi.nlm.nih.gov/25194428/, (February 2015)

4. Chamomile tea: Source of a glucuronoxylan with antinociceptive, sedative and anxiolytic-like effects—Pedro Felipe Pereira Chaves, Palloma de Almeida S. Hocayen, Jorge Luiz Dallazen, Maria Fernanda de Paula Werner, Marcello Iacomini, Roberto Andreatini, Lucimara M.C. Cordeiro, https://www.sciencedirect.com/science/article/pii/S014181302034126X, International Journal of Biological Macromolecules, (1 December 2020)

5. A meta-analytic review of the effects of mindfulness meditation on telomerase activity. Psychoneuroendocrinology—Schutte NS, Malouff JM, https://pubmed.ncbi.nlm.nih.gov/24636500/, (April 2014)

Pillar 6: Movement

1. Effects of different exercise modalities on inflammatory markers in the obese and overweight populations: unraveling the mystery of exercise and inflammation—Guo Y, Qian H, Xin X and Liu Q, https://www.frontiersin.org/journals/physiology/articles/10.3389/fphys.2024.1405094/full?utm, Front. Physiol, (12 June 2024)

2. Exercise and the lymphatic system—Heather Alexander, https://www.mdanderson.org/publications/focused-on-health/exercise-and-the-lymphatic-system.h20-1592991.html?utm, The University of Texas, MD Anderson Cancer Center, (November 2019)

3. Health & Wellness: Blood Glucose and Exercise, https://diabetes.org/health-wellness/fitness/blood-glucose-and-exercise?utm, American Diabetes Association

4. Exercising to relax: How does exercise reduce stress? Surprising answers to this question and more, https://www.health.harvard.edu/staying-healthy/exercising-to-relax?utm, Harvard Health Publishing, Havard Medical School, (07 July 2020)

5. The Effect of Physical Activity on Sleep Quality and Sleep Disorder: A Systematic Review. Cureus—Alnawwar MA, Alraddadi MI, Algethmi RA, Salem GA, Salem MA, Alharbi AA, https://pmc.ncbi.nlm.nih.gov/articles/PMC10503965/?utm, National Library of Medicine, (16 August 2023)

6. Staying Healthy: Exercise and Bone Health, https://orthoinfo.aaos.org/en/staying-healthy/exercise-and-bone-health?utm, OrthoInfo, (July 2020)

7. Interleukin-1beta system in anorectic catabolic tumor-bearing rats. Curr Opin Clin Nutr Metab Care—Turrin NP, Ilyin SE, Gayle DA, Plata-Salamán CR, Ramos EJ, Laviano A, Das UN, Inui A, Meguid MM, https://pubmed.ncbi.nlm.nih.gov/15192445/, National Library of Medicine, (July 2004)

8. The underappreciated role of muscle in health and disease—Robert R Wolfe, https://www.sciencedirect.com/science/article/pii/S0002916523290450?via%3Dihub#note1, The American Journal of Clinical Nutrition, (December 2006)

9. Resistance training increases total energy expenditure and free-living physical activity in older adults—Gary R. Hunter, Carla J. Wetzstein, David A. Fields, Amanda Brown and Marcas M. Bamman, https://journals.physiology.org/doi/full/10.1152/jappl.2000.89.3.977, Journal of Applied Physiology, (01 September 2000)

Index

A

ablation 11
acai
    berry antioxidant frappé 317
    chia and acai split bowl 158
acne 6, 14, 18, 23, 38, 73
adhesion 10
aging 124–5
alcohol 19, 43, 91–3
allergies 9, 65
amino acids 53
anxiety 18, 23, 55, 57, 71
apples
    the 2-minute craving crusher 270
    baked apple, cinnamon and pecan oats 150
    fruit and nut breakfast bars 269
    loaded apple tea cake 277
    morning zinger green smoothie 154
asparagus: salad Niçoise 204
autoimmune conditions 9, 18, 26, 34, 46
avocado
    avocado matcha smoothie 314
    beet falafel bowl 174
    elevated poached eggs 186
    grilled chimichurri chicken salad 173
    marinated salmon bowl 182
    peri peri chicken thighs 227
    rich and creamy chocolate mousse 239
    stuffed avocado 177
    ultimate omega breakfast toast 146

B

bananas
    banana and chocolate pancakes 169
    berry antioxidant frappé 317
    fruit and nut breakfast bars 269
    loaded apple tea cake 277
beans: Tuscan bean and kale soup 185

beef
    fragrant beef rendang 207
    rich and nutritious zucchini Bolognese 203
    smoky chorizo beef 208
beet falafel bowl 174
berries
    berry antioxidant frappé 317
    chia and acai split bowl 158
biscotti: chocolate, hazelnut and orange biscotti 281
bloating 10, 14, 18, 23, 46, 64–5, 71
blood sugar 14, 26, 30, 32, 35–9, 52–3, 57–9, 65, 74, 81, 104, 113, 115, 124, 130
BLT lettuce wraps 189
blueberries: lemon and blueberry pots 166
Bolognese 203
bone density 29, 124, 128–9
Bostock, Sophie 101, 104
bowel movement 27, 79–80, 93, 96–7
brain fog 6, 14, 18, 29, 38–9, 46, 87
bread 55
    grain-free seeded bread 258
    ultimate omega breakfast toast 146
breakfasts 54–5
    baked apple, cinnamon and pecan oats 150
    banana and chocolate pancakes 169
    breakfast nests 153
    chia and acai split bowl 158
    green shakshuka 162
    lemon and blueberry pots 166
    morning zinger green smoothie 154
    one-pot brunch 145
    salted maple and cinnamon granola 165
    shakshuka 149
    spiced carrot cake overnight oats 161
    ultimate omega breakfast toast 146
    whipped tahini 157
breakfast bars: fruit and nut breakfast bars 269
breathwork 112, 118
brownies: salted caramel swirl brownies 274

buckwheat and chickpea salad 228
butternut squash: roasted vegetable salad 178

C

cabbage
    crunchy slaw 193
    fermented rainbow kraut 291
    grilled chimichurri chicken salad 173
    marinated salmon bowl 182
    Thai salmon cakes 197
caffeine 99, 104, 106–7, 115
cakes
    loaded apple tea cake 277
    rich chocolate sandwich cake 285
    salted caramel swirl brownies 274
caramel sauce 294
carbohydrates 19, 37–9, 49, 55–8, 66
carrots
    crunchy slaw 193
    fermented rainbow kraut 291
    marinated salmon bowl 182
    rich and nutritious zucchini Bolognese 203
    roasted vegetable salad 178
    spiced carrot cake overnight oats 161
    Tuscan bean and kale soup 185
cauliflower: harissa cauliflower steaks 223
cauliflower rice
    fragrant beef rendang 207
    high protein cauli egg-fried rice 211
celiac disease 9
cheesecake: no-bake vanilla cheesecake 244
chemicals, environmental 74, 94, 113
chewing 72–3, 81, 84
chia
    chia and acai split bowl 158
    easy sugar-free raspberry and chia seed jam 303
    lemon and blueberry pots 166
chicken
    chicken karahi 224
    grilled chimichurri chicken salad 173
    high protein cauli-egg fried rice 211
    peri peri chicken thighs 227

chickpeas
    beet falafel bowl 174
    chickpea mash 223
    elevated poached eggs 186
    grilled chimichurri chicken salad 173
    marinated salmon bowl 182
    quinoa salad 194
    roasted chickpeas 255
    roasted vegetable salad 178
    zesty buckwheat and chickpea salad 228
chimichurri
    chimichurri sauce 292
    chimichurri steak 220
    grilled chimichurri chicken salad 173
chocolate
    the 2-minute craving crusher 270
    banana and chocolate pancakes 169
    chocolate, hazelnut and orange biscotti 281
    chocolate soufflés 247
    cocoa and almond energy bars 286
    coconut, chocolate chip and macadamia cookies 273
    healthy chocolate spread 295
    healthy hot chocolate 320
    no-bake nut and seed bars 282
    no-bake chocolate tart 251
    rich and creamy chocolate mousse 239
    rich chocolate sandwich cake 285
    salted caramel swirl brownies 273
    soft coconut macaroons 264
chorizo
    smoky chorizo beef 208
    spiced lentil and chorizo soup 190
circadian rhythm 101–2, 107, 114, 129
Claire, Mary 25
coconut
    caramel sauce 294
    coconut, chocolate chip and macadamia cookies 273
    coconut macaroon thumbprints 265
    fragrant beef rendang 207
    grilled chimichurri chicken salad 212
    mango and lime coconut pots 248
    natural live coconut yogurt 299
    no-bake chocolate tart 251
    soft coconut macaroons 264

coconut (*cont.*)
    sticky toffee pudding 236
    velvety vanilla custard 304
cod: pistachio-crusted cod 231
cold showers 112
constipation 9, 14, 18, 75-6, 79, 80, 91, 112
cookies
    coconut, chocolate chip and macadamia cookies 273
    oaty cookies 278
cortisol 24-5, 37-40, 50, 77, 99, 101-2, 110-11, 115, 119
crackers: flax and chia crackers 259
cravings 23, 37, 39, 43-4, 51, 76
crumbles
    rhubarb, strawberry and elderflower crumble 240
    savory soft crumble 300
cucumber
    beet falafel bowl 174
    marinated salmon bowl 182
    zesty buckwheat and chickpea salad 228
curries
    chicken karahi 224
    fragrant beef rendang 207
    spiced red lentil dahl 216
custard: velvety vanilla custard 304

D

dairy intolerance 9, 64, 67
deficiencies 90, 96
depression 6, 26, 71, 114, 125
desserts
    caramel sauce 294
    chocolate soufflés 247
    mango and lime coconut pots 248
    maple spiced poached pears 235
    no-bake chocolate tart 251
    no-bake vanilla cheesecake 244
    raspberry and pistachio panna cotta 243
    rhubarb, strawberry and elderflower crumble 240
    rich and creamy chocolate mousse 239
    sticky toffee pudding 236
    velvety vanilla custard 304

detoxification 7, 15, 20, 76, 86-97
digestive system 18, 58, 72-3
drinks
    avocado matcha smoothie 314
    berry antioxidant frappé 317
    ginger lime electrolyte cooler 310
    ginger shots 309
    gut-friendly lemon, turmeric and ginger switchel 318
    healthy hot chocolate 320
    morning zinger green smoothie 154
    quick and easy homemade lemonade 311
    spiced golden latte 321

E

egg freezing 6, 12
eggs 145
    baked apple, cinnamon and pecan oats 150
    breakfast nests 153
    chocolate soufflés 247
    elevated poached eggs 186
    gourmet high-protein Scotch egg 181
    green shakshuka 162
    high protein cauli-egg fried rice 211
    salad Niçoise 204
    shakshuka 149
    Spanish tortilla and romesco dip 198
    sun-dried tomato frittata muffins 194
    whipped tahini 157
eggplant
    chimichurri steak 220
    Greek style lamb chops 219
endometriosis 6, 10-12, 14-15, 18-19, 34, 40, 71, 101, 128
endorphins 115, 124
estrogen 24, 28-9, 38, 50, 76-9, 88
excision 11
exercise 20, 93, 96, 114, 120-31

F

falafel: beet falafel bowl 174
fatigue 6, 9, 18, 23, 25-6, 38, 87, 91
fats 49-51, 63, 66, 68, 88
fermented foods 82
    rainbow kraut 291
fertility 12, 24, 28, 50
fiber 58-60, 74, 80, 82
Finally Found podcast 84, 101

fish 54–5
    grilled spiced salmon 212
    marinated salmon bowl 182
    pistachio-crusted cod 231
    salad Niçoise 204
    stuffed avocado 177
    Thai salmon cakes 197
    ultimate omega breakfast toast 146
flatbreads 216
food 42–69
    carbohydrates 19, 37–9, 49, 55–8, 66
    diets 44–6
    and emotions 43–4
    fats 49–51
    intolerances 18, 46, 64–6
    and stress 115
    ultra-processed 38, 43–4, 46–7, 54, 68, 73
    what to eat 48–69
    wholefoods 81–2

G

gallbladder pain 87
genetics 18–19
ghrelin 76, 85
ginger
    ginger lime electrolyte cooler 310
    ginger shots 309
    gut-friendly lemon, turmeric and ginger switchel 318
    morning zinger green smoothie 154
gluten 9, 14, 64–7
granola: salted maple and cinnamon granola 165
Greek style lamb chops 219
gut health 20, 45–6, 70–85
    and detoxification 88, 93
    gut-brain axis 75, 77, 82
    and hormones 76–7
    improving 80–5

H

ham: sun-dried tomato frittata muffins 194
hormones 14, 21, 22–35, 111
    and blood sugar 37–40
    and food 49–50, 52, 57
    and gut health 76–7
    imbalances 91
    and sleep 101–2
hot flashes 29–30, 32
Huberman, Dr. 104–5, 115
hydration 81, 91, 94
hysterectomy 11–12, 14

I

IBS 18, 34, 64, 76
immune system 73
inflammation 6, 14, 17–21, 47
insulin 24–5, 37–8, 52, 111, 129
iron 62

J

jam: easy sugar-free raspberry and chia seed jam 303
Jardim, Nicole 29
joint pain 18

K

kale
    kale crisps 254
    Tuscan bean and kale soup 185
kidneys 89, 96

L

lactose 9
lamb: Greek style lamb chops 219
lemon and blueberry pots 166
lemonade 311
lentils
    roasted vegetable salad 178
    spiced lentil and chorizo soup 190
    spiced red lentil dahl 216
leptin 51, 76
libido 28, 30, 50, 76
liver 87–8, 91, 92–3, 96
lungs 89, 97
lymphatic system 87, 90–1, 94, 96, 124

M

macronutrients 49, 52, 66
magnesium 60, 75

mango and lime coconut pots 248
massage 91, 94
meat 46, 54–5
melatonin 101–2, 104, 106–7
menopause 23–9, 29–35, 39, 128–9
menstrual cycle 23, 25–9, 39
    and gut health 79
    and movement 127–8
    pads and tampons 94
    period pain 6, 9, 10, 14, 23, 34
    phases 25–28, 79
microbiome 59, 73–4, 81–2
micronutrients 60–2
mood swings 6, 14, 18, 26, 32–3, 125
movement 14, 20, 54–5, 91, 96, 120–31
    too little 91, 125–6
muffins: sun-dried tomato frittata muffins 194
muscle mass 30, 54, 125
mushrooms
    gourmet high-protein Scotch egg 181
    high protein cauli-egg fried rice 211
    rich and nutritious zucchini Bolognese 203

N

nuts 50, 58, 82
    baked apple, cinnamon and pecan oats 150
    chocolate, hazelnut and orange biscotti 281
    cocoa and almond energy bars 286
    coconut, chocolate chip and macadamia cookies 273
    fruit and nut breakfast bars 269
    gourmet high-protein Scotch egg 181
    healthy chocolate spread 295
    loaded apple tea cake 277
    no-bake nut and seed bars 282
    no-bake chocolate tart 251
    no-bake vanilla cheesecake 244
    pistachio-crusted cod 231
    rhubarb, strawberry and elderflower crumble 240
    rich and nutritious zucchini Bolognese 203
    salted maple and cinnamon granola 165
    savory soft crumble 300
    the ultimate nut roast 215

O

oats
    baked apple, cinnamon and pecan oats 150
    fruit and nut breakfast bars 269
    oaty cookies 278
    spiced carrot cake overnight oats 161
omega fats 50–1, 54, 60
osteoporosis 128–9
ovulation 28–9, 79, 127–8

P

pancakes: banana and chocolate pancakes 169
pancetta: rich and nutritious zucchini Bolognese 203
PCOS (polycystic ovary syndrome) 6, 23, 27, 34, 40, 101, 128
pears: maple spiced poached pears 235
peppers
    beet falafel bowl 174
    fragrant beef rendang 207
    pistachio-crusted cod 231
    rich and nutritious zucchini Bolognese 203
    roasted vegetable salad 178
    shakshuka 149
    smoky chorizo beef 208
    Spanish tortilla and romesco dip 198
    Tuscan bean and kale soup 185
peri peri chicken thighs 227
perimenopause 22, 29–32, 39, 128–9
periods *see* menstrual cycle
    periods 23
pilates 122, 124, 129
the pill 9, 14
pistachios
    pistachio-crusted cod 231
    raspberry and pistachio panna cotta 243
plastics 94
pneumonia 9
potatoes: salad Niçoise 204

prebiotics 59, 81–2
probiotics 82
progesterone 25, 28–30, 38, 50, 57
protein 52–5, 66, 68, 92

Q

quinoa
    chicken karahi 224
    sun-dried tomato frittata muffins 194

R

radishes
    crunchy slaw 193
    grilled chimichurri chicken salad 173
raspberries
    easy sugar-free raspberry and chia seed jam 303
    raspberry and pistachio panna cotta 243
resetting 132–41
resistance training 124, 128–9
rhubarb, strawberry and elderflower crumble 240

S

salads
    beet falafel bowl 174
    BLT lettuce wraps 189
    grilled chimichurri chicken salad 173
    quinoa salad 194
    roasted vegetable salad 178
    salad Niçoise 204
    zesty buckwheat and chickpea salad 228
salmon
    grilled spiced salmon 212
    marinated salmon bowl 182
    Thai salmon cakes 197
sardines: ultimate omega breakfast toast 146
saunas 93, 116
screen time 104, 106, 110–11, 116
seeds
    flax and chia crackers 259
    fruit and nut breakfast bars 269
    grain-free seeded bread 258
    loaded apple tea cake 277
    no-bake nut and seed bars 282
    rhubarb, strawberry and elderflower crumble 240
    roasted vegetable salad 178
    salted maple and cinnamon granola 165
    savory soft crumble 300
    the ultimate nut roast 215
selenium 62
sex, painful 10–11
shakshuka 149, 162
skin problems 6, 14, 18, 38, 73, 87, 89
sleep 10, 20, 30, 32–3, 57, 74, 82, 94, 98–107, 114, 124
    deprivation 99, 101–2
    and hormones 101–2
    improving 104–7
    schedules 102, 104–5
    and sunlight exposure 104, 107
    wind-down routine 105, 107
smoothies
    avocado matcha smoothie 314
    morning zinger green smoothie 154
snacks, savory
    flax and chia crackers 259
    kale crisps 254
    roasted chickpeas 255
snacks, sweet
    the 2-minute craving crusher 270
    chocolate, hazelnut and orange biscotti 281
    cocoa and almond energy bars 286
    coconut, chocolate chip and macadamia cookies 273
    coconut macaroon thumbprints 265
    fruit and nut breakfast bars 269
    loaded apple tea cake 277
    no-bake nut and seed bars 282
    oaty cookies 278
    rich chocolate sandwich cake 285
    salted caramel swirl brownies 274
    soft coconut macaroons 264
social media 43, 94, 109–10, 116
soups
    spiced lentil and chorizo soup 190
    Tuscan bean and kale soup 185
Spanish tortilla and romesco dip 198
spices 82

steak
- chimichurri steak 220
- minute steak 193

STIs 10-11

stools *see* bowel movement

strawberries: rhubarb, strawberry and elderflower crumble 240

strength training 128-9

stress 14, 17, 20, 38, 91, 94, 108-19
- causes 113-14
- and gut health 73, 75-7
- and hormones 111
- reducing 113-15
- symptoms 109-10

stretching 129

supplements 62-3, 75

sweet potatoes 145
- elevated poached eggs 186
- grilled spiced salmon 212
- Spanish tortilla and romesco dip 198

sweet corn
- peri peri chicken thighs 227
- zesty buckwheat and chickpea salad 228

T

tahini: whipped tahini 157

tampons 94

testosterone 24, 28, 30, 50

Thai salmon cakes 197

thyroid 38, 52, 57, 77, 85, 91

tiredness 6, 14, 18, 23, 39, 91

tomatoes
- beet falafel bowl 174
- chicken karahi 224
- Greek style lamb chops 219
- grilled chimichurri chicken salad 173
- rich and nutritious zucchini Bolognese 203
- shakshuka 149
- spiced lentil and chorizo soup 190
- Tuscan bean and kale soup 185

toxins 74, 88-9, 92-4, 114

tuna
- salad Niçoise 204
- stuffed avocado 177

Tuscan bean and kale soup 185

U

ultra-processed foods (UPFs) 38, 43-4, 46-7, 54, 73

V

vaginal dryness 30, 32

vagus nerve 112-13

Van Tulleken, Chris 43

vegan diet 44-6

vegan recipes
- the 2-minute craving crusher 270
- beet falafel bowl 174
- caramel sauce 294
- chia and acai split bowl 158
- chimichurri sauce 292
- easy sugar-free raspberry and chia seed jam 303
- fermented rainbow kraut 291
- flax and chia crackers 259
- fruit and nut breakfast bars 269
- harissa cauliflower steaks 223
- healthy chocolate spread 295
- kale crisps 254
- lemon and blueberry pots 166
- mango and lime coconut pots 248
- maple spiced poached pears 235
- morning zinger green smoothie 154
- natural live coconut yogurt 299
- no-bake chocolate tart 251
- no-bake vanilla cheesecake 244
- oaty cookies 278
- raspberry and pistachio panna cotta 236
- rhubarb, strawberry and elderflower crumble 236
- rich and creamy chocolate mousse 236
- roasted chickpeas 255
- roasted vegetable salad 178
- salted maple and cinnamon granola 165
- savory soft crumble 300
- spiced carrot cake overnight oats 161
- spiced red lentil dahl 216
- Tuscan bean and kale soup 185

    the ultimate nut roast 215
    zesty buckwheat and chickpea salad 228
vegetarian recipes *see also* vegan recipes
    baked apple, cinnamon and pecan oats 150
    banana and chocolate pancakes 169
    breakfast nests 153
    chocolate, hazelnut and orange biscotti 281
    chocolate soufflés 247
    classic shakshuka 149
    coconut, chocolate chip and macadamia cookies 273
    elevated poached eggs 186
    green shakshuka 162
    loaded apple tea cake 277
    no-bake nut and seed bars 282
    salted caramel swirl brownies 274
    soft coconut macaroons 264
    Spanish tortilla and romesco dip 198
    sticky toffee pudding 236
    velvety vanilla custard 304
    whipped tahini 157
vitamin B 62
vitamin D 61

W

walking 129
water 81, 94
weight gain 6, 14, 18, 32–3
wholefoods 81–2
work-life balance 116

Y

yoga 115, 127, 129
yogurt: natural live coconut yogurt 299

Z

zinc 61
zucchini
    breakfast nests 153
    chimichurri steak 220
    grilled chimichurri chicken salad 173
    marinated salmon bowl 182
    rich and nutritious zucchini Bolognese 203
    roasted vegetable salad 178

Acknowledgments

To my community . . . this book is for you. None of it would exist without the people who've followed my journey, shared their stories, and trusted me enough to listen. You've been my biggest source of motivation, and this book is my way of giving back.

To my mum and dad: thank you for supporting me through my health journey, without you I wouldn't have had the resources to be well enough to even dream of writing a book, let alone finishing one. I may not be a farmer (and, to your disappointment, I won't be marrying one either), but I think we can all agree women's health is where I'm destined to be!

To Dillon: My bald queen partner in life, in chaos, and in endless conversations about periods, inflammation, and, yes, poos. Thank you for letting this book take over our lives, for tasting every recipe, and for your endless patience when I've been obsessively talking women's health 24/7.

To Zoe Hindle: thank you for being my sounding board and lending your incredible knowledge and expertise. I'm so grateful to have leaned on you during this book and all our other projects together.

To Rebecca: my organizational rock. Thank you for keeping me on track, listening as I read chapters aloud, and proofing things a hundred times without complaint. I honestly don't know how I would've done this without you.

To Sarah and Oscar: I owe you both so much. Sarah, thank you for helping me see that I could turn my story and passion into a book in the first place. Oscar, thank you for helping make it happen. Together, you gave me the confidence and guidance I needed to bring this dream to life, and I'm endlessly grateful.

To Ione, Sukhmani, and the entire Michael Joseph and Penguin team, including Rebecca for the beautiful design and Claire, our brilliant photographer—thank you for making this book a reality, for guiding me through every step, and for capturing its spirit so beautifully. You gave me the confidence to bring it together, and I couldn't have asked for a better team.

To Sevs: thank you for being my rock in every way. For the hours on FaceTime, for letting me sense-check everything, and for proofreading until your eyes crossed. You deserve a medal (or at least a holiday).

To my cousin Jess: thank you for handing me *"The Secret,"* which changed my life and gave me the confidence to start sharing my health journey. You're still my cheerleader to this day. And yes, sorry again for giving you too much magnesium . . . I hope you can forgive me one day!

To Kirsty Smith: thank you for introducing me to the AIP, which set me on the path of researching women's health and inflammation.

To "*my loves*": my best friends from uni who've been with me through every high and low, and still are today. Thank you for making everyday so special, and for supporting me in everything I do.

To Emily Foort: The most chaotic and wonderful person I know, thank you for inspiring me to quit my job and go all in on women's health. Your courageous plans and outlook on life reminded me that we only get one shot, and it's meant to be lived fully. I'll forever be grateful.

And finally, to you, the reader—thank you for picking up this book, for being open to learning, and for trusting me with your health journey. Without you, none of this would be possible.

This book contains advice and information relating to health care. It should be used to supplement rather than replace the advice of your doctor or another trained health professional. If you know or suspect that you have a health problem, it is recommended that you seek your physician's advice before embarking on any medical program or treatment. All efforts have been made to assure the accuracy of the information contained in this book as of the date of publication. The publisher and the author disclaim liability for any medical outcomes that may occur as a result of applying the methods suggested in this book.

Without limiting the exclusive rights of any author, contributor or the publisher of this publication, any unauthorized use of this publication to train generative artificial intelligence (AI) technologies is expressly prohibited. HarperCollins also exercise their rights under Article 4(3) of the Digital Single Market Directive 2019/790 and expressly reserve this publication from the text and data mining exception.

THE ANTI-INFLAMMATORY 30-DAY RESET. Copyright © 2026 by Sophie Richards. All rights reserved. Printed in Canada. No part of this book may be used or reproduced in any manner whatsoever without written permission except in the case of brief quotations embodied in critical articles and reviews. For information, address HarperCollins Publishers, 195 Broadway, New York, NY 10007. In Europe, HarperCollins Publishers, Macken House, 39/40 Mayor Street Upper, Dublin 1, D01 C9W8, Ireland.

HarperCollins books may be purchased for educational, business, or sales promotional use. For information, please email the Special Markets Department at SPsales@harpercollins.com.

hc.com

Originally published in the United Kingdom in 2026 by Penguin Michael Joseph, an imprint of Penguin Random House.

FIRST U.S. EDITION

Design and illustration by Rebecca Hills
Photography by Clare Winfield
Recipe support by Sarah Flower

Library of Congress Cataloging-in-Publication Data has been applied for.

ISBN 978-0-06-349643-9

26 27 28 29 TC 10 9 8 7 6 5 4 3 2 1